Contemporary Clinical Practice with Asian Immigrants

Many first and second generation Asian immigrants experience acculturation challenges to varying extents. These challenges, such as language barriers, racial discrimination, under-employment, the loss of support networks, and changes in family role and structure, may exacerbate myriad mental health issues. In addition, their help-seeking behavior, as shaped by a general adherence to a collectivistic worldview and indirect communication style, often creates challenges for the practitioners who are trained under a Western practice modality.

Drawing on literature from English-speaking countries with sizable Asian immigrant populations such as the United States, Australia, New Zealand, Canada, and the United Kingdom, this text is designed especially for clinicians and students working with Asian immigrant populations. It discusses the therapeutic process in psychotherapy and counseling with these clients, exploring both key psychodynamic constructs and social systemic factors. Building on contemporary relational theory, which emphasizes the centrality of the helping relationship and sensitivity to the client's subjective realities, the book demonstrates how Western-based concepts and skills can be broadened and applied in an Asiacentric context, and can be therapeutic even in social service and case management service settings. There are chapters on issues such as domestic violence, intergenerational conflicts, depression amongst elders, and suicide, discussing the prevalence and nature of the mental health issues and each containing case vignettes from various Asian ethnic groups to illustrate the application of relational approaches.

This book is an important cross-cultural reference for practicing social workers and counselors as well as for social work students undertaking clinical practice courses.

Irene W. Chung is Associate Professor at the Silberman School of Social Work at Hunter College, City University of New York. Formerly Chair of Clinical Practice with Individuals and Families practice concentration at the School, she is currently President of the New York Coalition for Asian American Mental Health, a non-profit, volunteer organization of mental health providers in the Asian communities of New York City.

Tazuko Shibusawa is Associate Professor at the New York University Silver School of Social Work and serves as the Associate Dean of Professional Programs and Director of the MSW Program. She is a Hartford Geriatric Social Work Faculty Scholar, and serves on the Executive Committee of the New York Coalition for Asian American Mental Health and the Board of the Japanese American Social Services, Inc.

Contemporary Clinical Practice with Asian Immigrants

A relational framework with culturally responsive approaches

**Irene W. Chung and
Tazuko Shibusawa**

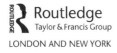

LONDON AND NEW YORK

First published 2013
by Routledge
2 Park Square, Milton Park, Abingdon, Oxfordshire OX14 4RN

Simultaneously published in the USA and Canada
by Routledge
711 Third Avenue, New York, NY 10017

First issued in paperback 2014

Routledge is an imprint of the Taylor & Francis Group, an informa business

British Library Cataloguing in Publication Data
A catalogue record for this book is available from the British Library
Library of Congress Cataloging in Publication Data
Chung, Irene.
Contemporary clinical practice with Asian immigrants : a relational framework
with culturally responsive approaches / Irene Chung and Tazuko Shibusawa.
pages cm
1. Asian Americans–Mental health. 2. Asian American families–Mental health.
3. Asian Americans–Mental health services. 4. Asian Americans–Medical care.
I. Shibusawa, Tazuko. II. Title.
RC451.5.A75C48 2013
362.196890089'95073–dc23
2013000011

ISBN: 978-0-415-78342-2 (hbk)
ISBN: 978-0-415-78343-9 (pbk)

Typeset in Baskerville
by Taylor & Francis Books

To Maeve
Irene W. Chung

To Vivian Matsushige and Laura Shiozaki Lee
Tazuko Shibusawa

Contents

List of illustrations

List of figures

List of tables

Preface

The idea for this book evolved from our experiences as social work educators, researchers, practitioners, and students of clinical practice over the last 30 years. When we were master of social work students in the 1970s, "multiculturalism" and "cultural competence" had yet to emerge as practice concepts, and clinical theories and skills were taught with little acknowledgment of the inherent dominance of Euro-American values and norms.

As Asian students, we felt compelled to meet the expectations of our Euro-American instructors and supervisors. We had to disown our ways of connecting with clients, which were largely shaped by our experiences growing up in Asian families and communities. In the classroom and supervision groups, we felt there was something wrong with us for not being as assertive as our peers in expressing our thoughts and feelings. Both of us experienced being penalized by receiving a B+ on a final grade because we had not participated actively in class even though we had received an A on our papers. From the perspectives of our instructors, we were too passive in our thinking and learning. In our clinical internship in predominantly Caucasian settings, our non-Asian supervisors questioned our ability to contribute in team meetings and apply clinical concepts and skills in the way they expected. Whether we had made the right decision to enter a clinical profession did cross our mind as well. We lived with a sense of inadequacy, shame, and feelings of anxiety about our professional capabilities.

Books and articles on clinical practice with Asian Americans had just started to be published at the time. According to the literature, Asians were difficult to engage in psychotherapy and counseling because of indirect communication styles, and reluctance to disclose personal problems, thoughts, and feelings. One of us was dismayed during her psychoanalytic training to hear a prominent psychoanalyst mention that Asians could not make substantial gains in psychoanalysis because they were not "individuated." As aspiring practitioners, we found these discussions both disappointing and discouraging. In fact, one of us distanced herself from clinical work for a while, interning and working in program development in non-Asian communities.

Upon graduation, we faced ongoing challenges to be accepted as Asians in the helping profession. We were often victims of the stereotype of Asians being quiet and compliant. Administrators and clinical supervisors continued to point out how we didn't speak up in meetings or were too indirect when communicating with clients. While we agree that there is always room for improvement in our communication skills, we have come to understand these stereotypes as a manifestation of subtle racism. Over time, we learned to respond assertively through the support and validation of our professional skills from our Asian colleagues. We have also engaged in our own personal work to understand the ways in which being stereotyped has left an indelible mark on us as individuals and practitioners. We now have a better understanding of how we, along with other colleagues of color, work under the pressure of being a Good Effective Mainstream Minority Therapist (GEMM) (Hardy, 2008). We know what it's like to be a GEMM, and the energy it takes to "smile and stay pleasant" regardless of racial slights or microaggressions and to "live with the implicit contradictory messages of our field that encourage differences but reward sameness" (ibid., p. 465).

After years of clinical practice, we both obtained our doctoral degrees and entered the academy. Our new careers gave us opportunities to reflect on the Eurocentric nature of clinical theories and to think about ways to be more discerning in applying these theories when practicing with Asian clients. We have been fortunate to serve as mentors to many students and professionals in the various Asian communities in New York City, and engage in discussions regarding their practice challenges. However, we have been dismayed that even after 30 years of progress in the field of culturally competent practice, the new generation of Asian and Asian American students and professionals continues to struggle with the challenges that we experienced, and often feel invalidated and unsure of their professional competence. When one of us helped with conducting a survey by the NYC chapter of the National Association of Social Workers on the professional challenges among Asian American social workers, "cultural dissonance" and "lack of culturally relevant training" were reported as the most significant challenges (Chung, 2006). In a focus group conducted with US and foreign-born Asian social work students, the most disconcerting feedback was the internalized feelings of inadequacy and helplessness over the dissonance between the Asian cultural and clinical professional values, as evidenced in the poignant remarks from one of the participants (Chung, 2006, p. 7):

> I want to learn more about "how to approach my supervisor" as an Asian student. I don't talk about my differences at all with my supervisor, because it might be a very sensitive issue, and I don't want to cause any problems, or I am afraid that I might appear to be "making excuses." I don't want to think that way because I feel that it is not a good attitude as a student. But sometimes I feel that I might have been taken advantage of because I am "quiet," and I don't stand up for myself when other American students might stand up for themselves. I am wondering if I could say to my supervisor "what is it like to have a Korean student?" or "what would you want me to improve in?" I am wondering if I've made some honest mistakes due to my cultural background. However, I will end up not saying anything …

This student's sentiments – the apprehension that he would "cause problems" if he brought up the issue of differences with his supervisor, and his sense of personal obligation to "learn and work hard" – are typical Asian collectivistic values that emphasize self-discipline and a harmonious relationship with others. This student was painfully aware that these values seemed to stand in the way of his becoming accepted in the profession, and he was at a loss as to how he could integrate his cultural values and emerging professional identity.

Over the years, we have also had to intervene when our Asian social work students receive negative evaluations from their clinical supervisors. Our students who come to us because of difficulties with their clinical supervisors are often devastated because the evaluations point to personal deficits, rather than cultural differences. For example, the following is an excerpt from a written evaluation by a clinical supervisor of Lin, a first generation Chinese social work student:

> Lin has acknowledged that to be more curious and open towards her clients is in conflict with her own cultural and personal values ... She does not demonstrate any interest in asking questions or exploring dynamics that might lead to a differentiated understanding of a client's difficulties. The emotional content with a client raises an anxiety level in Lin that interferes with her clients' concern. There is little indication that Lin can tolerate the expression of grief or anger or any other range of "difficult" feelings from a client.

At the beginning of the evaluative statement, the clinical supervisor acknowledges that Lin has told her that she is experiencing cultural conflicts about being "curious and open" toward her clients. Yet the supervisor proceeds to conclude that Lin is not curious because of her anxieties and is not able to tolerate expressions of grief or anger. We see how the supervisor applies a Eurocentric psychodynamic interpretation of the student's behavior and performance, and concludes that the student does not have the emotional capacity to engage in clinical work.

Those of us from a non-White background and who are familiar with Eurocentric clinical training can no doubt relate to the struggles of students like Lin. Our major concern is that through such interaction with supervisors, students end up burdened with feelings of inadequacy. We believe that supervisors and instructors can lift this burden when they understand how to bridge the issues of cultural dissonance and share the responsibility of helping Asian students make sense of two different sets of values and norms. We hope this book will help strengthen the capacity of our readers to explore modified and alternative perspectives that are consistent with successful multicultural practice with clients.

We are also concerned with the assumption that Asian practitioners can automatically work with Asian clients because of the mere fact that they share the same ethnic background. The Asian immigrant community is diverse and there are many cases in which practitioners of one Asian group work with clients of a different Asian background. For Japanese practitioners to provide culturally sensitive services to Chinese, Korean, and Filipino clients, they need to be aware of the historical legacy of the atrocities committed by Japan during World War II and how this may influence their client's reactions toward them. Not only do practitioners who grew up speaking Cantonese in Hong Kong have to study Mandarin when working with clients from mainland China, they also have to understand the socio-cultural background of their clients. Although practitioners from Hong Kong and clients from China share the same Chinese culture, the former grew up in a capitalistic and *laissez-faire* state under the sovereignty of the UK, while their clients grew up in a Communist state. Indian Hindu practitioners have to learn to decipher the differences between "cultural," "personal," and "religious" issues when working with South Asians who are Muslim. Although Vietnam became a unified nation in 1976, second generation Vietnamese practitioners whose parents emigrated from the former South Vietnam in the 1970s need to be aware of how their worldview differs from that of clients who are recent immigrants from the former North Vietnam.

Among non-Asian professionals, there is little awareness of the complexities of working with Asian clients using a Eurocentric practice framework. All too often we receive questions from Asian practitioners who wonder if they are stepping out of the clinical boundaries in responding to their Asian clients in culturally relevant context. For example:

> If I respond to my client's request for advice instead of exploring her thoughts and underlying feelings, would that be considered as colluding with the client?
> If I engage in small talk with clients as a way to connect, would this be deemed as breaching professional boundaries?
> If I accept a gift from my client on major Asian ethnic holidays, do I have to explore the underlying meanings associated with giving gifts?

These and many other difficult questions result in a sense of marginalization among Asian practitioners who work in immigrant communities. Practitioners who are supervised by non-Asian supervisors sometimes make a conscious choice to not share their interventions with their supervisors because they know that the supervisors will be critical or disapprove of their interventions. Unfortunately, these practitioners pay a price because they squander the opportunity for supervision and receiving validation for their work. We believe that ongoing clinical supervision is crucial to support Asian clinicians in redefining the clinical process in a culturally relevant context, as well as understanding the complexities of ethnocultural transference and countertransference in their relationship with clients.

Objectives

We often hear about the high turnover and shortage of clinicians in Asian immigrant communities. We cannot help but wonder how much of this issue is related to the lack of support and culturally relevant supervision which is needed to help practitioners cope with the emotional intensity of clinical practice with Asian clients, and to build a sense of competence and professional belonging and identity. One of the objectives of this book is to support the professional identity and development of Asian practitioners who work in our immigrant communities.

Over the past two decades there has been a proliferation of literature on multicultural practice, which emphasizes the need to understand different cultural values and norms, and the client's subjective realities from a social constructivist perspective. While we are heartened by such recognition, we believe that existing literature does not delve sufficiently into the cultural assumptions that are embedded in traditional Eurocentric concepts and skills in clinical practice. For example, the time-honored practice of the "talking cure," which entails clinical skills of exploring the client's thoughts, desires and/or feelings, is a reflection of the Euro-American cultural beliefs of individualism and direct communication styles. Our profession has always embraced these practices as universal truth and a benchmark of our effectiveness as practitioners. On the other hand, recent literature on clinical practice with Asians emphasizes culture-specific issues such as help-seeking behavior and communication styles without illuminating the actual process and clinical skills. Practice recommendations generally focus on culturally relevant strategies such as taking an expert and directive stance, working toward symptom-relief and problem-solving, avoiding confrontation and probing for disclosure of feelings. Such development is an important step in documenting the need for alternative practice models. However, we agree with contemporary theorists who posit that culture-specific knowledge is not a sufficient factor in effective clinical outcome with clients, and that culturally competent practice requires an empathic connection with the client that is based on the clinician's skills and professional use of self. In this book, we would like to take a step further in offering a paradigm that will help clinicians develop a deeper understanding and ownership of how clinical theories and skills can be modified in an Asiacentric context, while taking into consideration individual and within-group diversity among Asian populations. We believe that this is a critical task in supporting the professional development of Asian practitioners who work in our immigrant communities. We also hope the book will benefit non-Asian practitioners who work with Asian immigrants and supervise Asian practitioners and students.

Content

A major focus of this book is to differentiate the *clinical* components of theories and skills from *cultural* beliefs in our practice. Currently, clinical practice is still predominantly informed by theories that focus on the dynamics of the individual's psyche, personality, and behavioral patterns, and augmented by systemic and post-modern perspectives that emphasize the individual's subjective experience and influences of her familial, social, and cultural environments. We believe that psychodynamic theories offer a good foundation in understanding the human psyche and behavior, but we need to revisit the concepts because they are filtered through a Euro-American cultural lens. In this book, we will apply some key clinical concepts to gain a deeper understanding of psychodynamic issues underlying Asian cultural values and norms, by addressing questions such as:

- Why does traditional Asian culture emphasize certain human emotions and behavior and de-emphasize others?
- What are the origins of culture-specific constructs of well-being and distress that often influence individuals' subjective experiences?
- What are collective defenses and what adaptive purposes do they serve?

In addressing these cultural issues, it is important to incorporate historical and anthropological perspectives to our discussion. The enhanced understanding of cultural issues will help the clinician make judicious choices of *when* and *how* to use culture-specific strategies, with a clear understanding and accountability of the clinical purpose and implications.

This book focuses on Asian immigrants as the client population in the helping process. Asians have consistently been one of the largest and fastest-growing ethnic groups in developed countries throughout the world. Changes in immigration policies in many countries have opened up opportunities for Asians to immigrate to be with family, seek refuge and asylum, fill the labor shortage, and to start businesses. Census data from English-speaking nations indicate that during the years 2000–2006, Asian populations ranged from 11 percent in Canada, 9 percent in Australia, 6.4 percent in New Zealand, 6 percent in the United Kingdom to 4.2 percent in the United States. The majority of Asians in these countries are first generation Asians who identify with traditional Asian cultural values and norms.

As mentioned previously, Asian immigrants are by no means a homogenous group. Increasingly, they are diverse in terms of ethnicity, country of origin, religion, language, culture, and history. We will focus primarily on first generation immigrants from China, Japan, Korea, the Philippines, South Asia, South East Asia who currently live in the aforementioned English-speaking countries, i.e., Australia, Canada, New Zealand, United Kingdom, and the United States. We recognize that the recent thrust of globalization has brought about many changes in values and lifestyles within Asian countries. The extent to which immigrants from Asia have embraced these changes depends on geographical areas of origin, e.g., urban versus rural, and their socioeconomic background. We believe that there is still a substantial difference in the coping and help-seeking behavior among the Asian immigrant populations in the Western world.

Research on Asian immigrant communities has documented significant problems including domestic violence, gambling and alcohol addiction, elder abuse, depression, and suicide across age groups. We devote the second part of this book to examining some of these issues. We will feature case vignettes shared by practitioners in the Asian communities to illuminate the depth and breadth of these issues and the way in which culturally relevant relational approaches are deployed. These case vignettes are translated into English and the personal identifying information has been altered to protect the clients' anonymity.

Guiding our discussion on the helping process with Asian immigrants is relational theory, which evolves from psychodynamic, systemic, and social constructivist theories, and which we believe offers great potential for practitioners to make cultural adaptations to existing modalities when working with Asian client populations. The theory's central tenet of using the helping relationship as the venue of change requires the practitioner to attune to and respond to the client's subjective experiences and emotional needs, and thus be creative and flexible in the use of engagement, assessment, and intervention skills. The framework posits that both practitioners and clients bring to the clinical encounter their personality traits, belief systems, and subjective experiences, and validates the importance of culture as a moderating factor in shaping the nature of the helping relationship. The emphasis on genuine interactions with the client challenges the practitioner to develop professional yet culturally relevant communication and boundaries. Essentially the relational paradigm provides a forum to infuse diversity into clinical practice in ways that are meaningful for the client as well as the practitioner. We believe that the working relationship is at the core of any modality, whether the practitioner is engaging in psychodynamic, cognitive-behavioral, family systems, or narrative therapies.

Organization

Part I of the book consists of three chapters that focus on the major premises of relational theory and how Western-based concepts and skills can be applied in an Asiacentric context. Part II of the book begins with a chapter on the demographic profiles of Asian immigrants in English-speaking countries. We then present chapters on specific mental health issues that affect Asian immigrants and families. In the first part of these chapters, we provide current scholarship about the issues; in the second part we present the experiences of practitioners whom we interviewed. We will discuss case vignettes and highlight the therapeutic approaches from a relational and cultural perspective.

Readers

This book is written for graduate-level students and practitioners who have some foundational knowledge of the helping process as well as concepts and theories in human behavior.

Terminology

In this book clinical practice refers to the process of helping individuals and families. Clinical practice is defined by the Council on Social Work Education (2009) as "the professional use of self and application of advanced clinical knowledge and skills to restore, maintain, and enhance the biological, psychological, social, and spiritual functioning of our clients." We believe that methods of clinical practice should extend beyond brief and long-term psychotherapy and counseling, and include client-centered advocacy, crisis intervention, information and referral services, and case management, which take place in a wide range of settings including behavioral health and primary care settings, geriatric programs, shelters, community agencies, and schools. All these methods have a therapeutic component because they are offered in the context of purposeful helping relationships.

In this book we use the term "practitioner" to denote the various roles in the helping profession, such as psychiatric nurses, mental health hotline workers, child welfare workers, mental health case managers, shelter staff, hospital social workers, and mental health clinicians.

We use the pronouns "he" and "she" interchangeably in our reference to practitioners and clients.

Acknowledgments

We are indebted to many individuals whose help and support were crucial to the completion of the book. First and foremost, we are grateful to the following practitioners who tirelessly shared their insights and experiences with us:

Juliana Jae Chong, LMSW
Sooknam Choo, LCSW
Hsiao-Ching Chu, PsyD
Niraj Delhiwala, LCSW, MBA
Mari Konno Economides, MSW
Fran Gau, LMSW
Yuen Ling Elaine Ho, LCSW
Chris Kam, LCSW
Mizue Katayama, MA
Inok Kim, LCSW
Shin Woo Kim, LMSW
Fanny Fai Lin Lau, MSW
Jiyeon Lee, LMSW
Ching Sum Leung, LCSW
Fei Kwan Li, LMHC
Jennifer Lim, LMSW
Tracy Luo, MSW
Yoko Naka, MSW
Fumi Raith, LCSW
Ellen Sampao, Ph.D.
Meghana Savant, MS, LMSW
Pamela Yew Schwartz, Ph.D.
Hyun Jung Shim, LCSW
Haein Son, LCSW
Mary Vu, Ph.D.
Hao Wang, MSW
Grace Wong, Ph.D.
Hong Zhang, LCSW
Steven Zhou, LCSW

Irene W. Chung – I wish to convey my appreciation to Dean Jacqueline Mondros, DSW, at the Silberman School of Social Work at Hunter College, for her ongoing support for faculty scholarship on cross-cultural practice, and granting me leave to pursue this book project. I would also like to acknowledge my colleagues for their encouragement and enriching dialogs that have sustained me through the challenging process of writing, especially Elizabeth Danto, Robin Donath, Paul Kurzman, and George Patterson. As always, my students are my greatest source of inspiration and impetus for learning. I would like to acknowledge my two clinical practice classes of 2012, who provided me with wonderful insights on relational theory and cross-cultural practice. Special thanks to Jenny Chung and Elizabeth Moore, who gave me feedback on the manuscript from the perspective of student readers; Jenny also provided valuable assistance in literature review and formatting for the manuscript.

Last but not least, I would like to thank my family and friends, especially Jeremiah, Art, Beth, Esther, Grace, Pam, and Robin, who have been most supportive and understanding during my preoccupation with the book project the last 18 months. Your smiles and presence in my life helped me keep a balanced focus on my work.

Tazuko Shibusawa – I would like to express my appreciation to Dean Lynn Videka, Silver School of Social Work at New York University, for her commitment to diversity and encouragement to pursue scholarship on cross-cultural practice. I am grateful to my colleagues and students who inspire me with their passion for learning. A special appreciation goes to Hao Wang for his assistance with the literature review. I would also like to thank Irene Chung, my co-author, for her commitment to this book and for her patience.

I am indebted to the late Takeo Doi, MD, from whom I had the good fortune to receive clinical supervision, and who helped me understand the limitations of my Western training in working with Japanese clients.

Finally, I would like to express my appreciation to my friends and family – to Ken Hardy, Gliceria Perez, Debra Chatman-Finley, and Karen Herrera for their encouragement, Vivian Matsushige and Laura Shiozaki Lee for their friendship, Jim Runsdorf for his support and reviewing portions of the manuscript, and my parents, Masahide and Fusako Shibusawa.

Part I

Intersections of culture and theories

1 Clinical practice with Asian immigrants

Unpacking and re-packing theories and meanings

Irene W. Chung

Introduction

What are clinical theories?

Clinical theories in the behavioral sciences are bodies of knowledge that attempt to make sense of the complexities of human nature and behavior. They inform the way we focus on the interplay of thoughts, emotions, and behavior in our assessment and intervention with clients. Over the years we have seen theories rise and fall, with new theories building on existing concepts and reflecting the social, political, and cultural ideologies of their times (Applegate, 2000; Berzoff *et al.*, 2011). With the advent of post-modern practice approaches that examine the social construction of meanings and identities in shaping human emotions and behavior (Anderson, 2005; Neimeyer and Bridges, 2003), there has been much recognition that clinical theories, influenced by Euro-American values, need to be deconstructed and reconstructed to better reflect the diversity of client populations who may adhere to drastically different worldviews and behavioral norms (Bonner, 2002; Hodge and Nadir, 2008; Lokken and Twohey, 2004; Manning *et al.*, 2004; Nye, 2005; Sue and Sue, 2003). For those of us who work with Asian immigrants in our clinical practice, the implication is that we need to be able to distill the inherent Western cultural values that are embedded in theories and redefine them in an Asiacentric context (Nagai, 2007).

How can we apply Eurocentric theories in clinical practice with Asian immigrants?

First of all, we need to understand the difference between *clinical* and *cultural* meanings. Ideally, clinical meanings provide us with a framework to examine and understand how human beings tend to think, act, and feel when they seek to fulfill their needs and desires, and how they cope with disappointments, losses, and traumas in their lives. However, clinical theories are generally infused with cultural meanings when theorists emphasize and de-emphasize certain foci in their theoretical elucidation. Maslow's (1954) hierarchy of human needs in characterizing human nature is a good case in point. Maslow postulated that our intrinsic human needs that seek and sustain survival, which include basic provisions, physical and psychological safety, social support and connection, self-esteem, and self-actualization, are forces that drive and shape human behavior. His theory is a source of clinical meanings that enhance our assessment of and intervention with *all* clients in our practice. For example, an appreciation of these needs would help us formulate a more in-depth assessment with a client who presents with complaints of anxiety or depressive symptoms and yet is unable to articulate insights and information other than her personal background and physical complaints. Listening to the client's narratives for themes of these human needs and posing relevant questions will help to illuminate the nature of her emotional distress around her circumstances. So if this client's responses indicate that she is disappointed at her inability to care for herself, we can explore further her sense of deficiency in the mastery of her life roles and tasks. Or if this client expresses her fear of criticism and rejection by others, we will explore circumstances in her family and social life that may undermine her sense of belonging. Such focused exploration will help us make reflections of the client's concerns and emotional needs. This is an important clinical intervention in initiating empathic connections with *any* client and sustaining her motivation to stay in the helping process.

What is the cultural meaning embedded in Maslow's theory that may interfere with working with culturally diverse clients? His postulation that there is a hierarchy among these human needs and the ranking of self-actualization needs as the most desired is essentially a reflection of the Western values of rugged individualism – self-reliance, autonomy, and so forth that have been celebrated throughout American history. Theorists from a collectivistic cultural background, on the other hand, will likely focus on social needs such as the sense of belonging and acceptance by one's reference group over self-actualization needs. Thus a practitioner's strict adherence to a culturally defined hierarchy of needs without an understanding of the client's belief systems may risk alienating the client by imposing irrelevant questions and making conclusions that are unsubstantiated.

Obviously there are no absolute truths in any clinical theory, and no single theory can afford sufficient insights in understanding the complexities of human emotions and behavior. As clinicians, we are drawn to certain theories based on our background and professional experiences. We can only strive to be aware of our own biases and the cultural relevance of the theories we choose to inform our practice. It is important to keep in mind that our use of theories should be driven by a differential and holistic approach that contextualizes client's thoughts, feelings, and behavior.

The interface of cultural and clinical meanings

How do cultural values evolve? What purpose do they serve from a clinical perspective?

Cultural and clinical meanings are invariably intertwined. As illustrated by our discussion of Maslow's theory, cultural meanings, rooted in specific belief systems, are the organizing principles of clinical information. They shape the clients' perception of their stressors as well as the practitioner's foci of assessment and intervention in the helping process. However, cultural meanings do not exist in a vacuum. From a psychological and anthropological perspective, values, norms, and conduct of life in each culture generally evolve from the group's historical experiences in coping with challenges in their environments, for example, prevalence of resources, natural disasters, intra- and inter-group conflicts, as well as their fears and aspirations as a group. So cultural meanings are reflections of how groups of individuals make sense of their experiences and adapt to their unique environment (Saari, 2008; Schamess and Shilkret, 2011). The universality of such human coping mechanism is "clinical" information, whereas the different paths each cultural group undertakes to pursue these needs become "cultural" values and norms (Hughes, 1993; Nye, 2005).

As an illustration of the intersection between cultural values and human coping mechanism and adaptation, we will briefly review the themes of American and Asian history and identify the collective psyche underlying the drastically different values and norms between the two cultures.

Since the overturning of British colonialism and the founding of the country in the eighteenth century, US history has been marked by expansion of its frontiers, victories in the pursuit of democracy, freedom of speech and equality for minority members of society, successful entrepreneurship by immigrants, and leadership in the world's arms and space races and our current information age (Tignor *et al.*, 2008). Such accomplishment is both a reflection and reinforcement of the ideology of individualism, whereby the actualization of one's goals and interests, as Maslow puts it, is of utmost importance. It is no surprise that the history of social policies in the US has always been a political struggle to define and balance individual and public responsibility for the underprivileged (Blau, 2010; Fraser and Gordon, 1994; Karger, 2003). Socially, direct expression of one's thoughts, desires, and feelings and the challenging of opposing views are valued as a desirable communication style (Hall, 1977; Roland 1996).

Asian values are substantially different from the mores of American individualism. Asian history, which spans 4,000 years, is punctuated by political strife, rebellions, wars, colonization, and natural disasters that led to widespread poverty, sufferings, and loss of family ties. Unlike Western countries, industrialization and modernization did not occur in most of these countries until the last 30 years. As agrarian societies that depended on collective labor forces to ensure successful harvests, the ideology of Confucianism and Hinduism, which emphasize the virtues of maintaining harmony with others, loyalty to a hierarchical structure within familial and social institutions, fulfillment of responsibilities and obligations defined by one's roles, and pursuit of the prosperity of collective welfare through self-sacrifice and discipline, became the logical core influence of Asian cultural values and norms that offer hopes of order and stability (Bhela, 2010; Kagitcibasi, 1997; Tignor *et al.*, 2008).

From a psychological perspective, American and Asian values and norms are examples of cultural organizing principles that shape individuals' perceptions of events in their lives, emotional reactions, coping mechanisms, and behaviors. Rooted in different historical experiences, they are unique sets of meaning systems that help to create continuity and cohesion for individuals to make sense of past occurrences and resolutions for the future. While clinical theories provide parameters to examine the human psyche and behavior, cultural meanings often play a key role in shaping, amplifying, or attenuating the foci of the theorists and practitioners as well as the experience of the clients (Roland, 1996; Chung, 2012).

In the following section, we will continue to focus on the interface of clinical and cultural meanings by reviewing major theoretical concepts that guide the helping process and discuss their relevance in an Asiacentric context.

The helping process as informed by clinical theories

The helping process begins when a client and a practitioner come together to review the presenting problem and to agree on a course of discussion and/ or action to address the problem. The presenting problem could range from concrete issues such as housing, childcare services, and nursing home placement to psychological distress such as interpersonal conflicts, loss of significant others, and setbacks in job or academic performance. However, as we well know, it is insufficient to focus on a presenting problem without understanding and addressing the underlying issues, which consist of myriad interactive psychosocial factors. To use the aforementioned examples, families or individuals who wish to apply for housing, or childcare, or nursing home placement for their elders, etc. may also be dealing with emotional issues that are compounded by social and cultural meanings associated with the circumstances, family dynamics, and accessibility to formal and informal support. So the process of linking these clients to resources often involves working with their ambivalent feelings and behavior as well as navigating them through a host of social systems. In this regard, theories that characterize the complex interrelationship of the individual's physiological and psychological attributes, as well as the nature of environmental support, offer a universal framework for understanding a client's presenting problem and her coping behavior. The ecological theory (Bronfenbrenner, 1979) adopted by social scientists, and social work's person-in-environment perspective (Greene, 1999; Woods and Hollis, 2000), offer an inclusive paradigm that guides the practitioner in making a preliminary and holistic assessment that in turn informs intervention foci for each client in the helping process.

A multi-dimensional framework for differential assessment

In reaction to an emerging problem, it is part of human nature that individuals will engage in activities to alleviate the distress associated with the problem. They could take steps to resolve the identified problem, enlist the assistance or emotional support of others, and/or resort to relaxation activities to alleviate their stress. The choice and specifics of these stress-reduction venues, i.e., problem-solving, help-seeking, and self-soothing behavior, are shaped by personality traits, the individuals' accessibility to external resources and support, and the pervasive influence of cultural belief systems. The outcome could be positive with the dissolution of the problem and stress, or it could be maladaptive and further undermine the individual's level of functioning and distress. Figure 1.1 is an application of the ecological and systems perspective that captures the dynamics of the various dimensions of general human coping mechanism in the face of stressors, as shaped by their affiliated group values as well as individual needs and proclivities. Theories of human behavior and development, family and group dynamics, as well as social and cultural belief systems illuminate these dynamics and help to create an in-depth understanding of an individual client's behavior and needs.

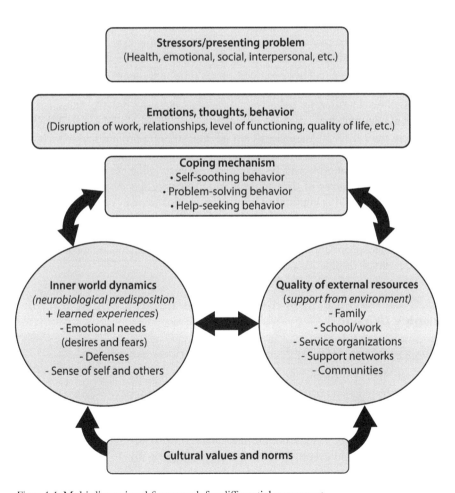

Figure 1.1 Multi-dimensional framework for differential assessment

Applying psychodynamic theories in an Asiacentric context

We would like to focus our discussion on the individual's inner world dynamics within this multi-dimensional framework. This is the mental process that consists of the interplay of desires, fears, emotions, and cognitions that are rooted in an individual's genetic predisposition as well as learned experiences, and plays a key role in shaping the individual's coping behavior. It is an area that tends to receive little attention in literature on clinical practice with Asians and Asian immigrants. Perhaps there is a tacit assumption that it is not possible or important to access the emotional life of Asians, who are often characterized as reluctant to share their inner thoughts and feelings and more interested in seeking concrete service and advice in the helping process. We believe that such a depiction, if indeed observed among Asian clients, is a clinical phenomenon infused with cultural meanings and values which needs to be understood in the helping process. Like everyone else, Asian clients do get angry or disappointed at their significant others and even their practitioners, sometimes over seemingly benign issues, and their silence or hostile responses are a manifestation of some underlying perceptions, emotions, and unresolved issues rooted in previous experiences. While it is beyond the scope of this book to delve into a thorough discussion of theories that offer insights into the human psyche, we believe that it is important for practitioners to be informed by some key psychodynamic concepts that illuminate the behavior of individuals as they cope with losses, disappointments, and stressful events in their lives. If Asian clients are hesitant in using professional services and could benefit from a more empathic and authentic engagement approach, psychodynamic concepts will be helpful in understanding their inner fears and desires, and the nature of their motivation in pursuing specific changes to reduce their stress. While it is important to distill the Euro-American values embedded in these concepts, we believe that there are universal aspects that can be applied and adapted to understanding human behavior in the Asian cultural milieu.

In the following section, we will discuss two major psychodynamic concepts and their relevance in practice with Asian immigrant clients.

Defense mechanism in the unconcious mind: a dimension of coping behavior

Concept of ego defenses from a Euro-American perspective

Like all clinical theories, the concept of the unconscious mind is infused with cultural meanings and has evolved with the values of the social world over the years. It originated in Europe during the late eighteenth century when Romanticism was the dominant ideology that emphasized individual expression of emotions and imagination. The concept subsequently gained much prominence through the writings of Sigmund Freud, the father of psychoanalysis. Under his classical drive-conflict model, Freud (1911; 1915) postulated that there are instinctual aggressive and sexual forces, wishes and urges that need to be discharged or gratified; those that are in conflict with the self and social norms are subsequently repressed and kept unconscious in the human mind. Freud believed that unresolved intrapsychic conflicts in the unconscious are the primary source of anxiety, neurotic behavior, and psychosomatic symptoms such as panic attacks and phobias. He argued that these conflicts needed to be analyzed and brought into the individual's consciousness. This core belief became the genesis of the "talking cure" and the predominant objective of psychotherapy practice in the Western world (Berzoff *et al.*, 2011; Roland, 1996; Borden, 2009).

Freud's postulation of the repression of drives and intrapsychic conflicts was expanded upon by ego psychology theorists as the cornerstone mechanism of ego defenses, whereby unacceptable thoughts, emotions, memories, and external threats that are too painful, shameful, or anxiety-provoking to process are distorted and replaced by less threatening forms of expression, such as projection, displacement, somatization, denial, and dissociation (Goldstein, 1995; Woods and Hollis, 2000).

While the mental process of defense mechanisms is a universal human phenomenon, the theoretical focus on intrapsychic conflicts has eventually shifted from Freud's biological perspective of a closed system's bodily functions that seek discharge and gratification, to those embedded in interpersonal contexts. As ego psychologists and object relation theorists recognized the intrinsic human needs for attachment ties to others and the role of society and culture in the complex layering of the human experience (Bowlby, 1969; Erikson, 1959), there has been less emphasis on aggression and sexuality as the roots of all intrapsychic conflicts and unconscious thoughts. This broadening of clinical focus of the nature of conflicts is evidently tied to evolving cultural meanings associated with human behavior, i.e., the importance of relationships over aggression and sexuality as driving forces. It is also a reflection of how contemporary Western culture views the latter differently from the nineteenth century Victorian era when sexuality received much attention in both public and private sectors, especially in Vienna where Freud lived most of his life. It was a time of sexual contradictions, when the ruling class and the Catholic Church emphasized the need to repress sexuality and yet sexual immorality was rampant across socioeconomic classes in Victorian society (Berzoff *et al.*, 2011).

Subsequently, additional conceptualizations of the unconscious mind have been formulated and applied in contemporary clinical practice (Kirmayer, 2007; Wachtel, 2008). For example, the unconscious is often referred to as the repository of an individual's forgotten memories, or automatic perceptions and thoughts, habitual behavior, etc. that are laden with meanings and may still be accessible to the individual's consciousness at a later time without much introspection. According to ego psychology, defenses that are more adaptive are generally in this realm of pre-consciousness (Goldstein, 1995; Woods and Hollis, 2000). For example, an individual who has been frustrated by an unresponsive employer may displace her frustration on her peers or loved ones, but there is a good chance that she is able to recognize the source of her anger upon reflection or discussion with others. On the other hand, someone who grew up in an unsupportive family environment and generally internalizes her anger toward others may have difficulties getting in touch with the repressed feelings.

What are the clinical aspects of unconscious defenses that can be applied across diverse client populations and human service settings?

The assessment of ego defenses is generally emphasized as a clinical task for mental health and counseling practitioners. As we discuss later, we believe that it is helpful for *all* practitioners to be able to identify their clients' defenses and issues that they are struggling with underlying their behavior. This requires ongoing observations of a client's thoughts, emotions, and behavior that are marked by some degree of rigidity and irrationality despite changes in circumstances, and an assessment of the nature and context of the defenses. In other words, the clinical observation has to corroborate with the client's current and past issues and circumstances that seem to have precipitated some form of conflict and distress for the client. Since the defense is largely unconscious to the client, it is the practitioner's professional responsibility to substantiate her assessment. Sometimes we hear practitioners describe clients as "defended against" or "in denial of" certain issues. We need to make sure that we are not conveniently labeling the behavior and overlooking our own biases and defenses. For example, how do we feel about working with an older client who seems to be complaining excessively about physical ailments but will not acknowledge her own fears of mortality when we try to broach the subject? Does that make us feel inadequate in the helping process or frustrated that she only focuses on her complaints that are unfounded? Is it possible that the client perceives her physical complaints as the only way she can get attention from others? How much does our own lack of interest in listening to her complaints perpetuate her need to dwell on those issues? These are a sample of questions that we need to consider before we can conclude that the client is avoiding the issue because it is too "threatening" to get in touch with her fear of dying.

When do we support the defenses and when do we try to modify the defenses?

It is important not to associate ego defenses with a negative connotation. Ego defenses protect the individual from overwhelming anxiety and intolerable thoughts, and they serve an adaptive purpose that supports the individual in his daily functioning. For example, it is not uncommon that we hear about individuals who channel or "sublimate" their grief or anger in regard to the loss of a loved one into social action that benefits others in a similar predicament. In doing so, these individuals allow themselves to be connected to the loss but not as much to the unbearable strong emotions. However, some ego defenses may require the practitioner's intervention if they interfere with the client's level of functioning and create further distress in the client's life (Goldstein, 1995; Woods and Hollis, 2000). For example, there are individuals who deny the impact of their substance abuse issues on their lives. The denial can jeopardize relationship ties and job security, undermine health and mental health well-being and negate overall quality of life. Intervention should then focus on weakening the denial defenses and supporting the individual's ego strengths of reality testing, judgment, and modulation of impulse control in initiating positive behavioral changes.

Ego defenses

In her seminal work, *Ego and the Mechanisms of Defense* (1946), Anna Freud outlined the way in which the ego's defenses help to protect against an individual's intrapsychic conflicts and support her level of functioning. Defense mechanisms are unconscious, automatic processes that keep threatening and intolerable experiences as well as feelings and impulses from one's awareness. It is important to recognize the protective and adaptive nature of defenses as a universal human coping mechanism in a complex social environment. Some defense mechanisms are more adaptive than others. Generally there is a host of defenses that come into play in an individual's behavior. In this section we discuss several common defenses separately for the purpose of clarity.

Table 1.1 Ego defenses

Defense mechanism	Definition	Example
Denial	Rejection of aspects of reality, such as one's perceptions or feelings.	A functioning alcoholic denies the severity of his drinking, maintaining that he drinks only as much as he needs for relaxation and enjoyment.
Reaction formation	Replacement of undesirable unconscious impulses with conscious behaviors or thoughts that are totally opposite in nature.	A person who is angry with and fearful of her supervisor is not aware of her negative emotions. Rather, she becomes overly compliant and eager to please her supervisor.
Projection	Attribution of unacceptable thoughts, feelings, or motives onto another person's behavior.	An individual who is upset with her significant other for not giving her attention is not able to be in touch with her anger. Instead, she perceives that her significant other is upset with her.
Displacement	Diversion of emotions or feelings from their original source to another target that is less threatening to the individual.	A young boy who is angry with his abusive father may instead express his hostility through bullying behaviors toward peers at school and his pets at home.

Table 1.1 (continued)

Defense mechanism	Definition	Example
Rationalization	Justification of behaviors, ideas, or feelings that are laden with intolerable meanings through inaccurate though common, reasonable, and plausible explanations.	An elderly man who experiences shortness of breath and fatigues easily decides not to seek medical consultation. He attributes his symptoms to aging and believes he will feel better if he cuts back on his activities.
Intellectualization	A form of rationalization; the avoidance of the direct experience of emotions through the use of discussion, reason, and logic to depersonalize the emotions.	A physician who just lost her father discusses the causes of his illness, treatment options, success rates, and other similar cases when friends offer condolences. She shows no evidence of emotion.
Repression	Keeping unwanted thoughts or feelings from one's awareness.	A person who experiences trauma may repress memories associated with the experience.
Sublimation	Redirecting socially unacceptable impulses into socially acceptable ones.	An angry and aggressive teenager channels his energy to become a brilliant baseball player on his school's team.

Source: Freud (1936) and Goldstein (1995b).

Why do we need to understand clients' defenses?

The practitioner's understanding of the client's defenses is crucial in her empathic connection and subsequent interventions with the client. For example, it is not uncommon that women who are victims of domestic violence are willing to go to a shelter with their children to ensure their safety and yet they are hesitant to file for divorce and cut off ties from their spouses. Evidently, cultural meanings of the women's role in the family, stigma regarding divorce, their ability to be financially independent, etc. are important sociocultural factors underlying their ambivalence, but the unconscious fears and desires of these women and their sense of self are interrelated psychological issues that also need to be understood and integrated into a client-centered collaboration and intervention. Or we can think of children who have been neglected or abused by their parents and yet generally have difficulties accepting that their parents have failed to be adequate caregivers. Some of them blame themselves for not living up to their parents' expectations, while others exhibit challenging behavior and take out their emotional distress on their siblings and peers. From the perspective of ego defenses, the child's self-blame behavior would be turning her unacceptable feelings toward the parents against the self, which relieves the guilt of harboring aggressive feelings, distracts from the pain of not being loved, and most importantly, maintains a sense of hope in eventually gaining love from the parents. On the other hand, the child who acts out his anger toward others would be considered as taking on the belligerent behavior of his parents and identifying with the "aggressor" to ward off his feelings of vulnerability and internal conflicts associated with the parental abuse. Thus using the theoretical lens of defenses will be helpful for the practitioner to look beyond the presenting behavior and empathize with the child's hidden psychological anguish, which includes the desire for unconditional parental love and fear of abandonment and rejection that have been repressed in the service of coping and adaptation.

Culture-specific defenses and individual coping mechanisms

Many theorists believe that each culture has its own unique form of unconscious that is deeply embedded in the individual's psyche. This cultural unconscious is a broad base of shared meanings and imprints that individuals of the same culture learned from their early experiences and internalized varying degrees of thoughts, emotions, and behavior (Hall, 1977; Robinson, 2010; Waldman and Rubalcava, 2005). Cultural values and norms with their specific beliefs and social etiquette, offer a glimpse of this collective unconscious. Herron (1995, p. 521) postulates that within an "ethnic unconscious," individuals' fears, defenses and wishes are shaped by "their cultural avowal and disavowal of beliefs, and shared by each generation with the next and with most people of that ethnic group." For our discussion here, we would like to examine how these cultural "disavowals" that marshal collective censorship against specific beliefs and behaviors within the family, the community, and social institutions affect individual coping mechanisms as well as practice implications. They can be considered as culture-specific defenses that serve as a powerful buffer to protect individuals from getting in touch with certain desires or conflicts, and shape their perceptions of distress and responses.

There are both adaptive benefits and drawbacks with being part of the collective unconscious. As individuals internalize the parameters of moral and emotional meanings in our activities, behavior and relationships, their coping mechanism is strengthened by an intuitive knowing of what is at stake in specific situations and circumstances and the range of appropriate responses. However, there are invariably conflicts created by idiosyncratic needs and environmental changes that do not fit into the scheme of the internalized unconscious. These are the times when individual coping mechanisms are challenged and maladaptive symptoms and behavior may emerge.

For example, if we look at American culture with the lens of collective defenses, we can speculate that the values of individualism that idealize freedom, choices, innovations, and improvisations, etc., are also defended unconsciously against the fears and disdain for mundaneness, conformance, and passivity, which represent a threat to the core beliefs of the American dream. As individuals acquire these values and defenses, they also internalize the associated positive or negative emotions (Chung, 2006). So individuals in American society who have internalized these individualistic values and yet do not fit into this cultural archetype due to environmental deficits and/or personality proclivities may experience a heightened sense of marginalization and failure and a range of negative emotions that may elude individuals in another culture.

We can also consider why sexuality is never extolled publicly, especially among women, as a pleasurable aspect of human life in traditional Asian societies (Le Espiritu, 2001; Lee, 2006). This can be viewed as a cultural defense to protect against promoting sexuality as an indulgence that undermines traditional values such as self-discipline, hard work, and fulfillment of the defined roles and responsibilities within the hierarchical and patriarchal structure of Asian societies. Thus individuals who have strong sexual drives constitutionally may unconsciously repress those desires, and instead lead an ascetic lifestyle. Or those who give in to their sexual urges may experience tremendous shame and guilt that can be manifested in physiological symptoms such as phobias and panic attacks (G. Wong, personal communication, 25 November 2012).

Sexuality and communication

The findings of a recent study of Asian American young women that explored their sex education experiences with their parents of Chinese, Japanese, Korean, Filipino, Asian Indian, and South East Asian origin affirmed the general reticence on the direct discussion of sex in the Asian immigrant family (Kim, 2009). Participants cited their parents' use of veiled and pejorative language in communicating their expectations of their abstinence from pre-marital sex, and concluded that their parents primarily transmitted cultural values that associate sex with the purpose of procreation, and illicit sex as shameful and bringing dishonor to the family.

The Asian hierarchical culture emphasizes individuals' deference to others and sanctions against verbal and physical aggression as part of the moral code. From an ego psychology perspective, this view toward aggression has been "sublimated" or channeled into the values of hard work and self-discipline in the service of the family, as well as fulfillment of obligations toward others in the Asian culture. Thus individuals in Asian societies are generally taught since early childhood to be polite and respectful to others, to be mindful and in control of their posture and movement and encouraged to engage in intellectual rather than physical activities. Those who transgressed against these norms may experience strong emotions of guilt, fear of retribution, and shame for encroaching upon the sense of self and belonging that has been defined by the collective unconscious. Some of these individuals may instead exhibit a host of defensive behavior, such as undoing and reaction formation, as a buffer against these intense feelings.

Somatization in the Asian culture

Asian clients are often characterized as focusing on somatic complaints when they are in distress. Does this mean they are defended against being in touch with their emotions? If so, how much is that a function of the internalization of culture-specific defenses? To address these questions and their implications for practice, we need to examine the origin and context of the concept of somatization from the perspective of both Western and Asian cultures.

According to psychodynamic theory, somatization has been defined as an individual's unconscious channeling of his repressed emotions into physiological symptoms in response to psychosocial stressors (Goldstein, 1995). This is a theoretical concept that is rooted in the dichotomous view of mind and body in modern Western medicine, specifically the notion that the mind is solely responsible for processing thoughts and emotions while bodily expressions of emotions are merely a fiction of the mind (McWhinney *et al.*, 2001). Thus somatization is perceived as a protective mechanism that comes into play when the individual is unable to cope with the psychological ramifications of an event. However, Chinese and Ayurvedic medicines, which are widely practiced in Asian countries, subscribe to the belief that emotions and bodily changes are interrelated through the circulatory channels of vital energies called *qi* or *prana* respectively. There is a long tradition of associating symptoms of organ malfunctions such as vertigo, abdominal discomfort, palpitations, and pressure in the chest as an outcome of imbalance of emotions (Ananth, 1984; Ots, 1990; Parker *et al.*, 2001; Tseng, 2004). As congruent with the Asian cultural value that emphasizes harmony in relationships and moderation in indulgences, excessive emotions are perceived as detrimental to an individual's health. So emotions are recognized as a key construct of an individual's sense of well-being, but emotional distress is manifested in somatic symptoms as per the cultural belief that discourages preoccupation with verbal expression of strong emotions.

It is important to note that recent neuroscience findings actually have substantiated this mind–body relationship perspective. By locating that emotions are generated by the limbic system in the brain, characterized by physiological changes associated with the fight or flight responses such as rapid heartbeat, numbing of the senses, churning sensations in the stomach, etc., neuroscience has established that emotional arousal is a universal human phenomenon that sets off bodily and hormonal reactions (Damasio, 2001; Le Doux, 1997). In addition, it has established that feelings, a product of emotions that are developed through an individual's cumulative experiences and learned perceptions of specific events, arise from the neocortical regions associated with cognitions, and may vary from culture to culture based on "the meaning humans assign to emotions" (Cappas *et al.*, 2005, p. 378). For example, feeling "depressed" is a common idiom of distress used among individuals in the Western culture to describe affective states of sadness, worthlessness, and hopelessness. In Asian cultures, these feelings states are associated with the stigma of mental illness and character weakness, and are seldom reported by individuals who exhibit symptoms of depression as characterized by Western psychiatry (Kleinman, 1988; 2004; Choi and Yeom, 2011; N. Delhiwala and M. Sawant, personal communication, 5 June 2012; M. Vu, personal communication, 8 June 2012). Studies indicate that Chinese individuals describe their distress in somatic terms as well as culture-specific feeling terms such as *hsin fan* that denotes "worry, unhappiness, annoyance, fretting and boredom" (Tseng and Lipson, 2007, p. 75). Mental health literature on Korean immigrant women has also documented that they generally use the term *Hwa-Byung* to describe their suffering of somatic complaints and emotional distress stemming from years of repressing their anger related to spousal abuse and interpersonal conflicts (Pang, 2000; Choi, 2006).

The aforementioned discussion offers a nuanced perspective of whether Asians are generally defended against their feelings because of their tendency to somatize their emotional distress. There are indeed layers of culture-specific defense associated with somatization. For example, the cultural value that emphasizes self-discipline of emotions and desires in the service of promoting individual health as well as harmony in the family and community is a strong deterrent against pre-occupation with one's emotions and feelings. Focusing on symptoms of physical illness, on the other hand, has the secondary gain of being able to take a socially acceptable respite from one's daily routine and responsibilities, as well as relationship obligations with others (Kleinman, 1988; 2004). In addition, the predominance of vocabulary in Asian languages that describe feelings is generally a mixed depiction of physical and emotional distress (Cheung, 1995; Lee *et al.*, 2007; H. Son, personal communication, 14 November 2012). For example, in the Chinese language, "heartache conveys sadness, fatigue or tiredness usually means hurt and despair." So one can argue that the Asian collective unconscious tends to protect the individuals from focusing on their emotions. However, findings from neuroscience and other medical schools of thought indicate that emotional distress can indeed give rise to somatic symptoms. Thus somatization can be considered as a rudimentary form of experiencing and expressing emotional distress, and not necessarily a "defense." We believe that whether the individual's episode of somatization is a defense rests on the nature and level of his awareness of the embedded emotional distress, and if there are any issues that he should be defended against.

We also need to remember that defenses may be adaptive or maladaptive. In the case of somatization, if the focus on illness symptoms can assuage the anxiety associated with issues that are more overwhelming to the individual, then it will serve an adaptive and valuable function for that individual. For practitioners who adhere to the Western model of practice that emphasizes verbal communication of the client's distress, working with clients who focus on their somatic symptoms can be challenging. It is important to understand the cultural context of somatization and appreciate its association with psychological distress.

Implications for practice with Asian immigrant clients

The theoretical concepts of individual and collective defenses as coping mechanisms provide another contextualized perspective for us to understand the client's thoughts, emotions, and behavior. An understanding of the relationship between Asian core values and norms and cultural defenses provides a context for practitioners to consider approaches to explore and address issues with Asian immigrant clients. Obviously, the defenses of the collective unconscious are modified as social, political, and economic changes impact on the belief systems of each culture. For Asian immigrant clients, there is the additional challenge of making sense of their host country's Western beliefs that may create stressors and conflicts. The coping mechanisms of each individual are indeed complex and multidimensional. The perspective of defenses can keep us focused on both the repressed fears and desires of our clients underlying their behavior and coping mechanisms. It will inform our approaches in creating a safe and trusting environment that resonates with their subjective realities, so that exploration of conflicts and concerns, sharing of psychological pain, and collaboration in problem solving can take place in a culturally relevant context. For example, awareness of culturally defended issues such as sexuality, aggressive feelings, and interpersonal conflicts may help the practitioner to be more observant of the client's focus of communication and consider more supportive approaches that minimize shame and blaming in raising those issues. While the Western psychodynamic approach emphasizes the articulation of intrapsychic conflicts and feelings as the antidote to the client's somatization, the practitioner's attention to the somatic symptoms or marshaling familial interest and care for the client as various forms of emotional support can be more meaningful and just as therapeutic to an Asian immigrant client.

Asian practitioners may also need to examine their own discomfort in initiating the discussion of culturally tabooed issues. Some Asian practitioners have acknowledged that it is difficult at times to make such inquiries, given the lack of appropriate vocabulary and idioms in the Asian languages to inquire about feelings, sexuality, and other culturally tabooed issues, as well as their own socialization experiences that reinforce this cultural norm. Other Asian practitioners have reported that they were able to explore these issues in a respectful manner and elicit responses from their clients after a trusting relationship was established (E. Ho, personal communication, 14 April 2012; M. Vu, personal communication, 2 March 2012). So the practice challenge essentially lies with *how* and *when* we can work around the clients' defenses and even modify their coping mechanism to improve their sense of well-being. The task begins with understanding the nature of defenses that we have to work with.

Case vignette: applying the concept of defenses

Mrs. Cao, a 50-year-old Vietnamese immigrant of Chinese descent, was referred by her family physician for counseling in regard to her depression symptoms. Mrs. Cao's chief complaints were insomnia, body aches, and general unhappiness about her life. Mrs. Cao was the only child in her family. Her father died when she was a young adolescent, and her mother, who never worked, sold congee as a street vendor to support the two of them. Mrs. Cao recalled getting up every morning at 3.00 a.m. to help her mother soak the rice and prepare the ingredients, and as an adult, would often still wake up around the same time with a great deal of anxiety. Mrs. Cao appeared to have a lot of regrets about how her mother never showed affection and appreciation for her. She shared with her clinician, Ching, that her mother never said anything to her even though she noticed that she was tired from sleep deprivation, and that she never had time to go out with friends. Mrs. Cao also disclosed that her mother rarely showed affection toward her, and did not remember her name when she was dying many years ago. Mrs. Cao showed little emotions as she narrated her childhood experiences and her relationship with her mother. However, Mrs. Cao complained bitterly that she had made a bad decision marrying her husband whom she did not find to be compatible with and physically unattractive. Mrs. Cao had two adult children, a daughter who was happily married and had a professional career, and a son who lived at home and appeared to be socially isolated. Mrs. Cao had mixed feelings toward her children. She complained that her daughter worked too hard, and worried that her son seemed to be unmotivated to pursue any interests in his life.

Mrs. Cao presented as a strong and independent individual who prided herself in overcoming the adversities in her life. When Ching initially tried to make comments about how she was neglected by her mother, Mrs. Cao would say, "I don't want to be mad at my mother." Yet she seemed to want Ching to know how much she suffered and would continue to bring up incidents to share with Ching. She finally started crying when Ching made validating comments that her mother should have paid more attention to her. Initially she would say, "Stop, I don't want to hear that. You are making me cry." As the relationship with Ching progressed, she would say, "I guess you are right, although I don't feel anything about my mother. Why is it that my body hurts all the time?" Ching tried to provide some psychoeducation about how Mrs. Cao's emotional distress was causing the physical symptoms, but Mrs. Cao would say, "No, it's just my body having problems." Mrs. Cao's crying episodes continued for a while, as she voluntarily brought up her childhood memories to elicit Ching's responses. But she would not accept any words of support from Ching. One subtle change was when Mrs. Cao accepted Ching's offer of tissues instead of using her own.

As an adolescent who depended on her mother, one can speculate that Mrs. Cao felt she had no choice but to get up in the middle of the night to help her mother to make a living, yet part of her unconsciously wished that her mother would relieve her from such a burdensome responsibility. The desire to be taken care of and "spoiled" by parents is universal among children. In Mrs. Cao's case, she had to repress her yearnings due to family circumstances and possibly the fear of further rejection by her mother. The anxiety that she still experienced as an adult could be a symptomatic indication of her internal conflicts and repressed feelings.

Growing up, Mrs. Cao appeared to be defended against her anger toward her mother and possibly the loss of her father, as evidenced in her adamant behavior of not wanting to revisit her strong emotions associated with her past. To Mrs. Cao, getting in touch with those feelings would mean the threat of breaking down the tough and fiercely independent façade that she built for herself all these years, which might very likely leave her feeling alone and vulnerable. Her own statement that she "didn't feel it" was a good illustration of a defense at work. Mrs. Cao also seemed to be unconsciously projecting her own feelings onto her children's circumstances: her resentment that her daughter was living the life that she would have desired for herself, and her pity for her son who seemed to be living a similar depressive life as hers. In addition, one could question if Mrs. Cao projected all her negative emotions as "unhappiness" about her marriage and her husband. For immigrant women of similar socioeconomic and cultural background, it was more common that they complained about the lack of concrete support from their spouses, which added to their hardships as married women, rather than incompatibility.

We can also speculate that the cultural values of family loyalty, self-sacrifice, and sanctions against harboring any negative emotions toward others also created another layer of defense that further buffered Mrs. Cao from experiencing those strong emotions.

However, one could argue that Mrs. Cao's defenses had modified with her clinician's interventions. Mrs. Cao's continued disclosure of her childhood experience and her subsequent crying was a discreet admission of her psychological pain. It appeared that she wanted Ching to bear witness to her suffering without condemning her parents. In doing so, she did not violate the cultural norms and her behavior would be deemed "acceptable". If Mrs. Cao had a parental transference toward Ching, her narratives and crying, followed by Ching's validation, would be culturally relevant and appropriate. In other words, Mrs. Cao would have found an empathic audience with her family without delving into deep feelings. If Ching had pressured Mrs. Cao to verbalize and own her feelings as per the Western modality, Mrs. Cao would have to live with the insights and those feelings which most likely she would not be able to share with her family and peers in her community and expect supportive responses.

The concept of an internalized sense of self and others

The development of an individual's sense of self and others is a vital and universal human task that evolves over one's lifetime. This sense of self is invariably tied to the individual's experience of other people, i.e., it is shaped by the nature of their interactions with her, her interpretations of their perceptions of her strengths and vulnerabilities and their expectations of her as a member of the group, etc. Her experiences with others – in the context of family, peer groups, and communities – create meanings, significance, and motivations for her sense of being. One could also view the individual as having multiple selves that are based on her varied social roles and affiliations, and thus the sense of self is an organization and integration of multi-faceted experiences (Kirmayer, 2007; Saari, 2008).

For the purpose of our discussion on the helping process, we would like to focus on the development of self representation in the formative years of childhood and adolescence that shapes the core structure of the human psyche and in turn, the personality, affect, social and interpersonal functioning, and dominant values of the individual. We will first examine the concept of internalized sense of self and others from a psychodynamic perspective and then discuss its applicability in an Asiacentric context.

How do individuals acquire "a sense of self and others"?

According to object relations theorists, the human psyche begins to take in its experiences with others, i.e., their attributes, thoughts, feelings, and emotions, from as early as infancy, and process them to become part of the psychological self. These "internalized" experiences from the past become representations that dominate the individual's inner world and shape her self-image as well as experience and perception of present relationships with others. The representations of others are called "object" representations because they encompass much more than the real person interacting with the self and are more compelling forces than the biological needs to discharge or gratify sexual and aggressive drives underlying human behavior (Cooper and Lesser, 2002; Greenberg and Mitchell, 1983; Flanagan, 2011). These internal representations of self and others are subjective and they are, at times, distorted belief systems about one's self and others. For example, there are individuals who believe that they have few desirable attributes to sustain any meaningful relationship with others, or that others will not be there for them when they need help. These schemas are partly internalized thoughts and perceptions based on the individuals' negative experiences with caretakers and others, the verbal and non-verbal messages of rejection that they received, and partly their proclivities to specific perceptions of themselves and others.

There are also internalized schemas and associated feelings, defenses, and behavior that are rooted in the socialization process of cultural values and norms, and together they form a relational template that is sustained and re-enacted over time in the individual's interactions with others. Markus and Kitayama (1994, p. 343) postulated the existence of a "collective emotional reality" whereby individuals of a given culture internalized "shared views of how and what to feel." So individuals learned to embrace or avoid certain emotions and feelings, cued by specific meanings that have been assigned to events and behavior. Shweder (1997) cited his ethnographic findings on how emotions were perceived and experienced differently by cultural groups that held divergent views on one's sense of self and others. Individuals from an individualistic culture viewed shame as diminishing their spirits while anger and happiness as strong feelings that could bolster their sense of self. On the other hand, individuals from a collectivistic culture viewed anger as "destructive of social relationships," and happiness and shame as "the glue of society," since shame is associated with the motivation to preserve one's respect by others and "an antidote to anger" (ibid., p. 157).

Clinical significance of this theoretical concept

We believe that the concept of internalized sense of self and others is an important dimension of the client's perceptions, reactions, and behavior in coping with the daily demands in their lives. Practitioners can utilize this conceptual lens to gain a better understanding of the client's subjective constructs of distress and well-being; in other words, her values and perceptions that will produce positive and negative emotions for her. Subsequently, practitioners can plan differential interventions that meet the client's concrete and emotional needs.

For example, the individual's sense of trustworthiness of herself and her sense of trust in others are generally played out in the nature of her interpersonal relationship and attachment patterns (Woods and Hollis, 2000; Goldstein, 2001). A client who has experienced rejections and abandonment in her early childhood and internalized a sense of unworthiness may encounter more difficulties in staying in an intimate relationship, and coping with the loss of significant others. Another client with a similar history who has also internalized a sense of helplessness may seek a lot of attention and reassurance from others to assuage her anxiety associated with her fragile sense of self and others.

These dynamics are also re-enacted in the helping process. We all know that even clients with similar presenting problems and background will relate to us differently. Some clients are more hesitant in seeking help from us, while others are more demanding, and some look for more reassurance and emotional support. Such varied behavior is rooted partly in the client's perception of the practitioner as a specific internal object representation, for example, an outsider who may judge them negatively for not being capable of taking care of their own affairs; a provider with resources who has a primary responsibility to take care of them; or a maternal figure who is compassionate and kind. These transferential thoughts, desires, and feelings shape the dynamics of the helping process, and illuminate the past history of the client's relationship with others. We believe that the concept of transference as it relates to the client's sense of self and others is important across all modalities of clinical practice. For our discussion here we would like to emphasize that understanding the client's interactions with the practitioner as re-enactment of his past relationships with others will be helpful to understand behaviors that may appear to be challenging and encroaching professional boundaries, and pre-empt empathic failures and power struggles in the helping process. (In Chapters 2 and 3, we will expand our discussion to examine the role of the practitioner in inducing and shaping the client's transference.)

What are the Eurocentric meanings embedded in the concept of "the sense of self"?

Object relations theorists primarily focus on the interactions of the maternal object with the infant and the child, and its impact on their developmental tasks that are defined as their ability to "separate" and "individuate" physically and psychologically from their caretakers. Aside from the discussion on the child's superego formation, which postulates that the child internalizes her parents' values, aspirations, and prohibitions, as well as social codes and moral standards in her environment, there has been little acknowledgment and interest on how diverse sociocultural factors are internalized as an integral part of the psychological self. Indeed, the focus of internalized materials by major object relation theorists such as Mahler and Winnicott, is rooted in the child-rearing practice of Western European and North American society, whereby caretakers tend to maintain some physical distance from their infants and children by providing separate sleep and play space for them and responding to their verbal cues for attention (Freeman, 1998; Shweder *et al.*, 1995). Their developmental goals are very much influenced by Western society's dominant ideology of individualism, i.e., autonomy, self-sufficiency, self-expression, etc. For example, Winnicott's widely used concepts of the "false self" (1960) and "capacity to be alone" (1958), and Mahler's seminal work on individuation (1975) are developmental benchmarks that underscore the importance of the child internalizing a sense of trust and security that is associated with autonomy and separation from undue influences or interferences from others.

What are the Asiacentric meanings that need to be considered in the development of the sense of self and others?

There is a marked difference in the process and nature of differentiation and individuation in children reared under traditional Asian cultural practice, which is centered on the development of an interdependent self and a heightened sense of others. As a major developmental goal, Asian parents strive to instill in their children the sensitivity to group norms and adaptability to function as social beings (Johnson, 1993; Roland, 1996). Thus Asian children are expected to acquire skills that will enable them to understand what is expected of them by their social environment and to meet these expectations. In Euro-American families, emphasis is placed on fostering the developmental goals of "self-determination" and "self-reliance." European-American children are encouraged to define who they are, and to shape their environment according to their interests and desires.

Traditional Asian child-rearing practice

In most Asian societies, it is not uncommon that there are multiple caretakers from the extended family to share childcare responsibilities. As befitting the Asian "total care" concept, Asian mothers and others tend to anticipate the child's needs without waiting for their cries or verbal cues. There is generally less physical separation with the baby and child – holding and sharing sleeping quarters and other chore activities are both an economic necessity and an acceptable form of indulgence. One can conclude that there is a prolonged period of symbiotic bonding, albeit with multiple caretakers, and that dependency in early childhood is encouraged as an expression of affection and attachment ties. However, differentiation in the Asian cultures also begins early by taking the form of the caretaker sensitizing the infant and the child to the impact of their behavior on others. The process often starts with the infant sensing the caretakers' subtle body language in reaction to her crying in front of others in public places, and continues with receiving direct cues when she is encouraged to minimize her crying or other affective expression as an older child to avoid being intrusive to others, or is reminded to pay respect to elders and other adults in a social encounter. Thus the social goal of differentiation in the Asiacentric context emphasizes the child's acquiring a keen awareness of the presence of others and internalizing the social code of relating in a hierarchical society (Roland, 2011).

These distinctive cultural patterns of child-rearing and social interaction invariably shape a specific sense of self and others that impact on how individuals perceive their stressors and problems and the cause of action to resolve them.

Choi and Kim (2012) and Roland (1996; 2011) characterize the central dimension of the Asian psyche as the "we-self" that emphasizes connection with others and reciprocal giving and taking as the major source of self-esteem. Roland (1996) also supports the notion that Asians often internalize a "public or social self" that is much more reserved and restrained but more dominant than and distinctly different from the "private self." This public self is a representation of the "we-self" that the individual is entrusted to preserve the honor and integrity of the family and kinship network. Thus any individual failings that endanger the image of the public self tend to trigger powerful feelings of guilt and shame. This public self also serves as a cultural censor in the individual's development of her super-ego, i.e., the parameters of when she can be assertive about her personal desires and when she needs to defer to the wishes of others. Appreciation of this cultural configuration of one's sense of self and others is important in our assessment of the Asian immigrant clients and their families. Practitioners have often struggled with Winnicott's concept of "the false self" when working with Asian clients, since the concept views the child's internalization of the need to hide her own self and complies with the expectations and wishes of others as a developmental detriment in her personality organization and functioning. We believe that the key issue lies with the fluid connection between the public and private self of the individual, and the predominant emotions that have been internalized. An individual with a "false self" generally lives with feelings of insecurity and fear of rejection and abandonment as a result of lack of nurturance and care in her early years, and her submissive behavior is driven by those negative emotions.

For individuals who internalized the Asian cultural values associated with interdependence, there is generally a sense of gratification and warm familial feelings when they are able to intuitively anticipate the needs of others and make compromises for the benefit of their family and group affiliations.

Our discussion on the divergent sense of self and others between Western and Asian cultures illuminates the distinctly different clusters of beliefs and behavior that are internalized and associated with a positive and negative sense of self and others among individuals from the two cultures. Such appreciation of the cultural layering of one's sense of self and others adds another dimension in understanding the subjective constructs of well-being and distress of our clients, and hence, enhances our empathic connection with them. For example, a Western-trained practitioner in a hospital setting who can support an older Asian client's wish to defer medical decision and after care options to her family as a positive and culturally relevant gesture to strengthen her ties with family, will be providing an intervention that gratifies her sense of being cared for by her children, who in turn, will also feel gratified that they have been entrusted with the opportunity to reciprocate care for her. Thus, even the concrete task of discharge planning can become a therapeutic experience for the client and her family.

In the following section, we will present a segment of a process recording by a Caucasian social work intern in regard to her work with a young gay man from Thailand seeking asylum in the United States. The intern's initial reflections and assessment, as informed by North American and Eurocentric values, characterized the client's communications and relatedness as traits of low self-esteem. Her impression in turn fueled her perception that she failed to engage the client in accepting services and developing trust in their working relationship. As the intern learned to examine her interactions with the client from an Asiacentric perspective, she had a much more positive understanding of the client's thoughts, behavior, and strengths, as well as his therapeutic gains from their relationship.

Table 1.2 Dialogs and reflections. Intern (Susan) and client (Chai) met up after Chai returned from a meeting with the lawyers working on his asylum papers. Chai reflected that he just took up three hours of the lawyers' time.

Dialog	Initial reflections	Final reflections
Susan: We've talked about this before, right? Are you still feeling the same way? **Chai:** Well I know when they have to deal with me they can't charge a cent, so that makes me feel useless. **Susan:** Hmmm.	I'm trying not to say a lot, to see where this goes, but I feel myself getting frustrated already. I try to focus hard on listening, trying not to interpret or react – just be there and validate what he's saying even if I've heard him say the same thing over and over again... By not asking questions I feel Chai tenses up and he looks at me, nervous, like there's something he should be doing to accommodate me – whether it's reporting the full details of something or divulging something – he often just looks at me with a face that I perceive to be incredibly anxious.	

Table 1.2 (continued)

Dialog	Initial reflections	Final reflections
Chai: It was a pleasant surprise to be showered with attention. **Susan:** A surprise? **Chai:** Yes I was surprised since it wasn't like I deserved it or anything. They ordered sandwiches and pastas and drinks for the meeting. It was a big conference room that was very nice. **Susan:** Hmmm. Besides money though, do you think they're getting something out of the work? **Chai:** Actually I asked them that, because that's the thing I'm most confused by. I asked them why they are working on my case. **Susan:** You did? And what did they say? **Chai:** They said they liked to help people. **Susan:** So they LIKE helping people… **Chai:** Yes and I know you told me the same thing. **Susan:** But you're skeptical… **Chai:** Yes but I guess I have to believe them. I try to focus on that. I don't want to annoy them.	He says this with heavy awkwardness and I don't take it as a joke – I'm worried about the fact he is putting himself down so much. I also felt that it was important to help him understand that he was not an imposition on others.	As someone from an interdependent culture, it is important for him to be able to reciprocate what others have offered him.

The conversation moved to Chai's life and his relationship with his boyfriend, Jim.

Chai: I think a lot about my work – will the jobs come in, will it still be busy, when will I get my paycheck. Outside from that, what we're going to cook tonight for dinner, what Jim wants to do for Christmas and how I can make that happen. **Susan:** You always think about how you can take care of Jim. **Chai:** (Surprised) Well, I don't know if I do that. I know that our rent is paid for this month, so that's good. But actually, should I be talking about this?	Is he still uncomfortable talking with me? Does he think that I don't understand him?	He actually trusts me. Confiding personal conflicts in me is an indication that I am in his private circle of trustworthy individuals. Checking with me is his way of showing respect and being mindful of boundaries.

Table 1.2 (continued)

Dialog	Initial reflections	Final reflections
Susan: Of course, if it's something you want to talk about we can talk about it. **Chai:** Well, I don't know if this is too personal but Jim and I got in a big fight a few days ago. Everything is fine now. **Susan:** You are saving to be able to take care of him. It's really amazing how much concern and care you show him. I can tell you're really worried about him. **Chai:** I don't know about that. **Susan:** That doesn't sound right to you? **Chai:** Well I don't want to take all the credit. He always took care of me when we were in Asia. Now it's my turn…		
After a brief silence:		
Chai: I just don't know if I'm bothering you with all this. **Susan:** Not at all. **Chai:** Okay, well, he says I skimp on things, even down to how I spread only a little bit of butter on a piece of bread. He thinks saving is just so embarrassing. He is embarrassed of me I think. **Susan:** Well, it's too bad if that's what Jim feels. I know you as someone who is incredibly resourceful. When I look at your life and what you have accomplished I am amazed at how much thought and planning, in the middle of a lot of pain and confusion, you were able to do. I think you have the ability to be able to see the big picture and plan ahead in order to survive, that is a real strength. **Chai:** I don't know about that. **Susan:** Well, it's just my opinion. But from where I'm sitting and from what I've heard	He doesn't seem to appreciate my highlighting of his strengths. Seems like he has a lot of self-doubts?	His not accepting my compliments directly does not necessarily mean he does not appreciate them. He is finally quite spontaneous when he said, "really?", and assertive when he said, "what do you mean?" That sounds more like the American way of relating! Perhaps he is becoming more bi-cultural! He actually said at one point, "I don't know what my mother would say if she finds out that I am seeing a therapist."

Table 1.2 (continued)

Dialog	Initial reflections	Final reflections
over the past few months, I think you care a lot about people and want to make sure they are going to be okay. I have noticed you doing it with me, even. **Chai:** Oh, really? No, wait, what do you mean?		

Discussion

Internalization is a complex and multi-layered mental process. It is not possible to find out how much Chai had internalized an Asian sense of self and others that shaped his behavior and emotions. However, the focus and style of his communication in the session certainly emphasized the interests of others over his, and contrasted sharply with the individualistic orientation of the social work intern. In a subsequent conversation with the student intern, Chai made reference to the fact that he was brought up to be "humble" and never "put himself on the pedestal," and that he had "never made a big thing out of everything" until he asked for assistance with his asylum application. On the other hand, he also acknowledged that his family rarely praised him or supported his interests, so he "never felt good about himself." We can argue that from an Asian perspective, Chai had a solid sense of self that revolved around anticipating and deferring to the wishes and needs of others, which in turn gave him a sense of belonging and purpose in the collectivistic culture of his home country. Although his homosexuality created a tremendous conflict between him, his family, and society and precipitated a crisis for his sense of self, one can argue that he would not have been able to get in touch with his sexual orientation and made the decision to leave his family without an intact agency of self. In other words, he had developed a "private" self that was cognizant of his personal desires and the ramifications of meeting his own needs at this point in his life. From a psychodynamic perspective, Chai was trying to configure a different sense of self and others. From a practice and relational model perspective, Chai would need the practitioner's support and acceptance of how much or how little change he was ready to initiate in this process. Chai, who was often insightful and articulate, offered a profound reflection as he acknowledged that he was "different" in his perceptions and reactions from individuals in American society, "It's a large part of who I am and it's not that it's good to be this way but it's who I am." This, paradoxically, would be the Western individualistic focus of the sense of self!

Concluding remarks

In this chapter, we discussed the importance of using clinical theories to guide our practice across all modalities in the helping process. We underscored the universal aspects of these theories to illuminate the complexities of human behavior in coping with stressors and the demands of different life roles in society. In our discussion of the key psychodynamic concepts of ego defenses and internalized sense of self and others, we delineated the Eurocentric values that shaped the development of these concepts and applied them in a context that resonated more with the core Asian cultural values and norms. The proposed perspectives are our own conjectures based on our practice, teaching, and research experiences and discussions with other practitioners in the Asian communities. They are illustrations of how theories can be deconstructed and reconstructed. As cultural values and norms evolve with the changing conditions and needs of society – a process that is becoming more evident with the increasing impact of a globalized economy and modernization around the world – we can anticipate theories and practice interventions to evolve as well.

Discussion highlights

The intersection of clinical theories and cultural meanings

Clinical theories are generally infused with cultural meanings when theorists emphasize and de-emphasize certain foci in their theoretical elucidation. (p. 3)

Ego defenses

Ego defenses protect the individual from overwhelming anxiety and intolerable thoughts, and they serve an adaptive purpose that supports the individual in his daily functioning. (p. 10)

Assessment of a client's defenses requires ongoing observations of a client's thoughts, emotions and behavior that are marked by some degree of rigidity and irrationality despite changes in circumstances, and an assessment of the nature and context of the defenses. (p. 10)

Whether the individual's episode of somatization is a defense, rests on the nature and level of his awareness of the embedded emotional distress, and if there are any issues that he should be defended against. (p. 16)

Somatization can be considered as a rudimentary form of experiencing and expressing emotional distress, and not necessarily a "defense." (p. 16)

Sense of self and others

The concept of internalized sense of self and others is an important dimension of the client's perceptions, reactions, and behavior in coping with the daily demands in their lives. Practitioners can utilize this conceptual lens to gain a better understanding of the client's subjective constructs of distress and well-being. (p. 21)

There is a marked difference in the process and nature of differentiation and individuation in children reared under traditional Asian cultural practice, which is centered on the development of an interdependent self and a heightened sense of others. (p. 22)

For individuals who internalized the Asian cultural values associated with interdependence, there is generally a sense of gratification and warm familial feelings when they are able to intuitively anticipate the needs of others and make compromises for the benefit of their family and group affiliations. (p. 23)

2 Relational theory

A two-person psychology model in the helping process

Irene W. Chung

In this chapter, we will discuss the major premises of relational theory in the context of how therapeutic changes for the clients take place in the helping process. In remaining true to its theoretical origin, we will utilize some of the key psychodynamic concepts and parlance in our discussion of relational theory as they are applied to an insight-oriented psychotherapy modality in the first half of the chapter. We will then expand our discussion to practice implications for other service models in the helping process. While counseling and psychotherapy services are often perceived as the major venues of psychological growth for clients, we believe that there are clinical and therapeutic aspects embedded in concrete service coordination and delivery. We agree with many relational theorists that even time-limited approaches that emphasize the support for and empowerment of clients have the potential to strengthen their interpersonal and coping capacities, as well as their social functioning (Borden, 2000; Floersch and Longhofer, 2004).

Theroretical background and discussion

Evolvement of treatment focus

Relational theory evolved from a host of theories that were rooted in a two-person transactional perspective. While classical Freudian theory focused on the individual's unconscious intrapsychic conflicts around biological drives of aggression and sexuality, subsequent psychodynamic theories have progressively adopted a broader orientation in understanding human growth and development in the context of relationship with others. Ego psychology, in its postulations of ego functions, defenses, and life roles, illuminated the adaptive capacity of individuals to meet the demands of family, community, and society (Erikson, 1959; Hartmann, 1939). Object relations theory, in examining the inner world and emotional life of individuals, emphasized the intrinsic human needs for attachment ties and connections with others over gratification of instinctual bodily needs (Bowlby, 1969), and provided elaborate insights on child development based on the quality of interaction with early caretakers (Fairbairn, 1952; Winnicott, 1965).

Object relation theorists also pioneered a treatment focus that facilitates the client's growth via a corrective experience within a "real" relationship between the practitioner and the client (Greenson, 1971; Levenson, 1985; Mitchell, 1988). Self psychology sharpened this relational focus and emphasized the active role of the practitioner serving as empathic and mirroring "selfobjects" to meet the specific emotional needs of the client. This highly attentive and responsive stance of the practitioner in connecting with the client's subjective desires and perceptions, marked the beginning of a mutually regulated relational paradigm in treatment (Kohut 1971, 1977). Recent object relations theorists in the United States elaborated on the dynamics of mutual regulation in the treatment relationship under the concept of intersubjectivity, which subsequently became a major underpinning of relational theory (Aron, 1996; Benjamin, 1998; Ogden, 1994; Stolorow and Atwood, 1992). Intersubjectivity is essentially a correlate of the reciprocal dynamics postulated under the ecological systemic theory (Bronfenbrenner, 1979) whereby units within a system both influence and shape each other, resulting in changes for all. Applied to the clinical relationship, intersubjectivity depicts the unique co-experience resulting from the interactions of the client and the practitioner. The recognition that there is a *meeting of two psyches* in the clinical encounter underscores the need to re-examine the concepts of transference and countertransference, as well as the applicability and effectiveness of traditional psychodynamic approaches in assessment and interventions. At the same time, the increased prominence of social constructionism in understanding the diverse complexities of human behavior from the subjective meaning systems of individuals, and its emphasis on co-construction of meaningful experiences within the clinical dyad in cross-cultural practice (Gergen, 1985; McNamee and Gergen, 1992), further affirms the belief that the practitioner cannot possibly be the detached observer in the clinical encounter and that a more active participatory style of relating has to emerge in the therapeutic process.

Several practice models have always emphasized the use of the therapeutic relationship as a milieu for the client's psychological growth before relational theory was fully coalesced and articulated in the last decade. The interpersonal school (Sullivan, 1953), the client-centered model (Rogers, 1951), and the feminist relational/cultural paradigm (Miller and Stiver, 1991, 1995) are proponents of the belief that human growth occurs within and not apart from relationships that offer empathy, support, and acceptance to clients. Last but not least, clinical social work practice has always viewed the social worker's use of self in cultivating a compassionate, authentic, and client's strength-based relationship as exemplary of its core principles and values in the helping process (Goldstein *et al.*, 2009; Freedberg, 2009; Woods and Hollis, 2000). Building on the relational characteristics espoused by these models, the work of relational theorists resulted in a paradigm shift in the way we understand how the change process takes place from an integration of psychodynamic and systemic perspectives.

Theoretical discussion

In this section, we will discuss how relational theorists dispute the traditional view of analyzing the client's unconscious as the key treatment approach and re-conceptualize major psychodynamic concepts. We will then illustrate how the two-person psychology approaches effect psychological growth for the client.

The traditional treatment focus on the unconscious

Uncovering the client's unconscious thoughts, feelings, desires, and fears has been the cornerstone of classic Freudian approach in psychoanalysis, and has had a major influence on psychodynamic-oriented psychotherapy and counseling. As discussed in Chapter 1, these unconscious materials are considered to be repressed drive derivatives of aggression and sexuality – the two major human motivational forces postulated by Freud – that are unacceptable to the client, and are roots of the individual's psychic conflicts and pain. Symptoms invariably emerge, as the inner conflicts remain repressed. Thus the ultimate goal of traditional treatment would be to bring these materials into consciousness through the client's introspection and subsequent renunciation and sublimation of these issues. This "talking cure" approach mandates that the practitioner maintain a neutral and objective stance, analogous to "the blank screen" in the process (Freud, 1912). It is considered an important clinical approach to facilitate the client's free association and enactment of those repressed materials based on her transferential experience of the clinician as a frustrating and non-gratifying object. In Freudian parlance, the client's transference is a crystallization of her subjective inner world representation of self and others that yields a wealth of information on her unconscious intrapsychic desires and conflicts. Thus the practitioner's observation and interpretation of the client's "distorted" transference is considered as the core treatment strategy, as the unconscious materials are rendered into the client's consciousness (Borden, 2009; Perlman and Brandell, 2011).

A contemporary view of the unconscious

Relational theorists argue that the traditional treatment approach is analogous to viewing the unconscious as a "frozen entity waiting to be discovered" (Wachtel, 2008, p. 48). In contrast, they emphasize that an individual's unconscious is a dynamic and fluid entity that is constantly evolving from interaction with others in the external world (Mitchell, 1988; Stolorow *et al.*, 1987). Adopting a transactional and system perspective, relational theorists postulate that pre-determined drives and unconscious fantasies, desires, and fears toward object representations of early caretakers are but *one* aspect of the individual's mental process, and that they, along with other repressed materials such as selective memories and feelings, are in a perpetual cycle of reciprocal influences with the individual's interpersonal life. Bromberg (1998) describes the human mind as a conglomerate of shifting states of consciousness that are somehow influenced by the individual's past and present experiences, projections into the future, and perceptions that *make sense to the individual at a particular time*. Fragments of repressed materials – partial memories of a scenario, conversation, or associated feelings may emerge and become incorporated into the individual's schema of self and others. Zepf (2007) discusses how the repression of unconscious materials is shaped by the demands of the individual's external world in defining the acceptability of her thoughts, feelings, and behavior, and how subsequently warded-off instincts take on changeable forms of distortion, omission, and substitution as the individual attempts to adapt to norms and values in an interactive environment.

By the same token, relational theorists regard the client's emerging intrapsychic issues and transference enactment in the clinical process as a layer of her unconsciousness that has been colored by her current life events as well as the interaction between the client and the clinician. The development of major events and circumstances in the client's current life naturally shapes the focus and subjectivity of the client as well as her motivation and capacity for introspection in the session. For example, a client whose estranged father just passed away might be more inclined to recall some good times she had with him, or get in touch with some longings that she had toward him that she had previously repressed.

In addition, relational theorists argue that the practitioner's "neutrality" is not a pure objective stance (Greenberg, 1991; Stolorow and Atwood, 1997). The presentation of a "blank screen" is nonetheless an action that triggers a reaction from the client's inner experience – for example, negative perceptions of the practitioner as a withholding, angry, or uncaring parent, etc. So the client's enactment and introspection possibilities are already skewed within a specific range of her subjective states. More importantly, the practitioner's observations and interpretations of the client's transference are essentially still her own organization of data and meanings based on her theoretical proclivity and subjective experience (Greenberg and Mitchell, 1983; Stolorow *et al.*, 1987; Wachtel, 2008). Hence the unconscious materials that are "uncovered" are those that emerge from a two-person interactive context in the clinical encounter. They are not "absolute truths" but subjective meanings influenced by the communication – verbal and non-verbal – between the client and the practitioner.

Implications for the change process: a relational perspective

This modified view of the unconscious and the practitioner's role in the therapeutic process greatly alters the landscape of the change process. Relational theorists postulate that the fluidity of the individual's unconscious in the context of interaction with others is an indication that psychological growth can occur in a purposeful relationship without delving into the individual's repressed materials. The implication is that a client who feels supported, cared for, and empowered in her interaction with her practitioner may experience a positive shift of her cognitions, emotions, her sense of self and others, and defenses. The client's positive experience may subsequently lend itself to reflection and introspection of her fears and vulnerabilities.

Dynamics of the change process under the relational paradigm

In traditional psychotherapy practice, exploration and interpretation are the major modes of intervention whereby the practitioner would pose questions, probe into repressed materials, and offer her observations for the client's intro-spection. Such insight-oriented approaches have been considered the hallmark mechanism that initiates the change process for clients. Under the relational paradigm, exploration, interpretation, and introspection occur in a seamless process within an interactive context of the clinical encounter, and become part of a therapeutic experience that promotes the client's psychological growth.

Exploration as empathic inquiry

Exploration begins with the practitioner listening attentively, responding affec-tively to the client's narratives, and engaging the client in discussing the nuances of his subjective experiences. Building on the concept of the "empathic stance" in self psychology (Kohut, 1957), relational theorists view the key objective of exploration as the practitioner being able to fully enter and understand the sub-jective world of the client, and making the client feel understood. The sense of trust and bonding that emerges from this empathic inquiry and understanding fuels the core dynamics of the change process in the relational context. In trans-cending the traditional psychodynamic approach of accessing and interpreting the client's inner process as the pathway to change, relational theorists adopt a more supportive and "present" focus in exploration. While the practitioner may note the defenses and hints of repressed materials of the client in this exploration process – her restricted affect and focus, etc. – these observations would serve as the parameter and *not* the focus of exploration and interpretation. Instead of viewing client's defenses as the underlying cause of resistant behavior that needs to be analyzed and interpreted, relational theorists adhere to the self psychology stance that any form of treatment-resistant behavior is the client's self-protective reaction to the fear of re-traumatization by past painful relationships with significant others that are marked by rejection, violation, and abandonment and re-experiencing the associated range of feelings – shame, guilt, hopelessness, and helplessness, etc. (Goldstein, 2001; Teitelbaum, 1991). Thus a direct inquiry and interpretation stance will most likely be experienced as harsh, interrogative, and judgmental, and most importantly, threatening to the client's self-esteem. The client's anxiety triggered by such an approach will actually be a deterrent for self-reflection.

Interpretation in the service of building self-esteem

It is important to note that relational theorists conceptualize anxiety differently from classical psychodynamic theory. Influenced by Sullivan's interpersonal theory (1953) and Kohut's self psychology (1971) that emphasize the central role of self-esteem in an individual's sense of well-being and capacity for change, relational theorists postulate that anxiety is primarily interpersonal in nature, rather than the outcome of intrapsychic conflicts of biological impulses in the indivi-dual's subjective inner process (DeLaCour, 1996; Wachtel, 2008). Influenced by Sullivan (1953), Fairbairn (1952), and Winnicott (1960), relational theorists posit that individuals learned to hide or disown parts of themselves – thoughts, feelings, and desires – as a result of their caretakers' dismissal or disapproval of those specific emotional needs. Unconsciously those split-off parts are associated with painful rejection by significant others and need to be repressed. Anxiety emerges when repression of those disavowed feelings and thoughts are challenged. Oftentimes, an individual's self-esteem and self-acceptance are compromised in the service of maintaining a conflict-free inner life, and she learns to resist integrating those ward-off parts at the cost of maintaining a negative image of herself. For example, it is not uncommon that some clients will experience unease and apprehension but not anger in situations where they have been rejected or slighted by significant others. Upon questioning they may agree that they have a right to be upset but will not be able to explain the source of their anxiety that appears to be irrational. It would seem that their anger has been repressed unconsciously as part of their coping mechanism. In the traditional psychotherapy process, the practitioner will generally explore and make interpretations of the client's anxiety and her self-esteem. It is not uncommon that the client will experience increased anxiety from such intervention that "threatens" her psychological equilibrium, resulting in missed appointments or a rupture in the therapeutic alliance.

Relational theorists believe that pre-empting the client's anxiety is more important than undoing their defenses and repression (Wachtel, 2008). Since defenses come in various interrelated forms and layers – for example, denial of one's feelings is often bolstered by acts of intellectualization and displacement of those feelings – interpretation of specific defenses would only threaten the underlying anxiety and trigger or reinforce other defenses, subjecting the client to a perpetual cycle of escalating anxiety, defenses, and restrictive functioning in the helping process. For example, a client coming late or missing sessions after the practitioner's interpretation of some repressed materials is likely an act of regression. Or the client could be marshaling the defense of intellectualization and dissociation when she marginally acknowledges an issue illuminated by the practitioner without allowing herself to experience the associated buried emotions.

Relational theorists posit that insights of the nature of anxiety have to be provided in opportune moments, and that the creation of empathic connections with the client through a supportive mode of exploration is a much more therapeutic approach to support the client in overcoming the underlying anxiety and move toward psychological growth. It is because of the sense of safety and feeling understood, communicated through such empathic bonding that the client may feel more inclined to reflect on her vulnerabilities and develop a more integrated sense of self-acceptance. Thus exploration, interpretation, and introspection is a two-person collaborative process, with the clinician paying heed to what is acceptable and meaningful to the client's self-esteem from moment to moment, and offering reframed perspectives for her consideration and introspection. As Wachtel (2008, p. 25) aptly puts it, "Change emerges from the process of exploration and interaction itself between two individuals – via deconstruction and co-construction of meanings, emotions and behavior."

Under the relational paradigm, the clinician's offering of support and empathic exploration are two crucial interrelated elements in the change process. When the clinician is able to immerse in the exploration of the client's subjective experience of stressors and challenges, she will be able to communicate genuine support through a more authentic discussion with the client in regard to her coping patterns, her vulnerabilities as well as strengths. Again, this serves to advance the therapeutic goal of providing a safe space and corrective experience for the client to develop a more cohesive agency of self and greater sense of self-acceptance – a healthy psychological base that energizes her motivation and capacity for change.

Interactive view of the client's transference

The client's re-enactment of her early relational patterns is inevitable in the helping process. As the client gains a sense of trust and safety in the therapeutic relationship and develops transferential feelings toward the practitioner, she will act out familiar desires and feelings, which traditional psychodynamic theorists think should be analyzed rather than gratified (Dewald, 1972; Friedman, 2002; Sarri, 1986). For example, a client who craves attention from his family may take up a lot of time in his session talking about his struggles and accomplishments in his life, and expecting the therapist, who he views as a parental figure, to listen patiently and validate his strengths. From the perspective of traditional psychodynamic theorists, the client's re-enactment of his early familial dynamics needs to be explored and interpreted as a major intervention approach. Relational theorists, however, would adopt a more expansive and interactive view of the client's transference. Instead of just focusing on the client's repetition of his past relationships and his projection of the associated feelings, relational theorists view transference as also being shaped by the practitioner's interaction that is filtered by her own inner experience with the client. So in the aforementioned example, the practitioner would need to consider her own responses to the client's excessive talking and expectation for her validation. Did she communicate some sense of boredom listening to the client? Did she fail to provide affirmation of the client's accomplishments and hence exacerbated the client's preoccupation in the session? These "here-and-now" dynamics have to be considered in characterizing the client's transference as re-enactment.

Processing versus interpreting transference

This modified perspective makes the re-enactment a two-person experience, starting with the client's familiar relatedness, thoughts, and feelings, and ending with insights from a new and real interactive experience with another person. The practitioner's objective interpretation is replaced by processing of the experience of re-enactment *with* the client. For example, a client who is sensitive to criticism by others in regard to his personality traits such as poor time management or difficulties in articulation of thoughts and feelings may perceive that the clinician's reminders of future appointments or assistance in the narration of past events as humiliating and patronizing. In taking a relational approach, the practitioner would examine her behavior and role in precipitating the client's transferential reaction, and engage the client in a dialog in understanding each other's perceptions and associated feelings. The experience of processing with the practitioner in a relational context affords the client an opportunity to understand the subjectivity of her transference and consider the potentiality of modifying that transference. Since both the practitioner and the client own the dynamics of inducing and responding to feelings and behavior in the clinical encounter, the client is also more likely to gain a broader perspective of the reciprocal dynamics embedded in his relational patterns with others, and appreciate a circular versus dichotomous view of interpersonal transactions. For example, clients who tend to feel self-righteous about their opinions and behavior may learn to be more tolerant of differences. Or clients who tend to internalize problems will feel more accepted and empowered in the introspective process of the repetitions, and may be able to work toward giving up some of the self-blaming in coping with relational issues.

As an outcome of the co-processing of the re-enactment, the client is also more likely to experience the practitioner as a fully-dimensional "subject" with divergent views and emotions versus a strictly "internalized" object of fears or desires (Benjamin, 1990; Flanagan, 2011; Goldstein, 2001). The practitioner's ability to manage the re-enactment and share her own reactions and hindsight of the interactions will be instrumental in providing a powerful corrective experience that can rework the unconscious relational schemas of the client. Rather than focusing on interpretation or confrontation of the client's re-enactment behavior, such as her unresolved need for attachment, validation and support, or hostile and hurtful remarks over perceived rejections, the practitioner's discreet and crafted response in maintaining authentic and supportive relational dynamics is a therapeutic intervention to reinforce a new schema of the client's sense of self and others, and positive help-seeking behavior. For example, instead of pointing out a client's tendency to ask for advice and opinions from the clinician and exploring the underlying transferential issue, the practitioner may continue to offer some form of advice while making empathic reflections in regard to her understanding of the client's lack of support in his past history, as well as commending his resourcefulness in seeking help. This relational approach would be congruent with the core idea of promoting the client's reflections of his behavior in the context of feeling accepted and empowered by the clinician, and initiating changes without verbal articulation.

Communication and interaction in the relational context

Authentic and spontaneous communication

The nature of communication and interaction in a growth-fostering two-person relationship provides a contextualized view of the re-conceptualized dynamics discussed in the preceding sections. Given the premise of mutuality between the practitioner and the client, communication and interaction within the therapeutic dyad are marked by a sense of authenticity and spontaneity. The practitioner is charged with the task of using herself differentially in responding to the client's narratives on a cognitive as well as an affective level. For example, instead of using the standard inquiry lines, "how do you feel about that?" or "what would you like to do about that?", the practitioner may infuse more of her concern about the client's well-being in her questioning. Or instead of using a scripted professional lexicon laced with interpretation to convey support – "It must be hard for you to express your anger ... Sounds like you felt abandoned ... ", etc. – the practitioner may share her spontaneous reaction with some nuances to let the client know she understands his subjective experience.

Practitioner's self-disclosure

Contrary to the asymmetrical stance of the traditional psychodynamic approach that discourages the practitioner's self-disclosure, relational theorists encourage the judicious use of such practice to create a more egalitarian and genuine relationship. Thus the practitioner may share some of her personal thoughts and feelings – positive and negative – in response to the client's discussion or behavior in the here-and-now context in the interest of the therapeutic growth of the client. Such disclosure may serve the purpose of providing a corrective experience for the client – in the forms of empathy from a caring person who understands her pain, feedback of the impact of her words and behavior on others in a supportive context, or validation of her sense of self from the practitioner's acknowledgment of failed empathy or misattunement to her emotional needs.

Relational theorists also sanction the practitioner's disclosure of appropriate personal information for the purpose of enhancing the therapeutic relationship, for example, the client's trust issue in the authenticity and expertise of the worker, or the client's need to identify with the worker. So it is not uncommon that clinicians will disclose background information such as immigrant or parent status to clients and personal understanding of the struggles and hardships experienced by the clients.

Permeability of professional boundary

Traditionally, practitioners are inclined to uphold a clear delineation of roles and functions that restricts their involvement with clients to preserve their objective and detached stance in the clinical encounter. Meeting the client's dependency needs, such as extending contacts beyond the counseling session, is considered a hindrance to the client's process of introspection and psychological growth, and should be avoided. Under the relational paradigm, physical and emotional boundaries are more fluid between the clinician and the client as stressors and needs wax and wane in the client's life. As a partner of a genuine relationship, it may be necessary that the practitioner respond to a client who is overwhelmed by life stressors via provision of concrete advice and support, or extension of session time spent with the client. By the same token, the practitioner also needs to accept the client's expression of appreciation or concern for the clinician's well-being. This reciprocal give-and-take quality of interaction provides another opportunity for a corrective experience whereby the client feels both valued and empowered.

Mutuality in the intersubjective space

According to relational theorists, all conscious and unconscious communication and interactions between the practitioner and the client – verbal articulation, body language, latent message, and exchange of affects, etc. – occur in a symbolic psychological field that came to be known as the intersubjective or "third" space in the clinical encounter (Benjamin, 1990, 1998; Ogden, 1994; Stolorow and Atwood, 1992). Influenced by Winnicott's concept of the transitional space (1971) where the child plays out her fantasies, thoughts, and feelings in adaptation to her external environment and development toward relative autonomy, the inter-subjective space is deemed as a safe space co-created by the client and the clinician to *explore and experience* the client's inner life as well as new ways of thinking, feeling, and being. It is a unique transitional space marked by a specific pattern of communication and interaction shared by the practitioner and the client as the relationship progresses, including a mutual awareness and sensing of each other's thoughts and desires. These dynamics are instrumental in helping the practitioner attune and attend to the fears, anxiety, and desires of the client. Through immersion in the relationship and the tracking of her own countertransference, the practitioner is able to experience a keener sense of the client's emotional needs, and responds empathically. For example, a practitioner who is mindful of intersubjective dynamics may experience a sense of awkwardness with her client who has become reticent as he discusses a specific troubled period in his past. She notices that her client starts to shift in his chair, checks his watch, and then abruptly changes the discussion to a mundane issue. Instead of interpreting the client's silence as resistant behavior and taking the stance that she should refrain from "colluding" with the client from a traditional psychodynamic perspective, the practitioner chooses to make eye contact and give a knowing nod, and trust that her sensitivity to the client's reluctance to discuss the issue is intuitively communicated to the client. This mutual yet unspoken recognition of each other's thoughts and feelings can be more therapeutic than the client's act of discussing his issue. Relational theorists posit that the tacit mutuality and empathic under-standing played out within the intersubjective space provides more opportunities of corrective experience for the client to feel valued, validated, and cared for.

"Moments of meeting" in the therapeutic relationship

As part of the intersubjective dynamics, relational theorists postulate that the "moments" when the practitioner and the client co-create new meanings and activities in the course of their relationship are powerful experiences in modifying maladaptive aspects of the client's internalized pattern of relatedness (Fonagy, 1998; Lyons-Ruth, 1998; Tronick, 2007). These changes are characterized as "altered domain of implicit relational knowing" (Tronick, 2007, p. 425), a concept that has been used to depict the movements of implicitly learned antici-pations and expectations during infant and caregiver interactions in the service of the infant's developmental growth (Sander, 1962, 1995; Stern, 1985). In the previous example, we can speculate that the client's reluctance to disclose sensitive issues to another individual stems from an implicit relational knowing that has been associated with a history of negative feedback or judgment from others. Thus the practitioner's response of acceptance is a corrective experience that creates a shift in this domain of the client's implicit relational knowing. It is a moment of meeting that is not based on interpretation and insights, but intuitive communication between two individuals who are bonded by authentic moments of humor, joy, tears, or frustrations in a real relationship. Changes from moments of meeting are indeed gradual and subtle, but cumulative and more lasting as they take place in an interactive process with a trustworthy and caring practitioner.

Empirical studies on the efficacy of relational approaches

Studies have indicated that strong therapeutic alliances are associated with positive treatment outcome (Horvath and Symonds, 1991; Lambert, 1992; Martin *et al.*, 2000; McCabe and Priebe, 2004). Recent findings of neuroscience, infant research, and child development have also elucidated the dynamics of psychological growth within the therapeutic relationship.

Siegel (2012, p. 40) characterizes the practitioner's attunement to the client's verbal and non-verbal communication as analogous to the highly interactive parent–child experience whereby the child "feels seen and enriched" and "will thrive in the moment." Over time, the child will internalize a positive self and other representation that she can access for self-soothing in times of distress. Schore and Schore (2008) utilize neurobiological findings such as brain imaging on the development of the right brain region to posit that the emotion processing and regulation capacity of the child is linked to the quality of early attachment communications between the parent and the infant, i.e., tone of voice, facial expression, posture, and other non-verbal affective cues. Similarly, they suggest that a nurturing and interactive relationship between the practitioner and the client can be a stimulus for growth in the right brain structure to regulate affect and strong emotions later in life as well. So individuals who suffer from the deleterious effects of childhood trauma can benefit from the shared experience of a therapeutic relationship and become better equipped in coping with demands and stressors in life. Finally, the evidence of the growth-inducing effect of right brain communication is also an affirmation of the value of implicit communication embedded in the relational model in the change process, for example, affective exchanges and eye contacts between the practitioner and the client (Lyons-Ruth, 2000; Scaer, 2005).

Practice implications and discussions

In the first half of the chapter, we focused on the two-person psychology of relational theory and how the paradigm charts a different pathway of the client's change process through a therapeutic relationship marked by a modified view of the use of the unconscious, transference, and countertransference. Rather than facilitating insight-oriented discussion with the client as the focus of change, the practitioner is charged with the task of creating a therapeutic space similar to Winnicott's concept of the "holding environment" (1965), whereby the client feels accepted and supported, and becomes motivated in exploring new possibilities of looking at herself and others from interactions with the practitioner. It is also similar to Kohut's postulation of the practitioner serving as "selfobjects" (1984) whereby the practitioner provides transferential experiences – providing valida-tion, partnership, advocacy, etc. – that meet the client's emotional needs for selective internalization and psychological growth. Indeed, relational theory is a logical progression and coalescence of theories that emphasize the two-person interactive perspective in the helping process. Its distinction lies with the focus of intersubjectivity, i.e., a relationship that is shaped by mutual influences between the client and the practitioner's subjective experiences, and marked by unique patterns of communication and interaction developed between the dyad. Such subjectivity includes myriad influences ranging from each individual's personality to class, racial, and cultural background, and thus accounts for why and how each therapeutic dyad is distinct from others, and how even the same client will have varied experiences with different practitioners. Most importantly, the inter-subjective perspective offers the practitioner a guiding principle to step out of the prescribed traditional role of communication and relating; it allows the practitioner to use herself differentially in the context of forging a purposeful and genuine relational space that emphasizes reflection and processing *with* the client on emerging issues. It is, however, a much more demanding task for the practitioner to be emotionally attuned to the client's cognitive and affective communication on different levels, and at the same time, be mindful of how her own words, presentation, and behavior are affecting the client in the treatment process. The practitioner has to be willing to take measured emotional risks in immersing herself in interactions with the client, taking responsibility for her own vulnerabilities and defenses.

In this section, we shall discuss how this intersubjective focus translates to practice implications for contemporary psychotherapy as well as service delivery in agency settings for specific client populations with mental health and health issues, which have been shaped by the short-term care mandate of managed care auspices and an increasingly diverse client population who hold different percep-tions and expectations of the help-seeking process. It is important to note that the approaches delineated here in the various phases of engagement, assessment, and interventions are highlighted for the sake of discussion, but should be used to enhance the therapeutic relationship throughout the helping process.

Engagement approaches

Communication of empathy

The issue of client engagement has become a significant topic of interest in the helping process, as non-compliance with treatment and premature termination of services are prevalent among involuntary clients and those who seek treatment as a last resort in resolving their life crises. Specifically, the practitioner's communication of empathy has been identified as a key factor in successful engagement as well as development of the therapeutic relationship (Meissner, 1996; Patterson, 1984; Jordan, 1991; Miller and Rollnick, 2002). The concept of empathy is generally defined as the practitioner's ability to step into the subjective experiences of the client and communicating her understanding of those experiences (Rogers, 1951; Kohut, 1957). The therapeutic purpose of the use of empathy is to elicit trust from the client who feels understood and accepted by the clinician's empathic responses. As per the traditional Western-based practice model, practitioners communicate empathy by mainly focusing on the client's thoughts and feelings in reaction to their circumstances. They make reflective statements based on the client's narratives so that the clients feel heard and understood. Some also communicate their understanding of deeper meanings behind the clients' communication that they may or may not be aware of (Freedberg, 2009; Clark, 2006). For example, a practitioner may indicate to a client who was extremely distraught over the preliminary findings of a lump in her breast that she had already gone through a lot of stressful transitions in her life, and that this latest occurrence might have added to her feelings of anxiety and frustration over the lack of control over her life. Such communication of empathy with an interpretation of the client's perception would then lead to a deeper exploration of the client's internalized coping mechanism that amplified her reactions. Thus the worker essentially uses empathy as an opportunity to reflect on and gain insights into the client's inner states.

From a relational perspective, the aforementioned approach of the practitioner proffering her assumptions would be considered as reflective of the ideology of the "one-person psychology" that we discussed earlier (Clark, 2006). Based on the premise of an egalitarian relationship that emphasizes the active participation of both the practitioner and the client, relational theorists would encourage the practitioner to share her thoughts and feelings as impacted by the presentation of the client's narrative in the session (Goldstein, *et al.*, 2009; Wachtel, 2008). So the practitioner in the aforementioned example would communicate empathy by disclosing her own thoughts and feelings to convey a sense of caring and support for the client, i.e., her shock and disbelief in hearing that the client had another setback, and her concern about how the client has been coping with the news, etc. Exploration of the client's underlying and historical issues associated with her distress would depend on the client's readiness and inclination for insights into her reactions. Thus relational theorists emphasize disclosure of the practitioner's personal reactions in the here-and-now context with the client to foster the authenticity of the therapeutic relationship and the relational component that the practitioner is genuinely concerned about and interested in the welfare of the client.

Indeed, given today's increasing diverse background of our clientele and their varied reasons and expectations for entering treatment, the practitioner's verbal articulation of her understanding of the client's experience may not be sufficient to elicit trust from the client. Vulnerable clients who have pressing dependency needs, such as the elderly who live alone with chronic health problems, individuals who struggle with parenting young children with special needs, immigrants who are marginalized and not fluent with the language of the host country, etc., may not remain in the helping process unless the practitioner makes an attempt to address their immediate concerns. In situations where the client's quality of life has been severely compromised by environmental stressors and inequitable resources, communication of empathy by action – whereby the practitioner goes out of her comfort zone to do for and with the client – can speak volumes of her understanding of the client's pain, as well as her stance as a trustworthy helping professional. With involuntary clients, the conveyance of empathy may need to be focused initially on their experience of being mandated to seek treatment, and not so much the circumstances that precipitated the presenting problem. For example, eliciting trust from an adolescent who failed school or parents who lost custody of their children due to alleged neglect and abuse would require the practitioner to demonstrate understanding of their resentment, fear, and shame associated with the mandated counseling. Again, the practitioner's communication of empathy may have to go beyond the verbal articulation of the client's distress, and include some offering of concrete support.

It seems that the need for the practitioner's flexible use of self in communicating empathy is more the rule than the exception. The challenge lies with the accountability issue of whether the flexibility meets the therapeutic objective of engaging the client in a purposeful helping relationship. Oftentimes, practitioners are faced with the delicate task of stretching their boundaries such as making phone calls to the client after work hours, visiting clients at home when they fail to make contact, or accompanying clients to appointments for benefit applications, etc. while setting a therapeutic structure for ongoing work with the client.

Since every client's needs, communication style, and help-seeking behavior are different, and there are complex agency protocols to contend with, it may not be easy to sort through myriad professional dilemmas in the engagement phase. In thinking through these circumstances, it would be helpful to bear in mind the concept of mutual regulation between the practitioner and the client under the relational paradigm. Relational theorists believe that the therapeutic relationship has to be co-created by the practitioner and the client, and shaped by their mutual influences on each other. From this perspective, the form of empathy communicated has to resonate with what makes sense *within* this genuine and unique relationship. For example, a practitioner who is attempting to engage an elderly client who talks excessively about her somatic complaints but feels intimidated by her medical doctor may agree to speak with him on her behalf to demonstrate her understanding of the nature of her anxiety. Thus the relationship would begin with the practitioner responding to the client's concerns. It would evolve as the client begins to trust the practitioner and reciprocate by confiding in her some of her inner thoughts and feelings. It may turn out that the client generally chooses to go into great details of her daily worries before she delves into troublesome interpersonal issues as prompted by the practitioner. Over time, a specific rhythm of the relationship will develop as both client and practitioner respond to each other's communication cues in regard to emerging issues in the therapeutic relationship. This would be the essence of mutual regulation embedded in the intersubjective dynamics of a genuine relationship. On the other hand, a practitioner who limits her involvement to offering information to a client, such as the symptoms of depression, the eligibility criteria, and the application process for benefits, etc. or direct the client to reflect on her underlying anxiety, would be utilizing approaches that focus more on reinforcing the professional and objective role of a practitioner and less on relational responsiveness and authenticity.

Addressing the issue of power differential between practitioner and client

Another engagement implication under the relational paradigm is the importance of leveling the power differential between the practitioner and the client to create a more egalitarian relationship. The treatment relationship, with the practitioner assuming the role of an expert with a specific body of knowledge and initiating the flow of discussion with the client, is asymmetrical by nature. In addition, practitioners who are in agency settings that administer benefits and resources, or monitor behavioral compliance of clients, are also viewed as authority figures with the capacity to take actions that will improve or disrupt the client's quality of life. Such power differential could affect the client's level of trust and comfort in sharing her thoughts and feelings. For clients who have a history of being marginalized and oppressed by mainstream society, the power dynamics in the helping relationship often trigger negative transferences that could become obstacles in the engagement process. Given the inherent inequitable distribution of power and privileges among population groups in our society, differences in race, class, gender, age, and other personal attributes between the practitioner and the client may also reinforce the perception of power differential in the relationship.

From the perspective of relational theorists, the aforementioned power issues need to be addressed as part of the engagement process. Applying the principle of mutual regulation that we discussed earlier, the practitioner would initiate different approaches to diffuse the power differential and shift the dynamics to bi-directional influences in the relationship. She would acknowledge the differences between her and the client and her position of power and authority when she senses distrustful reactions of the client, especially those who are mandated to seek treatment and from less privileged backgrounds. Relational theorists believe that the intersubjective space marked by authenticity and spontaneity within the therapeutic relationship is a good potential venue for the practitioner and the client to process the sensitive issues of power and privileges inherent in many societies and would provide for corrective experiences to work through cultural differences and impasses between the therapeutic dyad (Mattei, 1999; Ogden, 1994). Adopting the social constructionist stance, the practitioner can assume a "not-knowing" position (Anderson, 2005; Clark, 2006) in pursuing ongoing dialog with the client and empower the client to give voice to her own narratives, rather than rushing to make assumptions, interpretations, and dispensing advice. In immersing in the client's narratives, the practitioner would help to identify the client's strengths and resilience in her history of coping with the presenting problems, so that the client will emerge from the engagement process with a more positive self-image and a sense of hope in the helping process. For example, individuals who suffer from mental disorders such as schizophrenia tend to be marginalized in their social and family life due to stigma regarding mental illness and lack of services to support their recovery. Many of these individuals have difficulties trusting the mental health system and subsequently are caught in a vicious cycle of treatment relapse and hospitalization. A case manager assigned by court mandate to work with a client who has a history of non-adherence to treatment and multiple hospitalizations will first need to establish a genuine relationship with the client using some of the aforementioned approaches. It would be important to listen and empathize with his struggles with mental illness before questioning him on his medication regiment or "educating" him on the importance of taking his medication.

In addition, the practitioner can be mindful of correcting any subtle and unintentional communication of his power, privileges, biases, and social prejudices through his interactions with clients of disadvantaged background. A Caucasian female student intern of this author recalled noticing some strained facial expressions of her African American male client when she left her office door ajar during their first session. Upon reflection, the student intern realized that she had acted on her learned impulse to avoid being alone with an African American male of low socioeconomic background who is negatively stereotyped as potentially violent. Another student intern described how her fellow inpatient psychiatric staff had given up on a non-English speaking client who refused to talk through an interpreter and spent most of her time praying on her knees, and yet the client made eye contact with her when she knelt down next to her and asked if she could pray along with her. The student intern's act was a powerful communication to the client that she was not forgotten even as a typically "difficult" and "marginalized" client. The spontaneity and authenticity of this engagement intervention and the reciprocation of the client in making eye contact was a "moment of meeting" that initiated a positive connection between the client and the student intern.

Assessment foci

Client's organizing principles

As the client's subjectivity is recognized as an important component under the relational model, contextualization of the client's presenting problem and underlying issues is highly emphasized in the assessment process. This means that it is important to understand the client's personal perception of issues that are important to her and the specific meanings that are distressful to her, based on the interplay of the client's personal history, belief systems, and patterns of interpersonal relationships. Relational theorists conceptualize these internalized schemas as "organizing principles" of the individual's cognitions, emotions, and behavior (Stolorow and Atwood, 1992; Stolorow *et al.*, 1994). These organizing principles are part of the individual's personality structure that reflect themes of the individual's sense of self and others, i.e., specific constructs that translate to fulfillment of affirmation, attachment, and other emotional needs, as well as pathways and behavior that will attain those needs. Individuals' organizing principles take many forms with varied nuances, for example, a continuum of "I'm not good at anything" (which may lead to despair or anger and resignation of responsibilities or anxiety and total dependency, etc.) or "I have to do everything myself" (which may lead to resentment and controlling behavior, or distrust of others and lack of intimate relationship). As another example, there may be a myriad issues underlying a male client who exhibits depression symptoms of lethargy, poor concentration, and insomnia but is reluctant to seek psychiatric treatment, such as the fear of stigma and ridicule among his peers and family of suffering from mental illness, or the concern of incurring additional expenses that he may not be able to afford, or the belief that the symptoms would eventually dissipate, etc. Each issue can be a reflection of this client's specific organizing principles, such as the need for acceptance and approval from others, the importance of planning for financial security, and the tendency to delay taking actions, respectively. While it may take some time for the practitioner to assess the organizing principles that reflect these nuances associated with the client's decision against seeking psychiatric treatment, they do offer a better glimpse of the client's unconscious fears and desires in relation to his sense of self and others, and hence a more contextualized view of the client's thoughts, emotions, and behavior. Such assessment will provide a road map for the practitioner to become more attuned to the client's emotional needs, and address these issues in the context of constructs that are important to the client. For example, in processing with the client in regard to his reluctance in seeking psychiatric treatment, the practitioner will make empathic inquiry that resonates with the client's subjective concerns and reality, such as his past experiences with eliciting concrete and emotional support from his family and peers, and his eligibility for supplemental medical coverage.

Unconscious materials in the here-and-now context

As discussed in the theoretical section, relational theorists postulate that an individual's unconscious materials often emerge as fleeting and subjective fragments that are evoked by interaction with others. Thus the practitioner's task is to process those thoughts with the client and help her make sense of those thoughts and feelings as they emerge within the context of the client's subjectivity. While it is also important for the practitioner to assess the client's defenses – from individual to the collective psyche – relational theorists would view this task as an understanding of the subjective reality of the client, and not the focus of intervention. For example, a client who, after discussing her childhood experience with her mother, commented that she should be angry at her mother for leaving her in the care of relatives as a young child, but somehow she did not feel the anger. Instead of probing for the feelings of anger and betrayal that have been defended against, the practitioner may inquire empathically about the client's perception of circumstances that precipitated her mother's decision. The practitioner would then shape her inquiry and response based on the client's rendering of her subjectivity. Since the focus of the change process is to partner with the client to strengthen her sense of self and motivation for change, it is more important to empower the client to search for meanings that are congruent with her organizing principles and subjective reality.

Client's strengths and resilience

As discussed earlier, it is important to identify the client's strengths as a resource in fostering the client's sense of self. This is an approach that was less emphasized in traditional psychodynamic practice but has been gaining prominence in post-modern and social work practice. Since clients – especially those from underprivileged and oppressed backgrounds – tend to focus on their internalized deficits and vulnerabilities in their narratives, the practitioner may need to listen for as well as elicit the client's input to reflect on their strengths and resilience (Glicken, 2004; Saleeby, 2006). For example, the client's tenacity in coping with her adversities, small steps of progress in the past, and her willingness to seek help are common traits of strengths that tend to be overlooked in the helping process.

Under the relational paradigm, assessment is an important ongoing and comprehensive process. Contextualization of the client's issues of distress begins with a holistic assessment of the interplay of biological, psychological, and social variables in her life, analogous to the social work "person-in-environment" perspective, and culminates to a more differential assessment that enables the practitioner to respond differentially to the client's emotional and concrete needs.

Corrective experiences as interventions

Relational theorists conceptualize the therapeutic relationship as an opportunity for the client to strengthen her sense of self and others through purposeful interactions with a practitioner, whose emotional attunements to and acceptance of the client's fears and vulnerabilities provide the crucial sustenance in the change process. From the perspective of relational theorists, the corrective experiences afforded by the therapeutic relationship are the major mode of intervention. In the previous section, we have discussed the various possibilities of corrective experience as the practitioner crafts her interactions with the client. They are summarized in Table 2.1. We will then examine how the practitioner can provide corrective experiences based on the here-and-now dynamics with the client.

Repairing ruptures in the therapeutic alliance

As a participant in an authentic relationship, it is inevitable that the practitioner, given her own subjectivity and vulnerability as well as limitation of her agency services, may interrupt, misinterpret, or overlook the essence of the client's

Table 2.1 The therapeutic relationship as corrective experiences

Characteristics of relationship	Characteristics of practitioner's approach
Supportive	• Empathic inquiries and communication – immersion in client's subjective experiences • Exploration and interpretation in the service of supporting client's self-esteem
Egalitarian	• Process issues of power differential in the relationship • Maintain permeable professional boundaries
Authentic communication*	• Purposeful disclosure of thoughts and feelings • Mutual sensing and influences
Safe space*	• Processing of negative emotions and interactions • Co-construction of new meanings and activities

*Intersubjective dynamics

communication, resulting in empathic failures and a temporary rupture in the therapeutic bond, or even an impasse in the treatment process. The challenge lies with how the practitioner handles these disruptions, and turns them into opportunities of learning and corrective experiences for both participants of the dyad. Some common occurrences in the helping process that may evoke boredom, impatience, or even a sense of inadequacy in the practitioner are excessive talking of seemingly irrelevant materials by clients, and incessant demands for or complaints of agency services by the clients. In these and other challenging situations, the practitioner will need to grapple with how she can preserve or repair the therapeutic bond. Practitioners may need to consider questions such as, "What would be 'spontaneous' and 'authentic' responses that serve a therapeutic purpose?" "What kind of message will the client be able to accept and reflect upon?" "How can the practitioner remain empathic – the essence of the change and growth process for the client – when her own subjectivity collides with that of the client?"

Since every client (and practitioner) is different, and every therapeutic relationship is unique, the questions need to be considered differentially and contextually. The important guiding principle is that the practitioner needs to own her role and subjectivity in the misattunement experience, and process it with the client. So the responses to the previous example can range from validating the client's subjectivity, such as "Sorry, I was not listening carefully to what you were saying", "You need a lot of services, and we have disappointed you many times" to infusing an intersubjective perspective, such as, "I know it was important for you to vent, but it was hard to follow your thoughts after a while. Can I tell you what I have heard so far?" or "I know it's hard not to get what you need. I don't want you to feel you are alone in this. Can we talk about looking at other alternatives?"

There are times that the practitioner may need to contain the client's anger and disappointment, and not push for insight that is beyond the capacity of the client. In such cases, the client's subjectivity needs to be respected in the service of providing a corrective experience whereby the client's feelings and thoughts are not dismissed. At the same time, the opportunity for the client to view the practitioner as a human being with flaws and failings and yet the ability to acknowledge them may help the client to accept her own vulnerabilities as well as enhance her trust in others.

Concluding remarks

Relational theory offers a model of practice that evolves around an authentic and purposeful relationship that is regulated by the client's subjective needs and the practitioner's genuine and therapeutic responses in the helping process. Its expansive perspective on the change process that goes beyond the traditional practice focus on verbal communication and its emphasis on the practitioner's creative use of self has opened a new venue for cross-cultural practice. In the next chapter, we will discuss how this model of practice can be applied in working with Asian immigrants.

Discussion highlights

A contemporary view of the unconscious mind

Relational theorists emphasize that an individual's unconscious is a dynamic and fluid entity that is constantly evolving from interaction with others in the external world. (p. 32)

Relational theorists adopt a more supportive and "present" focus in exploration. (p. 34)

Relational theorists postulate that anxiety is primarily interpersonal in nature and emerges when repression of those disavowed feelings and thoughts are challenged. Oftentimes, an individual's self-esteem and self-acceptance are compromised in the service of maintaining a conflict-free inner life. (p. 34–35)

The change process for clients

Psychological growth can occur in a purposeful relationship without delving into the individual's repressed materials. (p. 33)

It is because of the sense of safety and feeling understood, communicated through empathic bonding that the client may feel more inclined to reflect on her vulnerabilities and develop a more integrated sense of self-acceptance. (p. 35)

Dynamics of transference and countertransference

Relational theorists view transference as also being shaped by the practitioner's interaction with the client … The practitioner's objective interpretation is replaced by processing of the experience of re-enactment with the client. (p. 36)

Intersubjectivity is a unique transitional space marked by a specific pattern of communication and interaction shared by the practitioner and the client as the relationship progresses, including a mutual awareness and sensing of each other's thoughts and desires. (p. 39)

It is important to understand the client's personal perception of issues that are important to her and the specific meanings that are distressful to her. (p. 45)

The practitioner needs to own her role and subjectivity in the misattunement experience, and process it with the client. (p. 48)

3 Applying the relational model in working with Asian immigrants

Irene W. Chung

In Chapter 1 we examined some key psychodynamic concepts and offered a different understanding of the development of the sense of self and coping behaviors from an Asiacentric perspective. We also discussed the practice implications for culturally relevant adaptations of assessment and intervention skills in the helping process. In Chapter 2 we presented the major premises of the relational model which emphasize the therapeutic value of a helping relationship that is built on empathy, mutuality, and authenticity to promote changes and psychological growth of the client. In this chapter, we will discuss the application of this relational paradigm in working with Asian immigrant clients. We will discuss communication between the practitioner and the client and the nature of the helping relationship in the context of Asian cultural values and norms and immigrant-specific circumstances. We will use case scenarios to support our discussion that relational theorists' attention to the client's subjective realities and help-seeking behavior as well the practitioner's use of self in forging therapeutic alliances can be an effective cross-cultural practice model in working with Asian immigrant clients.

Therapeutic communication in the helping process

Characteristics of the Asian communication style

Engaging Asian clients in conversations about their thoughts and feelings has always been perceived as challenging by practitioners who are trained under the Western clinical model. Unlike Western cultures, the introspection and articulation of emotions is generally considered to be detrimental to one's health and harmonious relationship with others in Asian societies (Ots, 1990; Tseng, 2004). Asian countries that are influenced by Confucianism, Buddhism, Hinduism, and Taoism have always placed a premium value on the virtues of being thrifty with words and intuitive in interpersonal communication (Chen, 2006; Kim, 2003; Saral, 1983). In traditional Asian cultures, communication reflects the Asian values of self-cultivation and discipline to eliminate ego-centeredness and reinforce a sense of interdependence and interrelatedness with nature, family, as well as the social and the spiritual world (Miike, 2007). Social and personal relationships are fostered by the reciprocation of obligations toward others and respect for each other's privacy rather than the Western norm of frequent expression of positive feelings toward each other (Pedersen *et al.*, 2008; Roland, 2011). Such cultural values are reflected in the various Asian languages whereby there is limited vocabulary in conversational lexicons to describe or explore emotions. In lieu of discussing emotions, native Asian language speakers use affective and somatic lexicons to indicate their distress or well-being, and tend to focus on the causes or consequences of their affective states rather than talking about how they feel (Bernstein *et al.*, 2008; Chung, 2008; N. Delhiwala and M. Sawant, personal communication, 5 June 2012; F. Raith and H.J. Shim, personal communication, 13 July 2012; E. Simpao, personal communication, 25 September 2012). These affective lexicons generally are not direct expression of emotions, unless keen attention is paid to the nonverbal cues of the speaker and underlying emotional content of the circumstances that are presented. For example, many immigrants of traditional Asian cultures tend to express apologies in their conversations as part of the social protocol even when they harbor personal feelings of hurt and disappointment. Or they may make self-deprecating remarks in response to compliments as an adherence to the cultural value of modesty instead of revealing their positive feelings. The minimizing of emotions in conversations is characteristic of the indirect and high-context communication style of Asian cultures (Hall, 1977; Leong and Lee, 2006), in which the subtext of the message is layered within the actual spoken words. High-context communication style is generally the norm in collectivistic societies as it supports the cultural emphasis on cohesive and interdependent relationships (Pedersen *et al.*, 2008).

Asian immigrants tend to adhere to the traditional high-context communication style. However, the level of their acculturation in their Western individualistic societies may influence their way of expressing their thoughts and feelings in the helping process. In applying the relational theoretical premise, we need to understand each individual client's internalized beliefs and norms in order to engage them in a therapeutic relationship that makes sense to them. For Asian immigrants who adhere to the cultural sanction against direct expression of strong emotions and assertion of individual needs, it is important to note that the therapeutic value of communication of one's thoughts and feelings is *not* limited to direct verbalization. Relational theorists believe that non-verbal communications such as subtle facial expressions, body postures, and movement patterns between the practitioner and the client can contribute to the "unconscious establishment of a safe and healing environment" (Scaer, 2005, pp. 167–8).

The challenge for practitioners in working with Asian immigrants who subscribe to the traditional cultural style of communication is essentially about *how* to make empathic connections with their clients. In the following section, we will make recommendations for practitioners to modify and contextualize their communication with clients under the relational paradigm.

Exploration of presenting problems and underlying issues

How can we explore with Asian clients in a culturally relevant and therapeutic context?

The task of exploration is a delicate balance between listening to the client's narratives to offer support and posing pertinent questions to gain a psychosocial perspective of the client's presenting problem and underlying issues (Kadushin and Kadushin, 1997; Woods and Hollis, 2000). In Chapter 2, we discussed the relational approaches of making empathic inquiries that follow the lead and pace of the client. In working with Asian immigrant clients who adhere to the traditional cultural norms of interpersonal relationship and communication, the practitioner may have to play a more active role in reflecting on the client's remarks and asking more direct questions to clarify the unspoken messages. In some cases, practitioners may have to make some suggestive inquiries to assemble a more cohesive narrative with clients who speak in a circular and repetitive manner, and are evasive with details (S. W. Kim, personal communication, 23 April 2012; E. Ho, personal communication, 21 April 2012). The challenge for the practitioner in taking this active stance is being mindful of when and how to probe in a respectful manner and when to accept the client's communication at face value.

The following segment of a dialog in the first session between a practitioner and an 80-year-old Korean woman who presented with panic attacks after her husband's death illustrates how the practitioner modified her exploration style in a culturally relevant and relational context:

MRS. KIM (CLIENT): I have this pain that comes up for no reason; it's like a little arrow that's cutting through here. (POINTING TO HER CHEST.) It's very uncomfortable. What can I do?

MARY (SOCIAL WORKER): (NODDING AND GRIMACING A LITTLE AT MRS. KIM'S FINGER GESTURE.) I understand you have seen our psychiatrist; he said you have what Western medicine called panic attacks, and he gave you some medication. Did that help?

MRS. KIM: I don't know. He told me to take it when I feel really bad.

MARY: So did you try taking the medication?

MRS. KIM: I take so many kinds of medication. (SIGHS.)

MARY: Yes, it's hard to keep track of all your medication. Do your children call you to remind you?

MRS. KIM: They are always busy. My daughter stops by after work every day.

(MARY PICKED UP ON MRS. KIM'S LEAD AND SHIFTED THE CONVERSATION TO THE LIVES OF MRS. KIM'S CHILDREN. AFTER A WHILE, MRS. KIM RETURNED TO THE TOPIC OF HER PANIC ATTACK.)

MARY: What do you do when you feel the little arrow coming through your chest?

MRS. KIM: I lie down in bed.

MARY: Does that help?

MRS. KIM: It really hurts when that arrow is pressing against my chest.

MARY: It must be frightening to get the pain all of a sudden, when you are by yourself and you can't do anything about it.

MRS. KIM (QUIET FOR A WHILE):   Do you have any advice for me to make the pain go away?

In this dialog, Mrs. Kim did not volunteer much information other than her vivid depiction of her panic attack in somatic terms. She did not respond directly to Mary's inquiry of how she had been dealing with the panic attacks. But the subtext of her communication did emerge as Mary tried different ways to gather information. Mrs. Kim's repeated references to her panic attacks, and the minimizing of support she got from the psychiatrist and her family appeared to be a statement of her fear and sense of helplessness associated with the panic attacks, and most likely, her current life circumstances. The dialog could be perceived as fragmented in how Mrs. Kim made cryptic remarks and did not appear to be engaged in the helping process. Contrary to the Western model of posing open-ended questions, Mary also had to ask concrete and detailed questions and even proffered her own interpretation of Mrs. Kim's affective state to elicit input from her. However, if we apply the relational lens, we can detect the non-verbal communication and the implicit alliance between Mary and Mrs. Kim as they moved from one issue to another with new layers of information. So it would seem that Mary's patience and resourcefulness in creating a dialog that was relevant in an older Asian immigrant woman's cultural reality paid off. Toward the end, Mrs. Kim began to view Mary as someone who could help her and appeared to be engaged in the helping process.

In the next section, we will discuss how Mary explored issues underlying Mrs. Kim's emotional distress as manifested by her panic attacks. While Mary adhered to a psychosocial and systemic perspective in guiding her exploration, she was sensitive to Mrs. Kim's possible reaction that she was being "interrogated" and her privacy was being invaded. Mary's initial approach was to inquire about Mrs. Kim's husband and her children to see if Mrs. Kim would disclose any issues with them. Mary started with asking about Mrs. Kim's life prior to her marriage. The use of a narrative approach that resembles the Asian indigenous conversation worked well with Mrs. Kim, who seemed to appreciate the attention. As Mrs. Kim reminisced, it became clear that she had regrets marrying her husband to appease her parents, since she had given up her vocational interest as a teacher and ended up working as a seamstress after immigrating to the US with her husband. Mrs. Kim also disclosed information implying that her husband did not treat her well, and her children were not on good terms with her.

MARY: Did your husband help you with raising the children?

MRS. KIM: He just went to work. I was stupid enough not to go to English classes after work. I rushed home instead to pick up the kids and cook dinner.

(MRS. KIM DISCLOSED INFORMATION THAT HER HUSBAND NEVER LIKED TO TELL HER WHAT HE WAS DOING BUT EXPECTED HER TO BE HOME A CERTAIN TIME.)

MARY: You were a good wife and good mother. You sacrificed for the family.
(MORE DISCUSSION OF HOW MRS. KIM TOOK CARE OF HER FAMILY.)
MRS. KIM: I should have taken English classes.
MARY: Why did you say that?
MRS. KIM: I would have been able to talk to the lawyer and find out more about my husband's will and how much he left me. My two daughters think I am hiding money from them.
MARY: That must be upsetting! You must have felt it was so unfair.
MRS. KIM: Sometimes when my chest is hurting me, I want to cry so I can feel better. But I can't cry. Can you tell me what to do?

In this dialog, Mary posed questions that were common conversational topics in the Asian immigrant communities, e.g., "How did you meet your husband – did he return to the home country to look for a wife?", "What did you do after immigration to the US?" These questions allowed Mrs. Kim to be as evasive or specific as she wished to be. Even the pointed question of whether her husband helped her with raising the children could be perceived as a benign cultural question since most Asian males of the older generation were not expected to help with household chores, and it would open up an opportunity to validate Mrs. Kim's hard work in raising her family. Thus Mary created a safe space for Mrs. Kim to confide in her if she felt ready. While Mrs. Kim did volunteer some personal information that seemed to be the source of her emotional distress, her disclosure was still delivered in the context of concrete issues, i.e., taking English classes, negotiating with the lawyer, etc. She did not respond directly to Mary's suggestive statement that it was upsetting that her daughters turned against her, and certainly did not reveal the nuances of her distress. Even the remark that had an overt reference to her dejected emotions – "I wanted to cry" – was infused with somatic meaning and turned into a request for advice from Mary.

One could question if Mary should have speculated on Mrs. Kim's reactions, but given the pattern of Mrs. Kim's evasive communication style, a direct probing of Mrs. Kim's feelings could have been perceived as inappropriate and invasive. On reflection, Mary acknowledged that her tone of concern in making the suggestion was an indirect way of communicating her own reaction and empathy for Mrs. Kim, and yet leaving the option for Mrs. Kim to dispute her statement. So both Mary and Mrs. Kim had developed a pattern of implicit communication and a safe space for Mrs. Kim to lead the pace and direction of the conversation.

From a psychodynamic perspective, Mrs. Kim's panic attacks would be perceived as stemming from her repressed feelings of hurt and rejection, and her desires for her husband and children to reciprocate the care she selflessly provided for the family. However, Mary was careful not to probe further and make any further suggestive statements in this session. Mrs. Kim's communication style indicated that she could be defended against processing any strong emotions directed at her family, since getting in touch with those feelings would have left her feeling more vulnerable both from a cultural and personal perspective. For example, she would need to reflect on: "Did she fail in her life role as a wife and

mother after all these years of sacrificing her self-interests to fulfill her obligations?" Or "how could she be angry at her children when as a mother she was
expected to offer them unconditional love?" And even if she defied cultural
values, she would have to face the question of "where did that leave her as an
older immigrant woman with no support network?" Such speculations based on
theoretical assumptions in regard to intrapsychic conflicts and defenses are helpful
in guiding the practitioner in the direction and depth of exploration. In applying
a relational perspective, Mary was able to explore Mrs. Kim's issues in a more
culturally appropriate and supportive approach.

In the following dialog, which involved a middle-aged Chinese immigrant who
was ashamed to inform his social worker that his wife had just left him and had
only disclosed the information to his psychiatrist who treated him for his depression,
the exploration was also crafted around respecting the client's defenses against the
rejection by his wife as well as showing concern in a culturally appropriate context.

LINDA (SOCIAL WORKER):   How have you been, Mr. Wong?

MR. WONG (LOOKING DOWN):   Not too bad.

(LINDA THEN POSED A FEW QUESTIONS TO INQUIRE ABOUT MR. WONG'S SLEEPING PATTERN,
APPETITE, AND HIS JOB. MR. WONG WARMED UP A LITTLE TO THESE QUESTIONS, AND
HINTED THAT "THINGS COULD BE BETTER.")

LINDA: How is your wife doing?

MR. WONG (SHORT PAUSE):   We have not been talking much.

LINDA: You two must be working long hours.

MR. WONG (ANOTHER PAUSE):   She has not been coming home much.

LINDA: Have you been able to reach her on the phone?

MR. WONG (LOOKING DOWN AGAIN):   She has moved out.

LINDA (LOOKING WITH CONCERN AT MR. WONG):   This is a major event. It must be
affecting your work and your life in general.

MR. WONG: Of course. I get agitated easily.

In this session, the social worker posed questions pertaining to Mr. Wong's
physical well-being and level of functioning, which were similar to inquiries made
by physicians in a medical or mental health consultation. She did not focus on
exploring his feelings, even after Mr. Wong finally told her that his wife had left him.
Instead she focused on facts and consequences that were not invasive but conveyed her
sensitivity to the enormity of the problem. Her benign speculation in response to Mr.
Wong's statement that Mrs. Wong had not been going home offered Mr. Wong
an opportunity to tell her the truth at his own pace, but her concern in his welfare came through, which made it safe for Mr. Wong to share the news with her.
In a subsequent session when Mr. Wong appeared to be more comfortable discussing
his life without his wife, Linda explored his feelings indirectly:

LINDA: Did you ever cry when you think about your wife?

MR. WONG: I was always told not to cry growing up. That's in our culture, don't
you know?

LINDA: You are right. So what do you think we should do? This is a big change in anyone's life.

MR. WONG: I told the group [*support group at the clinic*] the other day. They were very concerned about me, and told me not to worry and not to think about it.

LINDA (NODDING): They really care about you.

MR. WONG (AFTER BEING SILENT FOR A WHILE): The love songs they play on the radio talk about having broken hearts after the lover left. I guess that's what's happening with me. As the songs go, I guess I will grow old alone.

From a cultural perspective, Linda was successful in eliciting Mr. Wong's input in discussing his feelings in a way that was not intrusive and yet meaningful to him. While Mr. Wong did not articulate his feelings directly, he was able to process them in the presence of Linda who was supportive and accepting of his circumstances. From a relational perspective, the exploration was a therapeutic intervention.

The task of exploration is a process in tandem with the evolvement of the helping relationship. Practitioners who work under time-limited and outcome-oriented mandates, may feel the pressure to compromise this process with Asian immigrant clients who are not forthcoming in discussing the nature of the presenting problem and their goals of seeking help. From a relational perspective that emphasizes the egalitarian dynamics in the helping process, the practitioner should inform the clients of agency protocol and timeline and enlist their cooperation and understanding in an expedited intake process that may otherwise feel inter-rogative and humiliating. The task of exploration, even reduced to a mundane task of completing paperwork, can be a therapeutic process. From the perspective of relational theorists, this therapeutic value is the "larger meaning" of the practitioner's message (Wachtel, 1998, p. 3), i.e., interest in the client's narrative and respect for her perceptions, that is being communicated to the client in the exploration process. For Asian immigrants who generally struggle with marginalization in their new countries and feel ambivalent about applying for benefits and utilizing services, such a message could be a corrective experience.

Communication of empathy

Carl Rogers (1951, p. 348), the first psychologist to emphasize the therapeutic value of communication of empathy in the helping process, defined this skill as the practitioner's ability to:

> assume, insofar as she is able, the internal frame of reference of the client, to perceive the world as the client sees it, to perceive the client himself as he/she is seen by him/herself, to lay aside all the perceptions from the external frame of reference while doing so, and to communicate something of this empathic understanding of the client.

As we discussed in Chapter 2, relational theorists believe that the communication of empathy involves the practitioner's ability to respond on an affective and cognitive level based on the here-and-now interactions with the client, and is part of the ongoing empathic dynamics that characterize the helping process (Gibbons, 2011). Going beyond the traditional mode of verbal articulation of empathy by the practitioner, relational theorists emphasize the importance of making empathic responses that are authentic and meaningful to the client's personal and social beliefs, and in a mutual context that encourages reciprocal exchanges with the client. Such postulations resonate well with the Asian interpersonal and communication norms. In the following section we will discuss the nature of empathy and emotions in the Asian culture and how empathy can be communicated effectively in the helping process with Asian immigrant clients.

How is empathy communicated in the Asian interpersonal context?

In Asian cultures where the collective sense of self supersedes the private self, communication of empathy toward others is considered an essential aspect of human relationships. Similar to the dynamics of intuitive sensing postulated by relational theorists in the therapeutic relationship, individuals develop a heightened sense of anticipating and understanding each other's needs and feelings through socialization. This reciprocal intuitive sensing among individuals is highly valued in Asian cultures and takes precedence over verbal articulation of thoughts and feelings (Ham, 1993; Roland, 1996; Shonfeld-Ringel, 2001). In our earlier discussion of Mr. Wong who was initially reluctant to share the news that his wife had left him, his concerns about how others would view him apparently superseded his need to be in touch with the nuances of his personal feelings. He felt supported when his social worker and group members inquired about his well-being and did not press him for further disclosure. One can speculate that the responses of the social worker and the group members were prompted by some intuitive understanding of Mr. Wong's sense of shame from the cultural stigma associated with his wife leaving him and the need to support his defenses against his vulnerable feelings. Mr. Wong's anxiety about how others would view him could be a culture-specific emotion common in collectivistic society and not necessarily an indication of poor self-esteem.

Culture-specific emotions

Anthropologists contend that individuals' emotional experiences are largely shaped by their social and cultural milieu (Oatley, 1993; Wong and Bagozzi, 2005). Markus and Kitamaya (1994) indicated that the predominant nature of emotions in individualistic cultures reflects the differentiation of the individual from others as an autonomous being and the importance of pursuing one's needs and desires. Thus anger and dejection would be on one end of such a spectrum of expressed emotions and excitement and happiness would be on the other end. In Asian cultures where the sense of self is defined in the context of interdependent relationship with others, the individual's inner feelings are given less attention than those associated with the needs and responses of others. Feelings of shame and humiliation, or connectedness and sympathy that stem from interactions with others are the "other-focused" emotions that generally dominate the individual's consciousness and shape her behavior.

Our discussion on the way in which the experience and expression of emotions are shaped by culture has several practice implications in the communication of empathy with the Asian immigrant client population in the helping process. The concept of culture-specific emotions affirms our earlier assertion that it may not be effective and therapeutic to explore Asian clients' inner feelings directly, and thus communication of empathy cannot rely on the traditional Western approach that focuses primarily on the articulation of the client's cognitions and affective states. In the following section, we will use the relational model's stance of contextualizing the client's behavior and communication as a framework to create a different repertoire of culturally relevant approaches. We will illustrate how we can communicate empathy through purposeful behavior, actions, and interactions informed by our intuitive sensing of the client's subjective experience of distress and perception of her needs.

Doing for and with the client. As we discussed earlier, the focus and expression of distress of Asian clients tend to be around concrete issues and physical complaints, which is often reciprocated by concrete responses from others within the client's kinship network. Thus empathy in an Asiacentric context is communicated through individuals attending to and responding to the distressed person's physical or concrete needs while intuitively respecting her privacy (Chung, 2008; Pedersen *et al.*, 2008). For example, a cup of tea with words like "please take care of your health" is generally offered to someone who is distraught, or advice may be dispensed in regard to a stressful situation. This social norm is often translated to the provision of concrete assistance for clients by practitioners across all service modalities as a way to foster an empathic connection (S. Zhou, personal communication, 18 June 2012; M. Vu, personal communication, 6 July 2012, and J. Li, personal communication, 6 June 2012). In addition to the inherent responsibility of agency practice to make collateral contacts for the purpose of consultation and collaboration, practitioners often make inquiries on behalf of their clients in regard to service delivery that they are not able to negotiate on their own due to language barriers, lack of knowledge about resources, and bureaucratic agency personnel. Practitioners often read the client's mail and medical or legal documents, help them with bill payments, and write letters to support their application for benefits and services. Some of them also accompany their clients to important appointments to lend concrete and moral support.

Being there for the client. It is not uncommon that Asian immigrant clients ask for concrete help from practitioners who are perceived as authority figures with expertise and resources even though the problem is more psychological in nature, as befitting the interdependent and hierarchical structure of Asian societies. For example, Mrs. Kim, who suffered from panic attacks and struggled with adjustment to widowhood and living alone in our earlier discussion, asked her social worker and psychiatrist if she could call them when she experienced panic symptoms. Her request, seemingly an emergency measure for medical help, was a communication of her feelings of vulnerability and desire for support. While this could also be potentially an issue of burden and imposition on professional boundaries for both practitioners, they both responded positively and did speak to Mrs. Kim the few times she reached out to them. So their willingness to communicate with Mrs. Kim was an implicit message that they understood her fears surrounding her circumstances and would be there for her when she needed them. Such an empathic response of "being with the client" is similar to the practitioner saying, "I'll be thinking of you" to clients from the Western culture. The difference lies with the venue of communication that is more covert in emotional exchanges in the Asian cultural context.

Giving advice to client. Asian clients tend to ask their practitioners directly for their opinions in resolving their presenting problems due to the ethnocultural transference that we discussed earlier. This often brings up professional issues such as the risk of reinforcement of client dependency, breaching of professional boundaries, and exertion of undue influence on clients (Woods and Hollis, 2000). These issues should be considered in the context of the subtext message underlying the request for advice. For example, is the client asking for feedback from the practitioner in regard to her reaction and behavior? Or is the client looking for the practitioner to tell her what to do? It is also important to differentiate the cultural meanings that have been infused in the communication. While individuals from an interdependent culture are socialized to seek affirmation from each other, those from an individualistic culture may certainly perceive such behavior as a reinforcement of their character trait deficit. The request for advice could also be an affective lexicon that communicates feelings of confusion, or helplessness, as in the case of Mrs. Kim that we discussed earlier. From a relational and Asian cultural perspective, it is important that practitioners craft authentic responses that address the clients' requests instead of being evasive as per the Western traditional model (Sue and Sue, 2003). The request for advice needs to be perceived as part of the communication and relationship-building process between the practitioner and client, and dismissing or minimizing it would be detrimental to the practitioner's trustworthiness. Advice from the perspective of the practitioner can be presented as a subjective opinion that needs further discussion with the client.

On the other hand, the practitioner's response of being at a loss for advice along with the disclosure of her thoughts and feelings can also be a genuine communication and a corrective experience for the client.

In summary, there is a key criterion for considering the nature of empathic response to a client's needs that may challenge the traditional boundaries of service provision: it is the message that is being communicated to the client underlying the specific response, and the implication and consequence of the response. The centrality of the response needs to communicate the practitioner's understanding of the nature of the client's distress, for example, his feelings of helplessness, marginalization, or shame, etc. and the practitioner's desire to alleviate the distress. For Asian immigrant clients who tend not to articulate these feelings, the practitioners' initiatives to help them in concrete ways are powerful responses that validate the unspoken emotions and kindle a sense of hope in regard to their circumstances. For clients who are not familiar with seeking treatment and services in Western societies, such culturally and immigrant-relevant responses are effective means to elicit their trust and engagement. The following case vignette captures the clinical significance of these dynamics:

Case vignette: Mrs. Nguyen

Mrs. Nguyen, a Vietnamese immigrant who suffered from schizoaffective disorder, was exhibiting psychotic symptoms and suicidal ideations when she came for her appointment with May, her psychologist. Mrs. Nguyen, who had been seeing May for a few months and seemed to be engaged in treatment, was willing to go to the hospital when May offered to accompany her. They ended up spending a good part of the day in the emergency room with May intervening on behalf of Mrs. Nguyen to expedite the admission process. May's act of empathy – a communication of her understanding that Mrs. Nguyen was scared of her own psychotic state and the uncertainty of navigating through the bureaucratic and English-speaking hospital system – made a significant impact on their therapeutic relationship and subsequent work together. Even though Mrs. Nguyen did not recall the details of her psychotic state and the conversations she had with May on that day, the memory of May's protectiveness toward her and her acceptance of her suicidal ideations and delusional behavior in the emergency room stayed with her. She was able to talk about that day with appreciation, and was receptive to May exploring the nature of her psychosis. She was able to confide in May about the voices she heard, and eventually identify her arguments with her husband as triggers to her auditory delusions.

Showing sustained interest in the client's narratives. Due to the nature of the client's problems, such as chronic illness, bereavement, or persistent mental illness symptoms, there are times when the practitioners may not be able to provide concrete assistance or advice that would otherwise come across as insensitive and patronizing. So practitioners can only develop empathic responses by showing interest and asking details about the clients' circumstances and how they are impacted by the presenting problems and their futile attempts to alleviate the problems. This would be akin to the traditional style of communication with parental figures in the Asian kinship network, and can evoke in the clients feelings of being cared for during times of illness and vulnerability (Chung, 2008). In our earlier discussion of Mr. Wong, the social worker communicated concern by assuming the role of a nurturing authoritative figure and inquiring about details of his functioning, and subsequently engaged him in talking about his source of distress. From a relational model perspective, empathy was implicitly communicated as an interactive process in a culturally relevant context that goes beyond the practitioner's active listening.

Insights, information and perspectives

What are the therapeutic values in offering advice and education in an Asiacentric context?

It is universal human nature that individuals strive to make sense of distressful events and experiences as an adaptive attempt to gain a sense of continuity and control over their lives. In the helping process, healing begins when the client is able to create a cohesive set of meanings that support his sense of purpose and resiliency and a plan of action to ameliorate the impact of stressors in his life (Greene *et al.*, 1996; Saleeby, 1994; Sarri, 1991). These meanings can come in the form of insights, information, or different perspective about the cause and nature of the presenting problem. From the relational model's perspective, it is important to elicit the client's input in the construction of these meanings so that the process becomes an empowering and therapeutic experience.

In working with Asian immigrant clients, we need to consider *how* the co-construction of meanings can be facilitated in a culturally and immigrant relevant context. As we discussed earlier, Asian clients tend to seek advice from the prac-titioner rather than provide introspection of their thoughts and feelings as per the cultural norm of communication and the power differential embedded in the helping relationship. Thus the act of advice-seeking can have multiple layers of meaning. Many of them lack access to information due to their disadvantaged socioeconomic background and language barrier, and depend on the practitioner to provide them with knowledge and options in regard to their presenting problem. On the other hand, those who identify with the Asian hierarchical values may not feel comfortable to disagree with the practitioners, and their silence or compliant responses may not truly reflect their thoughts and desires. Or as we discussed earlier in our case vignette of Mrs. Kim, seeking advice may just be an affective lexicon to communicate distress and solicit support. So the challenge for the practitioner is to maintain her stance as the expert on general issues of mental health and social services and a cultural broker to Western societies, and at the same time, address the client's subjective needs.

How can psychoeducational approaches help to address emotional distress?

Psychoeducational approach is based on the notion that education is empowering. By gaining information about their problems, clients can consider constructive steps to alleviate or manage their deleterious effects (Kim, 2005). Psychoeducation approaches can also include skill training in specific areas such as socialization and stress relief to enhance the client's self-efficacy and level of functioning. Most importantly, psychoeducational approaches emphasize the process of the practitioner, client, and family members working together to come up with meanings and solutions that make sense to them (Bae and Kung, 2000), which is compatible with the premises of the relational model.

Psychoeducation approaches have been widely used in the Asian communities among families with mentally ill members with positive outcomes (Bae and Kung, 2000; Kim, 2005). The key functions of psychoeducation that are especially important for Asian immigrants who feel stigmatized by their mental illness is the normalization of their problems and the inculcation of culturally relevant knowledge and skills. We believe that these approaches can be integrated into working with Asian immigrant clients who struggle with interpersonal and life transitional issues. In the following section, we will discuss how the use of a psychoeducation approach can be used in addressing Asian clients' emotional distress in a culturally relevant context.

As we discussed in Chapter 1, Asian clients tend not to delve into their emotions in their communication and somatization becomes a culturally sanctioned venue to express their emotional and psychological distress. Sometimes, the history and nature of the problems that beset the individual and his personality traits may undermine his coping mechanism, and somatization may exacerbate the distress rather than serve the adaptive purpose of taking the focus off the underlying issues and eliciting support from others. In the case vignettes presented earlier, the clients all faced major life transitions that severely compromised their mental health. From a psychodynamic perspective, their anger toward others had been turned against themselves, and their anxiety, depression, and even their psychoses, were possibly symptoms of repressed and displaced aggression that in turn, had diminished their level of functioning. Unfortunately, depression symptoms, ranging from anxiety, insomnia, to chronic physical complaints, have been widely reported in Asian immigrant communities (Bhugra, 2003; Hwang *et al.*, 2008), and there is a great need for practitioners, across all agency settings, to offer psychoeducation about the clients' emotional distress in a context that respects clients' defenses against the cultural stigma of personal and familial failures associated with mental health issues.

From an Asian cultural perspective, "worrying about problems and the well-being of self and others" is part of daily life struggles and is associated with the individual's responsibility for the welfare of the family and kinship members, whereas expressing "anger at others" is deemed as improper conduct and an impediment to one's moral development as per the teachings of Confucianism and Buddhism (Ino and Glicken, 1999; Ishii, 2004). While worrying has a more positive connotation and is more readily acknowledged by clients, both behaviors are considered as detrimental to one's health and thus "letting go of the anger and worries" would be a common premise between clinical theory and cultural meanings. The use of a psychoeducational approach would focus on *how* this objective can be attained. Theoretically, both feelings have to be first identified and accepted by the client before they can be "given up," which is a practice encouraged by the traditional psychodynamic model. Western-trained practitioners will make an interpretation of the client's underlying anger and educate the client by telling him "he has a right to be angry." In many Asian languages, "worries" is a common concrete term used as an inclusive reference to emotional distress since the introspection of one's feelings, especially anger toward others, is not culturally appropriate (H. Son, personal communication, 27 November 2012; P. Yew-Schwartz, personal communication, 24 November 2012). Oftentimes, Asian clients will respond to the practitioners' attempts to help them process their thoughts and feelings around a specific stressful event with a fatalistic attitude, such as "What's the use of talking? It can't reverse the situation," or with annoyance at the practitioner's probing, "What's done is done. You can't help me anyway." From a psychodynamic perspective, there is a good possibility that these clients are either still angry at the situation and displacing the anger onto the practitioner, or they have resigned to the fact that they are helpless in the situation and are unconsciously angry with themselves and others. However, their resistance to explore the issue will merely perpetuate the depressive symptoms.

In our earlier discussion of the various case vignettes, the practitioners engaged the clients by focusing on the events and their impact on their well-being and functioning, and not their implicit anger toward their significant others. They continued to adopt this concrete approach in their subsequent use of psychoeducation on their clients' anxiety and depression symptoms. Tapping into the Asian traditional medical perspective, the practitioners characterized the negative emotions as general "pent-up frustrations" that disrupt the circulatory flow of vital energies and need to be released to preserve their physical and mental well-being. The "release" was defined in self-care behavioral terms such as deep breathing, or talking with the practitioner, but not the Western norm of communicating thoughts and feelings to the individuals who caused the distress. This psychoeducational approach objectified the anger as something that was deleterious to one's health and needed to be purged, and offered a medical perspective that resonated with the Asian cultural belief on the integration of mind and body. It took the focus off the culturally sensitive issue of whether the individual client had the right to express anger at others and avoided the risk of drawing attention to estranged relationships and being scrutinized within the kinship network.

To ensure that the clients were genuinely receptive to the content of the psychoeducation, the practitioners in the aforementioned case vignettes also included a problem-solving discussion to co-construct strategies with their clients to "release" their tensions. Eventually, Mrs. Kim talked about how she could take a walk every day in the park to get her mind off her "worries" and keep her body in shape. Mr. Wong decided to tell members of the support group about his wife having left him and asked them to keep the information confidential. Mrs. Nguyen promised to talk to her psychologist whenever she had an argument with her husband to preempt the auditory delusions. While these "plans" were not directly addressing the underlying anger, they were acknowledgment by the client that their symptoms were linked to their stressful interpersonal issues, and affirmation of their desires to take charge of their well-being. The psychoeducational approach was therapeutic in the sense that the clients' distress was validated by the concerned responses of the practitioners and they were able to regain a sense of efficacy with a broader and meaningful perspective of their issues provided by their practitioners. Relational theorists would attribute this to the intersubjective and safe space co-created by each practitioner and her client that fosters intuitive communication of the fears and desires of the client. As the helping relationship evolves, the client and the practitioner may co-construct further meanings of the presenting problem as the practitioner facilitates more reflection. In the afore-mentioned examples, Mrs. Kim later reported to her social worker that she "yelled" at a shadow that looked like her husband and "it had not returned." She also agreed to a brief family meeting with her daughter but would like the social worker to use the rest of the session to meet with her daughter and "educate" her in her absence. The psychologist who worked with Mrs. Nuygen finally made a gentle suggestion that perhaps she should be upset at her husband who did not reciprocate her care for him, which was a breach of his obligations as per the cultural norm. Mrs. Nuygen was silent for a while and then said she would like to practice the teaching of Buddhism to let go of others' transgression against her, which indicated that she accepted the interpretation of her underlying feelings. In working with Mr. Wong, the social worker was able to educate him further on how thoughts could affect an individual's "moods" – a more culturally acceptable term – and behavior, and Mr. Wong agreed to keep track of how this might apply to his work performance. When Mr. Wong agreed that there was a correlation between these variables, the social worker asked Mr. Wong how he could better take care of his "moods" and different aspects of his life. Mr. Wong, after giving it some thought, said "I guess I will have to take one day at a time and not worry so much." Again, these would not be considered significant "insights" gained from psychoeducation under the traditional psychodynamic practice model. However, from a relational model practice perspective, positive changes have taken place in how the clients view themselves and their ability to cope with their distress through therapeutic conversations with an empathic and skilled practitioner.

The nature of the helping relationship

As discussed in Chapter 2, the relational model views the nature of the helping relationship as an evolving process characterized by collaborative, reciprocal, and intersubjective dynamics between the practitioner and the client. This essence of mutuality serves the therapeutic purpose of providing a corrective experience for the client who feels accepted and supported by an empathic practitioner, and an opportunity to acquire new thoughts and feelings in the interactive process. Our discussion on communication between the practitioner and the clients in the first half of the chapter highlighted some of these dynamics. Despite the tendency of Asian immigrant clients to communicate in concrete behavioral and somatic terms in the helping process, we demonstrated how practitioners utilized their intuitive sensing of the clients' unspoken emotions, desires, and fears to make empathic connections through creative use of lexicons, cultural meanings, tasks, information, and being with the client. From a relational theory perspective, these intersubjective moments of connection make a more lasting impact on clients than verbal interpretations as they *experience* a deepening of the relationship and a positive sense of self and others during those moments (Fonagy, 1998; Tronick, 2007).

The helping relationship in working with Asian immigrant clients

In Asian cultures, interpersonal relationships are greatly valued and defined by mutuality and reciprocity between individuals. These interdependent interactions enhance the development of trust and the acceptance of each other into more intimate relational circles (Pedersen *et al.*, 2008; Roland, 2011). Such dynamics resonate with the characteristics of the helping relationship under the relational model. In the following section, we will discuss some common interaction dynamics between the practitioners and Asian immigrant clients that are informed by cultural norms and immigrant-specific circumstances, and how they shape the nature of their helping relationship from a relational theory perspective.

What are the common boundary issues that need to be examined in an Asian cultural context?

In working with Asian immigrant clients, the boundaries in the helping relationship tend to be much more permeable (Ito and Maramba, 2002; Shonfeld-Ringel, 2001; Sue and Sue, 2003). For example, it is not uncommon that personal questions are posed to the practitioners, generally about their life roles, i.e., marital status, care taking responsibilities, etc. and their history in the host country. While practitioners trained under the traditional Western model may be inclined to ask the clients to verbalize the underlying intentions and desires for further discussion, it is important to consider if the questions are posed in the context of good will as befitting the traditional Asian interpersonal norm, and if the client interacts with the practitioner as a trustworthy member of her kinship network. As the relationship progresses, some clients may make other inquiries based on their observations about their practitioners, i.e., they look busy, or under-dressed for the weather, etc. Some Asian clients also like to bring food items or small gifts to their practitioners. Again, practitioners need to consider if these are reflections of cultural norms that show care and appreciation in the context of a developing relationship. It is not uncommon that Asian clients are short on verbalizing their appreciation or feedback about their relationship with the practitioner. Thus the client's curiosity about the practitioner or the presentation of a gift can offer an opportunity to review the helping process with the client. For example, a practitioner recalled that a client once presented her with a jar of pickled cumquats after she had provided her with counseling and case management services for a period of time. Instead of inquiring why the client brought her a gift or talking about agency protocol in regard to gifts from clients, the practitioner thanked the client and half-jokingly asked why the client decided to give her cumquats. The client replied that her family always made a beverage with pickled cumquats for throat ailments, and she thought the practitioner would need to soothe her throat for all the talking she had to do in the session and phone calls she had to make on her behalf. The practitioner was pleasantly surprised by the client's remarks and expressed her appreciation for the client's thoughtfulness. The gift and the ensuing discussion enhanced the helping relationship and brought the participant and the client closer in their communication and understanding of each other. The practitioner noted more spontaneous exchange of personal thoughts between the two of them, and the cumquat beverage became a favorite metaphor that they shared in their conversation whenever stressful situations emerged.

The practitioner's appreciation of the client's reciprocation of care and thoughtfulness is especially therapeutic and empowering for Asian immigrant clients who are often marginalized and feel they have to be dependent on their English-speaking children or providers to navigate the systems in their host country. It is also important that the practitioners are mindful of opportunities to reinforce the sense of mutuality in the helping relationship. Even the most vulnerable clients, by virtue of their resilience to losses, stressors, and hardships, have something to "teach" the practitioners. Offering opportunities for clients to reminisce about their life experiences or share their life skills and knowledge, such as traditional ethnic cooking, gardening, cultural folklores, etc. can give clients a stronger voice in the relationship, and allow the practitioners to see the clients in a more holistic perspective.

What are some ethnocultural transference and countertransference issues that can enhance or impede the helping process?

The dynamics of transference and countertransference are a key construct in the helping relationship across all practice settings. From a traditional psychodynamic perspective, they are unconscious feelings, attitudes, desires, reactions, and defenses that originated from the practitioner's and client's significant people in their early childhood that are projected onto each other during the helping process (Woods and Hollis, 2000). Such perceptions and ways of relating are often distorted and become the issues of introspection for the practitioner as well as exploration with the client as the helping relationship progresses.

From a relational model perspective, it is important to examine the responses of both practitioners and clients in the context of the circumstances associated with the help-seeking process, their commonalities and differences as individuals in terms of age, gender, cultural background, beliefs, personality traits, etc., and ultimately the reciprocal dynamics of their interactions. These are inherent transferential issues based on social and cultural role expectations that shape the nature of all helping relationships, and could be addressed or resolved by the practitioner modifying the dynamics of these role expectations. For example, it is not uncommon that Asian immigrant clients believe that practitioners of their own ethnic background have a deeper understanding of their struggles and needs and thus expect more support from them. These clients are attributing the trustworthy qualities of the cultural kinship network to their relationship with the practitioners, and at the same time, evoking in the practitioners the cultural feelings of obligation toward the clients (Comas-Diaz and Jacobsen, 1991; Chin, 1993). Some practitioners feel pressured to do more for these clients, while others may be cautious of such dynamics and avoid extending themselves and reinforcing the client's dependency on them. However, as with all transferences, ethnocultural transference and countertranference can be modified within each relationship as it progresses. For example, Asian practitioners will more likely be influenced by the cultural expectation of taking care of the elders when they begin working with older clients, but they can also elicit different dynamics in the relationship if they validate their strengths and offer them opportunities to assume the role of being the benevolent elder in a kinship network. The key issue is to consider which aspect of the re-enactment of ethnocultural transference is therapeutic for the client. Some older immigrant clients may cherish their independence and feel empowered when the practitioner enlists them as collaborators in resolving their problems, while others who feel neglected by their children and family may feel supported when the practitioner assumes the role of a caretaker.

There is also a common perception that Asian clients generally view practitioners as benevolent authoritative figures with resources and knowledge, and they will be receptive to advice dispensed by the practitioners when the practitioners play up this transference that resonates with the hierarchical structure of Asian societies (Chin, 1993; Ito and Maramba, 2002; Sue and Sue, 2003). This author believes that this is one dimension of Asian clients' transference toward the practitioner that is more relevant in the engagement phase to help the client establish trust and a sense of optimism in the helping process. There are inherent risks in making cultural assumptions or reinforcing such transferential dynamics without understanding what the client is looking for from the practitioner in the context of agency setting and the nature of the problem. There are many Asian immigrant clients whose help-seeking objectives are to acquire advice and services around short-term, life transition issues. They perceive this process as similar to seeking consultation and treatment from physicians who, along with educators, are highly revered in the Asian cultures (Ito and Maramba, 2002). Thus the authoritative transference may help these clients feel taken care of and hopeful about their circumstances. However, for clients who suffer from a poor sense of self and others that compromises their interpersonal relationships, and who will benefit more from a nurturing and mirroring transference, the authoritative transference may deter them from getting their needs met through a more intimate relationship with the practitioner. Another consideration is the challenge of working with involuntary clients who are mandated to receive counseling, such as those with substance abuse issues, or parents accused of child abuse and neglect. While Asian clients may not directly articulate their negative reactions toward the practitioner because of this hierarchical transference, they can offer conflicting information, become evasive in their responses, fail to follow through with agreed tasks, arrive late to appointments, and ultimately terminate their services as a result of their resentment. For Asian practitioners who are already charged with the authoritative role of ensuring compliance of their clients with treatment or the protocol of residential and medical settings, the aforementioned behavior may trigger strong ethnocultural countertransference in regard to their clients' "resistance" to fulfill their obligations and responsibilities, resulting in impasses in the helping relationship. In instances when these clients do express their anger and resentment in regard to the practitioners' apparent lack of support and understanding toward their plight, such as filing reports on suspected child or adult protective cases, the sentiments that are expressed are usually laced with cultural meanings of disappointment and betrayal and could be more unsettling for the Asian practitioners.

Our discussion on intersubjective dynamics illustrated the challenge of navigating relational dynamics of two individuals coming together in the helping process. Asian immigrant clients are no different from other clients. They are individuals with unique personality traits, emotional needs, coping mechanisms that are shaped by the interplay of their history with significant others, experiences with their external worlds, nature of life stressors, and belief systems. In the following case vignette, we will discuss the evolvement of a long-term helping relationship, the mutual influences between the practitioner and the client, and how they created a unique safe space for connection and disagreement, and most importantly, therapeutic growth for the client.

Case presentation: the evolvement of an authentic relationship in an Asiacentric context

Case vignette: Ms. Yu

Ms. Yu, a recent single parent in her forties and an immigrant from China for over 15 years, was referred for counseling by her children's pediatrician. Ms. Yu stated her presenting problem as feeling overwhelmed and inept with raising her pre-adolescent children and would like to seek guidance and advice in regard to parenting skills. While the presenting problem appeared to be fairly direct, there were a multitude of underlying issues that created obstacles in the engagement process.

Ms. Yu never showed up for her first appointment. When Mei-ling, the social worker assigned to work with Ms. Yu and her children, called the apartment, Ms. Yu sounded very lethargic and disorganized, and claimed that she had forgotten about the appointment. Sounding surprised that Mei-ling would call her, she expressed appreciation and interest to re-schedule the appointment. In the weeks that ensued, Ms. Yu would arrive for her appointment substantially later than the scheduled time. Ms. Yu would apologize and settle for a shorter session with no complaint. Mei-ling started to call Ms. Yu the morning of her scheduled appointment, and would also apologize if she could not extend Ms. Yu's session. This pattern persisted for a few months. It appeared that while Ms. Yu had difficulty organizing her time, her long commute also posed additional hardships for her. But Ms. Yu always managed to attend her sessions, and eventually she would arrive within a few minutes of her appointment time. Ms. Yu would still apologize for her "tardiness," but she would smile when Mei-ling pointed out that she was not late given the long commute she had to make. On reflection, Mei-ling realized that Ms. Yu's "apology" was her way of drawing attention to the fact that she managed to arrive on time, and it was something that she was proud of. Mei-ling's intuitive response in giving Ms. Yu credit was recognition of the progress Ms. Yu had made in regaining a sense of control over her life, and something that Ms. Yu wanted from her. The ritual of apology at the beginning of their session thus became a subtle way of exchanging positive feelings between Mei-ling and Ms. Yu.

Ms. Yu indeed related to Mei-ling as an authoritative figure initially and presented her with scenarios of her interactions with her children for feedback and advice. However, it appeared that Ms. Yu was struggling with some depressive symptoms that included feelings of self-blame, sadness, and anxiety that often immobilized her. These symptoms were manifested in Ms. Yu's excessive worries and frustration in regard to her ability to prepare meals that her children would enjoy, or supervise her children to finish their home work and daily chores and go to bed at a reasonable time. Ms. Yu only talked briefly about her ex-husband who divorced her when he met another woman, and the fact that he had criticized her parenting and housekeeping skills. Ms. Yu described her own mother and sister as having their own lives and much more "capable" than her. Ms. Yu had a part-time job as an accountant's assistant but felt her job performance was disappointing her supervisor, and her peers did not like her because of her lack of social skills.

Mei-ling did not actively explore Ms. Yu's background and her relationship with her family, but stayed primarily with the current issues that were troubling Ms. Yu. She asked for clarifications and contextual information when Ms. Yu presented her concerns. While she provided information about behavioral norms of children attending school in the US, Mei-ling communicated her understanding of the cultural expectation of Ms. Yu's role as a mother, compounded by the social stigma of being divorced by her husband. In listening to Ms. Yu's narratives, Mei-ling also made a point of identifying Ms. Yu's strengths and resilience in her struggles as an immigrant parent. Ms. Yu initially would smile shyly and made some self-deprecating remarks such as, " I really don't know what I am doing," "I am a very slow learner." As Ms. Yu and Mei-ling got to know each other better, Mei-ling realized that Ms. Yu actually had a good sense of humor, and she would respond with a frown and an emphatic nod when Ms. Yu made those remarks. Ms. Yu's face would then light up with a broad smile. Underlying the verbal and non-verbal exchanges, there was an implicit mutual acknowledgment that Ms. Yu indeed had some positive attributes despite her self-perception, and that a deep understanding had developed between Ms. Yu and Mei-ling.

Over time, Ms. Yu also seemed to have made some progress in regard to handling interpersonal issues at work. Instead of ruminating over insensitive remarks from her co-workers and complaining that they were scapegoating her, Ms. Yu seemed to be able to let go of those incidents after discussing them with Mei-ling. Generally Ms. Yu would present these incidents as dilemmas that needed advice from Mei-ling, who would make suggestions in regard to how she herself would have handled the situations. However, Mei-ling would also speculate how Ms. Yu must have felt, and Ms. Yu was able to make some reflections and add her own perspective. Most of the time, it did not seem that Ms. Yu followed through with Mei-ling's suggestions, but the fact that Mei-ling was willing to problem-solve with her and listen to her narratives really seemed to have helped her. Ms. Yu would report that she was able to sleep better and concentrate at work. During one of those discussions, Ms. Yu volunteered some information about her childhood and made a connection between her experiences of being ostracized at work to her earlier years during the Chinese Cultural Revolution when she was being criticized during political study group meetings. It seemed that Ms. Yu was feeling stronger with the support from Mei-ling and thus was able to recall some painful and frightening experiences. Ms. Yu made reference to this incident several times after this, adding new details and perspective. She also seemed to have developed more vocabulary to express herself. With the new insight about the impact of her past experience, Ms. Yu began to ask reflective questions such as "Am I paranoid about other people's intentions?" and "Am I too hard on myself?"

Evidently Ms. Yu's depression had lifted, and Mei-ling brought up the issue of planning for termination. Ms. Yu agreed that she had been doing better, and would not mind taking a break from counseling. However, she wanted reassurance that she could see Mei-ling when she needed help. She indicated that she understood Mei-ling had to see other clients, but it seemed "such a big loss to have to cut off a precious relationship that took so long to develop."

Ms. Yu indeed came back a few times to see Mei-ling over the next two years. Sometimes she would bring her adolescent children along when she felt she needed someone to mediate their conflicts and offer some advice. While Ms. Yu usually had good insights about the issues that emerged, apparently it was important for her to be able to talk to Mei-ling and get her input and validation.

Then Ms. Yu had a setback. She was diagnosed with stage-two breast cancer and went through a horrific experience with getting tests and consultation with scant feedback and support in a bureaucratic medical system. Her poor command of English limited her choice of medical care and she had to rely on interpreters or her children to communicate with the doctors in terms of her prognosis and options. However, Ms. Yu surprised Mei-ling with her resilience. She was very focused and persistent with following through with doctors' appointments and test procedures on her own. When she finally came in to speak with Mei-ling, she was fairly clear about her decision to undergo mastectomy and which surgeon she would pick to perform the procedure. On the other hand, Mei-ling sensed that Ms. Yu was not ready to process her shock and fear in regard to her cancer diagnosis and her impending surgery. She realized that at that point in time Ms. Yu really just wanted her to bear witness to how she tried to navigate herself through the chaos in her life. So she mainly listened to Ms. Yu, and asked about how her children were coping with the news. It appeared that Ms. Yu was comforted by the fact that her children had stopped arguing with her and had been compliant with their school and household respon-sibilities since they found out that she had been going frequently to medical appointments. However, Ms. Yu had decided not to disclose the severity of her illness and the nature of her impending surgery to her children as well as her mother. She believed that it was a good practice in the Asian culture to protect the young and the elders from disturbing news, and that it was something that she should do for her family. While Mei-ling felt that Ms. Yu needed her family's support at this critical time, she told Ms. Yu that she understood her selfless intentions. Mei-ling then disclosed her own feelings of concern for Ms. Yu, and asked Ms. Yu to consider eliciting more support from her family to gratify her own "selfish" needs to make sure that Ms. Yu would be cared for after the surgery. Ms. Yu was quiet at the time. At the end of the session, Mei-ling offered Ms. Yu her cell phone number and told her to call if she needed help. Ms. Yu eventually left a message on Mei-ling's cell phone to tell her that her surgery went well, and that her mother had come by to help her with cooking and taking care of the children.

Ms. Yu returned to see Mei-ling a few weeks after her surgery. She was wearing a hat to cover her thinning hair from chemotherapy. She smiled awkwardly and started to apologize for her appearance. She looked down at her chest and said softly that she should go to the bathroom to straighten out her mastectomy bra. Mei-ling looked at her and said emphatically, "You look fine." Ms. Yu lowered her head briefly, and there were tears in her eyes when she looked up at Mei-ling. Upon reflection, Mei-ling realized that there were a lot of mixed emotions that were exchanged in those initial moments. Ms. Yu's self-consciousness and apology about her appearance was laced with anger about her situation. It also seemed that Ms. Yu was glad to see Mei-ling but was feeling vulnerable. With Mei-ling's firm message of acceptance, she was able to allow herself to get in touch with some of those vulnerable feelings. After some conversations about how Ms. Yu has been doing with her recovery, Ms. Yu suddenly shook her head and said, "I'm a damaged person." As Mei-ling tried to explore and question Ms. Yu's perception, she sensed Ms. Yu's anger from her stubborn stance that she was a "damaged person." However, Ms. Yu would not delve into her feelings. So Mei-ling switched to sharing her own thoughts and feelings as someone who witnessed Ms. Yu's ordeal. She balanced her disclosure of her anger that life was so unfair for Ms. Yu with respect and admiration for Ms. Yu's courage and stamina during this period. Ms. Yu initially listened and then filled in some details of the narrative. She did not talk about her anger, but seemed comforted by Mei-ling's depictions of her strengths. In her usual self-deprecating way, she said wistfully, "I had no choice ... I worried about who would take care of my children." There were similar discussions in the ensuing weeks. Ms. Yu went through a period of insecurity but eventually agreed to join a support group for cancer survivors for Chinese immigrants that Mei-ling found for her.

In presenting this case vignette, we focused on the interactions between the practitioner and the client that fostered the growth of a therapeutic relationship. As the practitioner used herself purposefully in engaging the client and helping her gain insights into her behavior, she was guided by the client's implicit communication of her emotional needs that were shaped by both cultural and personal influences. The spontaneous exchange of thoughts and feelings through various modes of communication and the practitioner's expansion of professional boundaries to convey support and empathy were memorable moments that made this relationship unique. Evidently the client's growth and adaptation to the stressors in her life did not result from interpretations and advice from the practitioner. It was the relationship with an individual who was genuinely caring, understanding, and accepted her vulnerabilities as well as appreciated her strengths that brought out the client's insights, resilience, and resourcefulness. It would be fair to say that the practitioner herself had also learned and gained something personal from this relationship.

Concluding remarks

In this chapter we discussed how the relational paradigm is a viable practice model in working with Asian immigrants who adhere to their traditional communication and interpersonal norms. In reviewing and illustrating how therapeutic relationships can be developed in an Asiacentric context, we also demonstrated the potentiality of this relationship in helping clients develop insights, enhance their self-esteem and coping mechanism, and make positive changes in their lives. There are tremendous challenges for practitioners who put more of themselves into the relationship and use themselves creatively in expanding the parameters of traditional Western practice in the helping process. We will examine these issues further in the chapters on the various mental health issues in the Asian communities.

Discussion highlights

Communication with clients

The therapeutic value of communication of one's thoughts and feelings is *not* limited to direct verbalization. The challenge for practitioners is essentially about *how* to make empathic connections with their clients. (p. 52)

The challenge for the practitioner in taking an active stance in exploration is being mindful of when and how to probe in a respectful manner. (p. 53)

We can communicate empathy through purposeful behavior, actions and interactions informed by our intuitive sensing of the client's subjective experience of distress and perception of her needs. (p. 59)

Ethnocultural transference and countertransference

Ethnocultural transference and countertransference can be modified within each relationship as it progresses. The key issue is to consider which aspect of the re-enactment of ethnocultural transference is therapeutic to the client. (p. 68)

There are inherent risks in assuming that cultural authoritative transference should be reinforced in the helping process. (p. 68)

Part II

Mental health issues in the Asian immigrant communities

4 Asian immigrants in English-speaking countries

A global perspective

Tazuko Shibusawa

Overview

In 2008, close to 214 million people, about 3.1 percent of the world population, lived outside of their birth country (United Nations Department of Economic and Social Affairs, 2008). If the world's immigrants lived in one country, they would represent the fifth largest nation in the world following China, India, the United States, Indonesia, and Brazil (Martin and Widgren, 2002). Among the 214 million immigrants are refugees or asylum seekers; in 2010, this group numbered 15.4 million worldwide (United Nations Department of Economic and Social Affairs, 2008).

Worldwide, it is estimated that 55 million people of Chinese ancestry live outside of mainland China (Ryan, 2002). Another large group of Asian immigrants are South Asians – 20 million people from India, Pakistan, Bangladesh, Sri Lanka, Nepal, Bhutan, and the Maldives live outside their country of birth (Rangaswamy, 2005). An estimated 7.5 million Filipinos and 2.5 million Vietnamese also live outside of their home country as immigrants (Hugo, 2005b). Though much smaller in number, in 2001, 5.6 million Koreans, or 8 percent of the total number of South and North Koreans, lived in 151 different countries (Yoon, 2005).

Asians constitute close to 50 percent of migrants to English-speaking countries (Hugo, 2005b). Table 4.1 presents the demographic characteristics of Asian immigrants in Australia, New Zealand, Canada, the UK, and United States. In Australia, Asians account for 45 percent of all immigrants, with the largest number from China and India. New Zealand accepts about 60,000 new immigrants annually, and, as with Australia, Chinese and Indians represent the largest group. Asians comprise 60 percent of immigrant admissions in Canada. In 2010–11, immigrants from the Philippines (13 percent) were the largest group followed by people from India and China (both 11 percent). In the UK, because of the history of colonization, the majority of Asian immigrants are from South Asia (India, Pakistan, Bangladesh, Sri Lanka), but there has been an increasing number of Chinese immigrants. In the United States, which admits the largest number of immigrants in the world, 35 percent are from Asia (United Nations Department of Economic and Social Affairs, 2011).

Table 4.1   Asian immigrants in English-speaking countries

Country	Percent immigrants	Percent Asians	Largest Asian groups (percentage)
Australia[1]	25 (2010–11)	45 (2010–11)	Of all immigrants arriving 2010–11[2] Chinese (17.5) Indian (12.9) Filipino (6.4) Malaysian (3) Vietnamese (2.8) Sri Lankan (2.7) Korean (2.5)
Canada[3]	8 (2010)	23 (2010)	Of all permanent residents in 2010 Filipino (13) Indian (11) Chinese (11) Korean (2) Pakistani (2)
New Zealand[4]	20 (2005)	9.2 (2006)	Of all immigrants: Chinese (13) Indian (10) Filipino (8)
United Kingdom[5,6]	13 (2007)	7.5 (2011)*	Indian (2.5) Pakistani (2.0) Bangladeshi (0.75) Chinese (0.6) Other Asian (1.4)
United States[7]	13 (2011)	28 (2009)	Of all Asian race-alone (2010) Chinese (23) Indian (19) Filipino (17) Vietnamese (11) Korean (10) Japanese (5)

[1](Australian Government Department of Immigration and Citizenship, 2012)
[2](Australian Government Department of Immigration and Citizenship, 2011)
[3](Citizenship and Immigration Canada, 2011)
[4](New Zealand Department of Labour, 2012)
[5](Papademetriou *et al.*, 2010)
[6](Office for National Statistics, 2012)
[7](US Census Bureau, 2012)
* England and Wales

Many Asian immigrants continue to maintain strong linkages with their families in their home countries, and provide financial support. In 2002, Filipino immigrants residing in Canada and the US remitted an estimated $4 billion dollars to the Philippines (Hugo, 2005a). The remittance by Bangladeshi migrants was equivalent to 35 percent of the export earnings in Bangladesh, and money sent to Vietnam from *Viet Kieu* (overseas Vietnamese) totaled 11 percent of the country's GDP (Hugo, 2005a).

Asian immigrants are a diverse population, migrating for different reasons. Circumstances that "push" people to leave their countries include poverty, unemployment, political unrest, discrimination, persecution, change in government regimes, and man-made or natural disasters (Loue, 2009). People can also be "pulled" to migrate by the receiving countries because of employment and educational opportunities, or to be unified with their families. For example, between 1966 and 1977, 85,000 scientists, physicians, and engineers immigrated to the US from India to fill a labor shortage in these areas (Subramanian, 2007). Currently, 5 percent of physicians in the US are of Indian origin (Pandey *et al.*, 2006). Large numbers of medical professionals also migrated from the Philippines during this period. In the 1980s, many immigrants arrived from India, China, Taiwan, and the Philippines because of demands for engineers in high-tech industries. During the same years, Korean immigrants entered the United States in large numbers because of political and economic instability in their country. Because their skills did not transfer to professional jobs in the United States, this group became small business owners and, consequently, the largest number of self-employed workers (Lee, 2007). Another large Asian group, Southeast Asians – Cambodians, Hmong, Laotians, and Vietnamese – initially came to the United States as refugees as a result of US military involvement in Vietnam and the surrounding area (Zhou and Gatewood, 2007).

Transnational migrants

Migration used to be viewed as a linear event – people moved from one country to another, disengaging from the home country as they assimilated into their host country (Falicov, 2012). During the last decade, however, there has been increasing recognition of transnational migrants who have family members residing in both home and host countries and who continue to maintain strong links to their home country (Levitt and Jaworsky, 2007). The increase in transnational migrants has been driven by globalization of the labor market and enhanced communication technologies (Ho, 2002). Women account for close to half of the migrant population, leading to the *feminization of migration* (Oishi, 2008; Ross-Sheriff, 2011). While many Asian women migrate as skilled professionals in medicine, education, and the technology sector, a larger number migrate to work as factory workers, domestic servants, and to provide other low-wage services. Asian female immigrants who work for low wages tend to leave their children in their home countries, migrate alone, and "mother from a distance" (Parrenas, 2005). For example, in the Philippines, 70 percent of emigrants are women, and 27 percent of children and youth have mothers who work abroad (Oishi, 2008).

Other examples of transnational family patterns among Asians include:

1　"astronaut families," where fathers live abroad for economic reasons while the rest of the family members stay home;

2   "parachute children," who are sent abroad on their own for education;
3   "goose families," in which mothers and children live abroad for the sake of the children's education while fathers earn a living in their home country;
4   parents who send their young child to their home country to be raised by the grandparents so that they can both work and earn a living; and
5   Asian elders who move between adult children who live in their home country and host countries.

(Cho and Shin, 2008; Ho and Bedford, 2008; Ho, 2002)

It is also important to note that some people migrate several times. For example, *huayi* (foreign nationals of Chinese descent) who initially migrated to Southeast Asia remigrated to Western Europe, North America, and Australia in the 1950s and after the war in Vietnam because of discrimination (Ryan, 2002). There are also a large number of Indians who remigrated from East Africa to Europe, and from countries including Fiji and Trinidad to Canada and the US (Gijsbert, 2007; Mishra, 2007)

Although not within the scope of this book, there are two other Asian immigrant groups in English-speaking countries. A group of Asian migrants in English-speaking countries who remain most invisible are "modern day slaves" – children and adults who are trafficked for labor, domestic servitude, and sex work. In the US, an estimated 18,000 to 20,000 people are trafficked every year, and the largest number of trafficked women is from Southeast Asia (Thailand and Vietnam) and China (Miko, 2003). In Canada, both men and women from China, India, the Philippines, and Thailand are transported illegally as domestic servants (Government of Canada, 2012). According to a 2011 UK government report, 62 children were trafficked from Bangladesh, China, India, Malaysia, Pakistan, and Vietnam. The majority were boys from Vietnam who were trafficked by Vietnamese criminal groups to work on cannabis farms (Child Exploitation and Online Protection Centre, 2011). The largest number of Asians who are victims of trafficking in Australia are women from Thailand (Larsen, 2010).

Another large Asian immigrant group in English-speaking countries are adoptees from Asia. The nine Asian countries who send the most children are China, Korea, India, Vietnam, Thailand, the Philippines, Cambodia, Taiwan, and Nepal (Selman, 2009b). While numbers of adoptees from Asia have decreased in recent years, in 2007, there were over 10,000 adoptees from China (8,753), Vietnam (1,692), Korea (1,265), and India (978) (Selman, 2009b) worldwide. Korean children were one of the first groups of Asian children adopted in the United States, where there are now more than 100,000 Korean adoptees (Huh and Reid, 2000). During 2010–11, the largest inter-country adoptees in Australia were from Asia (80 percent). The three largest countries of origin of the adoptees were China (24 percent), the Philippines (17 percent), and Taiwan (12 percent) (Australian Institute of Health and Welfare, 2011). In Canada, in 2004, 1,955 children were adopted internationally of whom 1,001 were from China (Human Resources and Skills Development Canada, 2011). The United Kingdom accepts fewer inter-country adoptees compared to other European countries (Selman, 2009a).

The following is a brief background of Asian immigrants in English-speaking countries that we address in our book. Asian immigration is characterized by:

- an increasing number of Asian immigrants following the liberalization of immigration policies in English-speaking countries;
- diverse occupational and socioeconomic backgrounds.

Australia and New Zealand

The first group of Asians to migrate to Australia and New Zealand were the Chinese who arrived during the gold rush in the 1850s. By 1881, there were over 38,000 Chinese in Australia (Guo, 2005). Immigration from Asia to Australia, however, was limited for a long period because of the White Australia policy. Immigration restrictions for non-Europeans were lifted in 1973, resulting in an increasing number of Asian immigrants. In the early 1980s, Asians became the largest immigrant population to Australia. Immigrants from Vietnam, Cambodia, and Laos arrived as refuges in the 1970s and 1980s and their families continue to migrate under the family reunion program (McNamara and Coughlan, 1997). Koreans began migrating due to poor economic conditions in Korea in the early 1970s, followed by skilled workers and business migrants in the 1980s and 1990s (Han, 2002). In recent years, there has also been an increase in the number of temporary migrant workers from Hong Kong, Singapore, and Malaysia (Collins, 1995). Since the 1960s, there has been an increase in the migration of Filipinas who marry Australian men (Thompson *et al.*, 2002). Currently, there are more than two million Asians in Australia (Colebatch, 2011). The largest Asian groups are the Chinese and Indians, and it is estimated that in the next few years, the number of Asian-Australians will outgrow the number of European-Australians (ibid.).

New Zealand has one of the highest number of immigrants in the world among Organisation for Economic Co-operation and Development (OECD) countries. In 2005, 20 percent of New Zealanders were foreign-born. Asian immigration to New Zealand increased dramatically following the Immigration Act of 1987, which based immigration preference on professional skills and potential capital investment to New Zealand (Ip, 2000; Rasanathan *et al.*, 2006). According to the 2006 census, Asians are the fastest growing ethnic group in New Zealand and are projected to increase to 14.5 percent of the population by 2021 (Ward, 2009). The largest number of Asian immigrants are Chinese (41.6 percent), Indian (29.5 percent) and Korean (8.7 percent) (Ward, 2009).

Canada

Like Australia and the United States, Canada had restrictive immigration policies until the late 1800s and early 1900s. The "White only" immigration policy was not lifted until 1962. Canada accepts about 200,000 immigrants every year (Martin and Widgren, 2002), and currently 23 percent are Asian. The majority of these are admitted as skilled workers and business investors, followed by those entering for family reunification, and as refugees (Martin and Widgren, 2002). The largest immigrant group are the Chinese (Wang and Lo, 2005). While the majority of Chinese immigrants used to be from Hong Kong, the largest group of immigrants since the late 1990s is from the People's Republic of China. Other large Asian immigrant groups include Indians, Pakistanis, and Filipinos (Martin and Widgren, 2002). South Koreans are also becoming a sizeable group in Canada, and it is estimated that there were over 150,000 Koreans in Canada in 2001.

UK

The largest group of Asian migrants in the UK is from India, who make up close to 1 percent of the UK population. They are followed by Pakistanis, Bangladeshis, and Sri Lankans. Together they make up 4 percent of the UK population. In British English, the term Asian usually refers to South Asian populations because of the British history of colonialism in those countries. Historically, immigration policy in the UK has tried to limit immigration. The Commonwealth Immigrants Act 1962 and Immigration Act 1971 largely restricted primary immigration except for family members. However, in practice, there has been an increase in immigrants, especially among those from the European Union (EU). In addition to South Asian immigrants, there was a sizable group of immigrants from Hong Kong. In recent years, there has been an increase in immigrants from the People's Republic of China. Currently, skilled immigrants are admitted on a points-based system, and low-skilled immigrants from non-EU nations are being phased out. It is anticipated that there will be a continuing decrease in the number of immigrants being admitted from non-EU countries (Papademetriou *et al.*, 2010) because of immigration policies that favor immigrants from EU nations.

USA

Asian Americans are one of the fastest-growing ethnic minority groups in the United States. While Asian Americans were just 4 percent of the total US population in 2000, by 2050 it is projected that they will constitute 11 percent, about 41 million people (US Census Bureau, 2008, 2012). The largest group of Asian immigrants are Indian, Chinese, Filipino, Korean, and Vietnamese. The first Asian immigrants arrived in the United States during the mid-1800s through the early 1900s from China, the Philippines, Korea, India, and Japan. The majority came in response to labor demands during an era of intense anti-Asian sentiment. While more than 27 million Europeans came to the United States during the 1880s and 1920s, the Asian population remained small because of exclusionary policies. It was not until the Immigration and Nationality Act of 1965, which abolished national quotas and national origin, race, and ancestry as a basis for denying immigration to the US, that Asians began to immigrate again. Immigrants were admitted based on three criteria:

1 family reunification;
2 occupational immigration; and
3 refugees and those seeking asylum from political persecution.

Asian immigrants – adaptation challenges

As noted earlier, Asian immigrants in English-speaking countries are diverse with regard to country of origin, reasons for migration, socioeconomic background, and demographic patterns. There are, however, some common factors among this population. When working with immigrant families, it is important to understand their presenting problems in the context of their experiences as immigrants and the way in which stress factors affect the process of their adjustment to a new country (Shibusawa, 2004). Immigrants face varying degrees of adaptation challenges. Some have pre-existing psychosocial issues that are exacerbated by immigrant-specific circumstances. Others may develop physical and psychological problems as a result of migration. It is important for practitioners to understand cumulative risk factors during all phases of the immigration process including pre-migration, peri-migration, and post-migration (Loue, 2009). Table 4.2 lists potential risk factors which contribute to the vulnerability of some immigrants.

In the following section we will discuss the risk and protective factors that affect immigrants post-migration.

Table 4.2 Risk factors against positive adaptation

Pre-migration	Peri-migration	Post-migration
Low socioeconomic status	Adverse migration conditions	Low socioeconomic status
Lack of education	Detention experiences	Lack of opportunities
Pre-existing health and mental health conditions	Trafficking	Lack of education
Lack of family support	Smuggling	Undocumented status
Lack of social support	Unsafe and traumatic experiences	Discrimination experiences
Stressful circumstances for migration		Significant gaps between culture of origin and that of receiving country
Age at immigration		Lack of social support and resources
		Lack of ethnic enclaves
		Extent of loss (social status, family ties, familiar environment, resources)
		Lack of knowledge of language of receiving country
		Lack of bilingual, culturally competent services
		Financial obligations
		Cumulative stress

Risk factors

Acculturative stress

Acculturation is the process of change in beliefs, values, and behaviors that take place among immigrants as a result of contact with the receiving society (Berry and Sam, 1997). The pressure to accommodate to the larger culture is a complex and powerful force in the lives of all immigrants (Berry, 2003). The similarity between the receiving culture and the migrant's heritage culture can help determine how much acculturation is required to adapt to the receiving culture (Potocky-Tripodi, 2002; Rudmin, 2003). Acculturation was initially viewed as a uni-dimensional process in an individual and was viewed as moving along a single continuum from conformity to the ethnic culture of origin to adaption of the receiving culture (Gordon, 1964). In recent years, acculturation has been understood as a multi-dimensional process, in which an individual holds on to his or her culture of origin while adapting to the values, attitudes, and behaviors of the dominant culture (Hwang and Ting, 2008).

Acculturative stress refers to the stressors that immigrants experience during the course of adapting to their new environment. One source of stress stems from the attempts to integrate one's own cultural values and beliefs with that of the receiving culture. Studies indicate that the majority of immigrants worldwide try to integrate into the receiving society and gain structural assimilation while maintaining their cultural heritage and traditional values (Ward, 2009). Trying to integrate one's own culture and that of the receiving society can create conflicts within an individual and in relationships with others. The process of acculturation, of course, is not confined to immigrants alone; the second generation born into families whose cultures are different from the dominant one also faces ongoing acculturation pressures. Generational conflicts due to differences in degrees of acculturation are common stressors among many immigrant families.

In addition to adapting to a new culture, immigrants face other stress factors that stem from losses such as the loss of a familiar environment, extended family members, social support, and social status. Lack of language skills and access to social resources is also a significant stress factor for recently arrived immigrants. Adapting to a new lifestyle can also be a source of stress for some immigrants. Another stressor is discrimination by the receiving society. Studies in the US indicate that immigrants who identify less with mainstream US culture are more likely to experience psychological distress (Hwang and Ting, 2008). Immigrants who are not able to integrate into the receiving society because of lack of language skills and/or because of discrimination are more likely to experience distress. Acculturative stress also includes experiences of discrimination, family conflicts, poverty, and trauma.

Discrimination

Immigrants often face discrimination in their host countries because of prejudice and perceived threat to the status quo and the job market. Discrimination occurs on institutional/structural, community, and individual levels. Attitudes toward immigrants on the part of the receiving country are often influenced by its relationship with the immigrants' home countries. For example, following the 9/11 terrorist attacks, ethnic and religious targeting of and discrimination against Muslims in the United States resulted in great stress among this population (Khan, 2006).

In Australia, the influx of Asian immigrants has resulted in their becoming targets of racial stereotypes and discrimination. Asians have been perceived by the majority culture as destroying the Australian way of life and taking jobs away from the native born (Betts, 1996; Collins, 1995). In recent years, there have been attempts by some government officials in Australia to restrict immigration from Asia (Fujimoto, 2004; Mak and Nesdale, 2001). In New Zealand, attitudes toward Asians, on the whole, are more positive compared to other English-speaking countries, but they are perceived less favorably than immigrants from Australia, UK, and South Africa (Ward and Masgoret, 2008) because they are not White, and are more likely to report discrimination than other immigrant groups (Ward, 2009). In the US, although a large number of Asians have high levels of education and hold professional positions, Asians hold fewer managerial or executive-level positions than non-Hispanic Whites. Asians, as a group, have higher rates of college graduates than non-Hispanic Whites; however, only 1.5 percent of executives of Fortune 1000 companies are Asian because of discrimination (Shibusawa, 2008).

Critical race theorists posit that the mental health status of minority groups including immigrants must be understood in the context of racial stratification, including the ways in which racial stratification or institutionalized racism results in social conditions such as poverty, unemployment, and experiences of discrimination (Brown, 2003). Miller and colleagues delineate six ways in which racism-related stress is experienced by Asians in the United States. *Transgenerational transmission* refers to the history of each immigrant or minority group such as exclusionary immigration policies; *collective experiences* are the way one's group is treated by society; *chronic contextual stress* includes the impact of institutional inequalities on individuals; *daily racism microaggressions* are subtle "demoralizing incidents" that can occur on a daily basis that have a cumulative negative effect; and *vicarious life experiences* are those that cause emotional distress through exposure to the experiences of others (such as witnessing or hearing about discrimination toward a member of one's immigrant group). The authors conclude that Asians in the US *are likely to expend a considerable amount of psychological, emotional, and physical energy coping with racism-related stress* (Miller *et al.*, 2011, p. 440).

In fact, there is increasing evidence that suggests an association between racial discrimination and health and mental health status among racially and ethnically diverse populations in Australia, Canada, UK, and the United States (Gee and Ponce, 2010; Gee *et al.*, 2009; Heim *et al.*, 2011; Miller *et al.*, 2011; Paradies, 2006; Tummala-Narra *et al.*, 2011). Experiences of discrimination are linked to heart disease, hypertension, respiratory illnesses, chronic health conditions, and depressive symptoms (Gee *et al.*, 2007). Discrimination is a stressor that increases the cortisol level, which in turn leads to physical illnesses. Substance abuse has also been linked to coping with racial discrimination (Yoo *et al.*, 2010). Discrimination often results in feelings of shame, and is something that people do not feel comfortable discussing (Laszloffy and Hardy, 2000). It is important for practitioners to be aware of the ways in which discrimination affects Asian immigrant clients and attend to what Laszloffy and Hardy (2000) call the "invisible wounds of oppression."

Family conflicts

Conflicts between immigrant parents and children can occur because of differences in acculturation levels among each family member (Rastogi, 2007). Immigrant parents typically acquire the host language and cultural norms at a slower rate compared to their children. Therefore, children of immigrant parents commonly serve as cultural brokers by assisting their parents, which may not be appropriate developmentally (Trickett and Jones, 2007). The reversal of roles can add burden on the family and exacerbate parent–child relationships (Kim and Choi, 1994).

Another source of family conflict among Asian immigrant families is the change in power balance between men and women. In the case of working-class immigrant families, women are often able to find work before their husbands. As a result, in some families, the husband may lose the social status that they had in their home country.

As stated previously, there has been an increase in "transnational families" in which families experience prolonged separation. While families that immigrate together have conflicts because of difference in acculturation levels, such conflicts can be pronounced when only one part of the family emigrates. Reunification can also be stressful when children have been separated from their parents for a prolonged length of time because of the lack of opportunities to develop and strengthen relational bonds (United Nations Department of Economic and Social Affairs, 2011).

Poverty

Poverty is a risk factor for immigrants, especially recent immigrants. Studies in the United States indicate that poverty rates are twice as high among Asian immigrants with a length of stay of five years or less compared to native-born Asians or those who are foreign-born with more than five years of stay (Takei and Sakamoto, 2011). A national study of Canadian children reports that foreign-born children are twice as likely to live in poverty compared to native-born children (Beiser *et al.*, 2002). A key factor that facilitates immigrants' integration into the receiving society is economic integration, i.e., labor force participation (Coughlan, 1997). However, immigrants often do not have access to the mainstream labor market because of lack of language skills. Limited language ability has been found as one of the causes behind lower employment and self-employment among the Chinese in Canada (Wang and Lo, 2004). Economic recession can also have a disproportionately negative impact on immigrants. In the UK, the unemployment rate for Pakistanis and Bangladeshis increased to17 percent in 2009 following the economic downturn in 2008 (Papademetriou *et al.*, 2010). Immigrants are also vulnerable during recessions since governments tend to cut back on public services, including immigrant integration programs (ibid.).

Poverty is associated with poor mental health among the general population (Kessler *et al.*, 2003). Factors associated with poor neighborhoods such as high rates of unemployment, crime, and violence, and social isolation are risk factors for stress among immigrant communities (McLaughlin *et al.*, 2009). Immigrants with low educational achievement are particularly vulnerable to poverty and mental health problems. For example, the Fuzhounese are an extremely vulnerable group. Most are undocumented workers from a rural area in China with barely an elementary school education. In New York City, the Fuzhounese live in the margins of Chinatown and are minorities within a minority community with little access to mental health services (Kwong, 1997; Law *et al.*, 2003)

Trauma

Fleeing a war-torn country, as was the case with South East Asian refugees after the war in Vietnam, can have traumatic impact on families. Studies of Vietnamese, Cambodian, Lao, and Hmong refugees have focused on depression and post-traumatic stress disorder (PTSD). The majority experienced tremendous hardship including incarceration, torture, physical abuse, starvation, and severe illness before and during emigration. They also lost their homeland, social status, and their possessions. In one study in the US, 73 percent of the refugees had experienced a major depressive episode and 14 percent had symptoms of PTSD shortly after arrival (Kroll, *et al.*, 1989). Pre-migration trauma is associated with prolonged psychological distress (Chung and Kagawa-Singer, 1993).

Protective factors

Demographic and socioeconomic factors

Age is a protective factor against acculturative stress. Quite often, the younger the immigrant, the fewer difficulties he or she experiences in adjusting to a new culture since it is easier for young children to acquire the language and cultural practices of the host culture (Falicov, 2011). People who migrate as adults have a more difficult time acquiring a new language, and older adults face the biggest challenges in adopting the lifestyles, values, and culture of their new country (Schwartz *et al.*, 2010). Adjustment to a new country can also differ according to gender. Studies in the US suggest that some immigrant women have an easier time than men in adjusting because they have more opportunities for financial achievement than they had in their home country. At the same time, it is important to note that women who immigrate alone are vulnerable to exploitation and abuse (Ross-Sheriff, 2011).

Personal characteristics such as optimism, self-esteem, and hardiness also facilitate adjustment to a new country (Mak and Nesdale, 2001). In a study of Chinese immigrants and discrimination in Australia, Mak and Nesdale (2001) found that internal resources, specifically ethnic self-esteem and personal self-esteem were important protective factors in addition to having Anglo-Australian friends. Studies among Korean immigrants in the US have reported that self-esteem and optimism are associated with overcoming adversity (Lee *et al.*, 2008)

Social support

People with high levels of social support tend to cope with stress better than those with low levels of support (Taylor, 1995). Interpersonal support has been reported to buffer depression among Korean immigrant women in the US (Ayers *et al.*, 2009). A study of Chinese immigrants in the US also identified support from family, friends, and community, as well as communication among family members, ability to balance their own and recipient cultures, and spiritual well-being as sources of family strengths (Xie *et al.*, 2004). At the same time, support from the host country is also important in the adjustment process (Boehnlein *et al.*, 1995).

Resilience

Despite the challenges of adapting to a new country, many Asian immigrants are resilient and able to thrive in the face of adversities. Resilience is the capacity to withstand or endure difficulties and to recover or grow in the face of disruptive life challenges and make positive adaptations (Luthar *et al.*, 2000; Walsh, 2010). Personal characteristics such as optimism, being extroverted, and having the ability to view change as inevitable have been associated with resilience (Aroian and Norris, 2000; Campbell-Sills *et al.*, 2006; Walsh, 2010). Building on a family systems perspective, Walsh (2010) has identified the following key processes that enhance family resilience:

- family belief systems – ability to make meaning of the adversity, have a positive outlook, and look to cultural and spiritual resources for strength;
- organizational patterns – flexibility and openness to change, connectedness among family members, and the ability to mobilize social and economic resources;
- communication processes – clear and consistent communication, sharing feelings and tolerating differences, and ability to problem solve collaboratively.

The applicability of these key processes for Asian immigrant families has not yet been examined. However, the concept of family resilience provides a useful framework for practitioners to help Asian families build on their strengths (Walsh, 2010).

Summary

This chapter presented a brief overview of Asian immigrants in English-speaking countries and discussed immigrant-specific challenges in the process of adapting to the receiving country. Stress factors as well as protective factors were presented. In the next chapters we will discuss specific mental health issues that Asian immigrant families encounter, and ways to address the problems using a relational framework.

Discussion highlights

Population of Asian migrants to English-speaking countries

Asians constitute close to 50 percent of migrants to English-speaking countries. (p. 77)

Adaptation challenges

It is important for practitioners to understand cumulative risk factors during all phases of the immigration process including pre-migration, peri-migration, and post-migration. (p. 83)

Immigrants who are not able to integrate into the receiving society because of lack of language skills and/or because of discrimination are more likely to experience distress. (p. 84)

Acculturative stress also includes experiences of discrimination, family conflicts, poverty, and trauma. (p. 84)

Strengths and vulnerabilities

Many Asian immigrants continue to maintain strong linkages with their families in their home countries, and provide financial support. (p. 78)

Immigrants with low educational achievement are particularly vulnerable to poverty and mental health problems. (p. 87)

Despite the challenges of adapting to a new country, many Asian immigrants are resilient and able to thrive in the face of adversities. (p. 88)

5 Working with Asian immigrant families

Parenting practices and intergenerational relationships

Irene W. Chung and Tazuko Shibusawa

In this chapter, we present clinical practices with Asian immigrant families with young and adolescent children. We will first focus on families with younger children and explore differences between Asian and Western parenting in the areas of:

1 parental expectations;
2 parent–child communication; and
3 the way parents expect their children to cope with distress.

We will also discuss discipline and the use of corporal punishment, which can be perceived as mistreatment and abuse in their host countries. In the second part of this chapter we will discuss families with adolescents and present issues specific to Asian immigrant adolescents, including identity, mental health, and inter-generational relationships. In the final section of this chapter, we present ways that practitioners can work with families using a relational perspective.

Cultural characteristics of Asian immigrant families

Immigrants from Asia, influenced by social and economic changes in their home countries, hold diverse values and beliefs about families. Traditional norms and expectations regarding family relationships in Asian countries have been in flux due to increasing urbanization (Hindin, 2005). In China, for example, family norms differ between those in urban and rural areas. In urban areas where the one-child policy has been enforced, there have been changes in parenting values and beliefs about child development. The one-child policy, with an ensuing family structure of four grandparents, two parents, and one child has resulted in more child-centered family parent–child relationships than in the past (Chuang and Su, 2009). As mentioned in Chapter 4, adaptation to host countries among immigrant families also varies according to factors such as educational background, social class, human and social capital, and receptivity of the host country (Landale *et al.*, 2011). Family composition is also diverse among Asian immigrants since some immigrants maintain transnational family arrange-ments in which one or both parents migrate while leaving their children to the care of the grandparents in their home country. Despite variation in expectations about family relationships, it is important to understand core structures and values, which are at the foundation of contemporary Asian immigrant families.

Core values and structures of Asian families

- Patriarchal family system
- Bilateral family system

There are two basic family systems in Asia, one that is patrilineal and based on patriarchal ideology, and the other, which is referred to as a bilateral system where the positions of men and women are more egalitarian (Mason, 1992). The patrilineal system can be found in East Asian countries such as China, Japan, Korea, and northern Vietnam, and in the northern part of South Asia including Bangladesh, northern India, Nepal, and Pakistan. The bilateral family system exists in South East Asian countries such as Thailand, Indonesia, the Philippines, and the southern areas of India, Sri Lanka, and Vietnam.

Patriarchal family structures are hierarchical and men have formal decision-making powers, greater independence, and greater opportunities than women (Chung, 1992; Min, 1998). Because men are accorded more privilege, preference for sons is stronger in patrilineal/patrilocal families than in bilateral families. In bilateral family systems, gender roles are more egalitarian than patriarchal families, and women, including those in Filipino families, command more respect than do women in East Asian and northern South Asian families (Root 2005). At the same time, *machismo* is an important part of the Filipino male culture because of the Spanish influence (Yap, 1986). Non-hierarchical kin networks are also important in bilateral family systems. In many Filipino families, extended family members such as second and third cousins are considered a core part of the family. Some families such as those in the southern parts of India are matriarchal and family lineage is succeeded through women (Mulatti, 1995).

Regardless of family structure, the goals and needs of the family take precedence over the desires of individual members in traditional Asian families. Personal identities are based on family membership and individuals are expected to sacrifice their desires for the sake of the family (Agbayani-Siewert, 1994; Lee and Mock, 2005). For example, in India, where over 80 percent of the population is Hindu, the notions of self and family are strongly influenced by Hinduism (Pillari, 2005), and the individual self is defined as an extension of the cosmic absolute and viewed as being part of a collective whole (Pettys and Balgopal, 1998). Indian families discourage autonomy, and studies indicate that Indian immigrants in Western countries continue to base their lifestyles on traditional collectivistic values and expectations many years after immigration (Jambunathan and Counselman, 2002). Filipino culture emphasizes loyalty and solidarity with family and kin groups. Individual interests or desires are sacrificed for the good of the family, and cooperation among family members is stressed over individualism (Agbayani-Siewert 1994). Filipino families also emphasize mutual support and the importance of belonging to the family (Wolf, 1997). The sense of self is highly identified with family in Filipino culture (Tompar-Tiu and Sustento-Seneriches, 1995). Filipinos emphasize family cohesiveness, honor, loyalty and gratitude (*utang na loob*), respect for authority and obedience (Woelz-Stirling *et al.*, 2001). Self is intertwined with identification with family, and the needs of family rather than the individual.

Traditional Chinese, Korean, Japanese, and Vietnamese cultures are heavily influenced by Confucianism, which dictates the position and roles of individuals within families. The sense of self is defined and expressed in relationship to others within a hierarchically structured family context. Expectations are placed on individuals to maintain social order and harmony by honoring the requirements and responsibilities of their family roles (Bond and Hwang, 1986). Family roles are clearly delineated, and children are expected to obey and respect their parents, and women are expected to submit to male members of their family (Kim and Choi, 1994). Since individuals are defined by their family affiliation, any wrongdoing on the part of an individual is considered to bring shame on the family as a whole. It is important, however, to note diversity within nation states that have been influenced by Confucianism. For example, in Japan, the extent to which Confucian norms dictated family ideologies differed according to social class. Confucianism was more entrenched among ruling class families than merchant class or agricultural families.

Families with children

Parenting practices among Asian immigrants

Parenting practices in Asian cultures differ in many ways from Western cultures. In order to work effectively with Asian immigrant families, we believe that it is important for practitioners to have some general knowledge of parenting practices and appreciate the cultural and immigrant-specific values that shape these differences.

- Expectations for child development
- Socialization of collectivistic values
- Emphasis on educational achievement

Parenting practices are guided by cultural norms and values, which, in turn, influence child development (Chuang and Su, 2009). To represent Asian and Western practices as monolithic and binary oppositions is, of course, to risk distorting the truth; nonetheless, some general differences are userful to note. Traditional cultural values that Asian immigrant families bring to the United States often conflict with the values of the host countries. The most common conflict stems from the difference between Western notions of individualism and Asian cultural values of group harmony. In Western cultures, children are trained from a young age to develop a sense of self; they are taught that they can change their environment, and that self-determination is important. Asians, on the other hand, are taught from a young age to be sensitive to their environment, to suppress one's wishes in the interest of the family and group, and to be able to mold oneself according to the demands of environment rather than individualism (Ho, 1994).

Sleeping arrangements in traditional Asian families reflect the sense of collectivism. It is common practice for many Asian families to have infants sleep in the same room or bed with the parents. Co-sleeping has been observed among Punjabi and Gujarati immigrants in the UK, and Japanese and Korean families in the US (Dosanjh and Ghuman, 1998; Hackett and Hackett, 1994; Jin *et al.*, 2010).

Most parents in English-speaking cultures encourage their children from a young age to develop a sense of self that is independent from others. While expectations may differ depending on the gender of the children, in general, children are expected to assert themselves. In contrast, children in traditional Asian cultures are taught to respect the family hierarchy and the authority of parents and grandparents. Children are also expected to honor their families by doing well in school and society (Chao, 1994).

In Western cultures, emphasis is placed on fostering "self-determination" and "self-reliance" as children are expected to grow out of a dependent state of infancy into autonomous individuality. In traditional Asian cultures, individuation and autonomy are not conceptualized as developmental goals. Rather, parents strive to instill in their children the ability to adapt to group norms. For example, studies in the United States indicate that Asian immigrant parents emphasize "good behavior" while Caucasian parents emphasize "self-directed behavior" (Maiter and George, 2003; Tajima and Harachi, 2010; Yang, 2009; Yee *et al.*, 1998).

Asian parents perceive self-control, obedience, helping with family chores, and achieving in school as "good behavior," and compared to Western parents, place less emphasis on fostering independent thinking among their children (Tajima and Harachi, 2010). Self-control and self-restraint are viewed in Asian cultures as signs of maturity (Chuang and Su, 2009). According to a study of Hong Kong parents, ideal children:

1 have good relationships with their parents;
2 fulfill family responsibilities;
3 do well academically;
4 are positive toward studying; and
5 are self-disciplined.

(Shek and Chan, 1999)

Indian parents emphasize character development, which is common among other Asian parents (Maiter and George, 2003). In Filipino families, if children do not do well, it is seen as a reflection of the parents, resulting in loss of face and shame (*hiya*) for the family (Agbayani-Siewert 1994).

Educational achievement is important for Asian immigrant parents because most Asian cultural traditions place value on education, and because they believe that educational achievement will improve occupational opportunities for their

Table 5.1 Cultural differences in parental expectations

Western	Asian
Conceptualization of selfhood	
Psychological self	Social self
Emphasis on individual dimension	Emphasis on collective dimension
Expectations for development	
Development of cohesive self	Development of non-egocentric self
Self-determination	Adaptability to groups
Independence	Interdependence
Self-expression	Impulse control
Leadership skills	Effective participation in groups
Emphasis on ability	Emphasis on effort
Self-enhancement	Self-effacement

children (Dugsin, 2001; Goyette and Xie, 1999; Wu, 2001). Parents tend to view academic success and obedience as a benchmark of their children's loyalty and competence as parents (Chung and Bemak, 2002). Asian parents also place more emphasis on effort than ability compared to Western parents and expect their children to do well in school if they exert effort regardless of their abilities (Shibusawa, 2001).

Because of language differences, structural barriers, and lack of transferable skills, many Asian immigrants who are educated end up taking jobs for which they are overqualified. The sense of demoralization and disappointment that follows is often projected onto their children, and can become the source of parent-child conflict. Although the academic achievement of many Asian immigrant children is touted as a visible sign of a "model minority," the pressure that accompanies these expectations can have severe negative impacts on the children (Larsen *et al.*, 2008).

Parent–child communication

- Expanding the understanding of Asian "authoritarian" parenting styles
- Implicit communication of love and affection

Researchers in the US distinguish between "authoritative" and "authoritarian" parenting styles (Baumrind, 1991). "Authoritative" parenting styles are characterized by expressions of warmth, acceptance of children for who they are, respect for children's autonomy and regulating children's behaviors through reasoning. Parents who are "authoritative" provide explanations and reasons for their decisions and include children's input in their decision-making (Kim and Ge, 2000). "Authoritarian" parenting styles, on the other hand, emphasize parental control of children and include verbal and physical coercion and lack of reasoning when regulating children's behaviors. In Western cultures, "authoritative"

Table 5.2 "Authoritative" and "authoritarian" parenting styles

Parenting style	Authoritative	Authoritarian
Characteristics	Warmth	Physical coercion
	Acceptance	High expectations
	Reasoning oriented	Verbal hostility
	Regulation	Non-reasoning oriented
	Autonomy granting	Regulation

parenting is considered to be more effective with positive outcomes for their children than "authoritarian" parenting styles (Steinberg *et al.*, 2006).

Asian immigrant parents are often perceived as being "authoritarian" because they are restrictive and expect their children to obey without providing any explanations, opportunities for negotiation, or emotional support (Baumrind, 1991). The applicability of the concepts of "authoritative" and "authoritarian" parenting styles, however, has been questioned for Asian families, because they do not fully describe Asian styles of parenting. Chao (2001), in her study of Chinese immigrant families, notes that the beneficial effects of "authoritative" parenting are not applicable to children of Chinese descent in the same way that they are for children of European descent because the notion of closeness in parent–child relationships is constructed differently (Chao, 2001). While research indicates that "authoritarian" parenting was negatively associated to closeness among children of European descent, authoritarian parenting was associated with closeness among Chinese students.

Parenting practices of Asian immigrants from East and Southeast Asian countries including China, Korea, Japan, and Vietnam, are influenced by the Confucian concepts of *guan* and *gin*. *Guan* is generally translated as "to govern" or "to teach and inculcate values" by the parents, but it is also associated with the demonstration of parental love, nurturance, and support. Chao (1994) characterizes this parenting style as "training," which denotes high parental involvement and physical closeness with the children. In South Asian cultures, Indian and Pakistani families also tend to view roles of parenting as "training" their children (Farver *et al.*, 2002). Parents believe that it is their responsibility to instill values of self-discipline, obedience, hard work, and academic success in their children. At the same time, parents are also expected to sacrifice their needs for the care and welfare of the children (Jambunathan and Counselman, 2002). The children, in turn, experience *gin*, or "closeness," through their parents' care and devotion, and are motivated to reciprocate by fulfilling their obligations (Wu and Chao, 2011). Once children reach school age, instead of expressing physical affection, parents communicate their love for each other and their children through fulfilling their obligations to the family, and sacrificing their own needs for their children.

The degree to which affection is displayed among Asian immigrant families depends on the extent to which the parents have incorporated communication patterns of mainstream culture of the host country. Asian immigrant children tend to compare images of parent–child interactions in the host culture as a measuring stick of their own relationships with parents and grandparents. While many understand the sacrifice that parents make on their behalf as love and caring, they can also perceive their parents as lacking in affection and this can result in increased distance in intergenerational relationships (Chao and Kaeochinda, 2010; Kang *et al.*, 2010).

Parental expectations toward coping with distress

There are two main ways that people respond to distress: by actively trying to change the source of distress or by trying to change themselves or their perception of the cause of distress. The first approach is known as problem-focused coping and the latter as emotion-focused coping (Tweed *et al.*, 2004). Researchers conclude that Asians, in general, use emotion-focused coping instead of problem-focused coping. Emotion-focused coping is a passive approach and is considered to be suitable with the collectivistic nature of Asian cultures. The hierarchical nature of Asian cultures also hinders individuals from actively resolving conflicts (Kuo, 2011). The passive coping style is also influenced by Buddhism which views suffering as unavoidable, and Taoism which places emphasis on people adapting themselves to nature and their environment (Tweed *et al.*, 2004).

After the 9/11 terrorist attacks in the US, studies found that compared to Blacks and Latinos/Latinas who engaged in religious coping, Asians emphasized accepting the attacks as fate (Constantine *et al.*, 2005). In a study comparing Japanese and Japanese American survivors of domestic violence, Japanese immigrant women used more passive coping strategies such as minimizing the problem or focusing on the positives of the abusers than American-born Japanese women (Yoshihama, 2002). Studies of South East Asian refugees in Canada also report that in response to racial discrimination, passive coping was more helpful in reducing depression than active, problem-focused coping (Noh *et al.*, 1999). Similar results are found among Korean immigrants in Canada, who use emotion-focused coping when the cause of the stress is out of one's control or is associated with interpersonal conflicts (Kuo, 2011). The findings, however, do not mean that Asians do not engage in problem-solving coping. Lee and colleagues report that emotion-focused coping was used when family conflict was perceived to be high, while problem-focused coping was used when family conflict was low among Asian college students in the US (Lee *et al.*, 2005). Furthermore, coping strategies are influenced by the level of acculturation. Problem-solving coping has been found to be helpful for acculturated Korean Canadians dealing with racial discrimination, but not helpful for less acculturated Korean immigrants (Noh and Kaspar, 2003).

Asian immigrant parents try to instill emotion-focused coping skills because they believe that their children need to learn to endure hardships because adapting to adverse circumstances builds character. For example, among Japanese immigrant families impulse control is viewed as a sign of emotional maturity and the children are frequently told by their parents that they have to endure or withhold ones' wishes (*gaman*) (Shibusawa, 2001). In Filipino families, value is placed on "smooth relationships," and conflicts between people are minimized. Children are discouraged from displaying anger or aggression and are expected to behave in a passive, cooperative manner (Agbayani-Siewert, 1994). Emotion-focused coping can also negatively affect Asian immigrant children in schools. Teachers often view Asian children as passive and lacking in autonomy. As the children grow up, guidance counselors can inadvertently encourage them to select academic disciplines that do not require an extroverted style of communication. Several large-scale studies in the United States report that in comparison to non-Asian children, Asian children tend to internalize their distress. Instead of acting out, they experience depression, sadness, and loneliness (Huang *et al.*, 2012; Nguyen *et al.*, 2004).

Discipline

- Cultural beliefs about discipline
- Beliefs about parental rights

The way Asian immigrant parents discipline their children must be understood in the context of cultural beliefs and norms. Children are highly valued in all Asian cultures, and disciplined in order to function optimally in a collectivistic culture. In many Asian cultures, young children are given a lot of latitude with regard to their behaviors because they are perceived as not being able to understand reasoning. When children reach the age of six, stricter discipline is used (Roland, 1996).

In East and Southeast Asian cultures, Confucian tradition emphasizes respect for authority figures, and children are expected to respect their parents. Cross-cultural studies comparing Chinese immigrant groups, Chinese Americans, and Caucasians on parental attitudes toward children report that Chinese mothers demonstrated the highest approval for parental control over their children (Lin and Fu, 1990). These findings may be influenced by the highly emphasized values and Chinese traditions of parental control of children, strict discipline, and filial piety (ibid.). Chinese parents believe that they have a right to discipline their children (Yang, 2009). It has also been noted that Chinese parents show little or no concern about damaging their child's self-respect and self-esteem (O'Brian and Lau, 1995). This perspective, however, is based on a Western lens, which focuses on the centrality of individualism. In a collectivistic culture, self-esteem is not considered as important as the ability to get along with others, or self-esteem is defined in the context of interpersonal relationships. South Asian parents believe in child indulgence, but emphasize strict obedience to ensure that their children are quickly socialized into adulthood and this accompanies stringent expectations, which can result in the harsh treatment of children (Segal, 1991).

Punishment

- Understanding verbal threats in a cultural context
- Traditional use of corporal punishment

Punishment, ranging from verbal threats to corporal punishment, is an integral part of disciplining children and there are cultural differences in the way parents punish their children. Verbal threats of abandonment, for example, can reflect the nature of parent–child relationships. For example, in Japanese culture, mother–child relationships are close and the threat of distance and separation are used as methods of punishment. Silence is used as a punishment, in which the mother ignores the presence of the child (Tomita, 1998). Verbal expression of disapproval also connotes threats of abandonment. For example, "A bad child like you does not belong to us" is a typical statement that is used by mothers in Japan. Childhood verbal humiliation and disapproval from parents are common themes that frequently come up among Japanese American adults in psychotherapy (Shibusawa, 2001). In traditional Japanese society, children were locked out of the home and not let in until they expressed regret for their actions (Johnson, 1993). This is in direct contrast to Euro-American children who are often grounded and not allowed to go out of the home. Threatening not to love the child, or threatening to send the child away has also been observed among Gujarati parents in the UK (Hackett and Hackett, 1994).

Although in recent years corporal punishment has become controversial in Western countries, and a number of countries including the US have passed laws banning the practice, some 94 percent of American parents reported that they used physical punishment (Gershoff, 2002). Corporal punishment has also been a source of debate among researchers as to its positive and harmful aspects. A number of countries including the US have laws that prohibit parents from using physical punishment (Gershoff, 2002), but it is important to note that in even in Western countries, it is only in recent years that the effectiveness of physical punishment has come into question.

Traditionally, Asian parents used to condone physical punishment. The practice is considered by Chinese parents as a means to instill discipline and integrity of the character of the child rather than a punishment (Kwok and Tam, 2005). Korean and Chinese parents traditionally used caning to formalize and control children's behavior (Yang, 2009). In general, corporal punishment was traditionally not considered to be excessive in Asian cultures. Discipline was seen as a sign of parental concern and love, and physical punishments at times were viewed as a necessary part of parental love. In a study of South Asian families in the UK, Irfan (2008) concluded that the majority of parents believe that they have the liberty and the right to use physical punishment to discipline their children. In most cases, parents who practice and are in favor of physical punishment as a form of discipline are those who have themselves experienced these traditional forms of discipline from their parents (Irfan, 2008).

Acculturation to Western culture also influences parental attitudes toward physical punishment. For example, Dosanjh and Ghuman (1998) point out in their study of two generations of Punjabis in the UK, that mothers who are second generation do not believe in physical punishment (*Dosanjh and Ghuman, 1998*).

Immigration-related stressors and physical discipline

- Parents' acculturation difficulties and experiences of loss
- Mental health issues
- Reunificiation issues for children sent back to home countries

When excessive discipline is observed among Asian parents, it is important to understand stressors associated with the immigration experience (Lau *et al.*, 2006). Anxiety and adjustment problems associated with migration can cause immigrant parents to rely on traditional methods of discipline, which they believe are effective to protect their children from undesirable influences in a new country (Kwok and Tam, 2005). Parents who are under undue stress can end up exerting excessive discipline, which in turn can be detrimental to their child's physical and emotional well-being. A study examining lifetime parent-to-child aggression in a nationally representative sample of 1,293 Asian American parents found that minority status including perception of discrimination and low social standing increased the risk of lifetime parent-to-child aggression (Lau *et al.*, 2006). Another study conducted in the US reports that Vietnamese children and adolescents are punished severely by their fathers who feel that Western culture guarantees too many rights to their children. This is because in recently arrived immigrant families, it is difficult for fathers to exert control as the head of the household (Long, 1997). A study of Korean immigrant mothers in the US also reports that greater levels of mother–child acculturation conflict were associated with stronger endorsement of physical punishment (Yang, 2009). Loneliness and depression may plague immigrants and refugees in their early years in the United States and can persist even longer. This is particularly significant for child welfare since parental isolation is frequently connected to child maltreatment (Harrington and Dubowitz, 1999). Poverty, social isolation, lack of social support, and inadequate housing add further stress to this population. Intergenerational conflicts, as well as the role reversal between parents and their children due to English skills, also increase the risk for maltreatment (Chang *et al.*, 2006; Pelczarski and Kemp, 2006; Xiong *et al.*, 2005)

Separation and reunification is common in immigrant families from a number of countries, especially those who are trying to establish themselves financially (Falicov, 2011). In some families, children are sent back to the home country to be cared for by their grandparents so that both parents can work. The children are then reunited with their parents when they are older. For some families, the separation is a natural part of their culture where extended families regularly care for children. Reunification, however, can be challenging, especially if the child has felt abandoned and is not able to bond with the parents. The lack of bonding can lead to parenting difficulties, which in turn can exacerbate conflicts and result in excessive physical discipline.

It is important to note that physical discipline differs from physical abuse. The ways in which Asian immigrant parents discipline their children, however, are often viewed as abuse by local authorities in their host country. This does not mean that child abuse is not recognized in Asian countries. In recent years, many

Asian countries have begun to recognize corporal punishment as a potential problem that can result in abuse and maltreatment and have implemented policies regarding child abuse. For example, laws against child abuse were established in both Japan and Korea in the 2000s (Goodman, 2002; Yang, 2009), and efforts to prevent child abuse in countries such as India and Vietnam are under way with the support of international organizations such as UNICEF (Kacker *et al.*, 2007). Although there is growing awareness of child abuse in Asian countries, many Asian immigrant families are unfamiliar with child abuse laws of their host country, and there are cases in which they are referred to child protective services (Fong, 1997).

Child welfare laws in English-speaking countries

Many host countries have laws to protect children from parental abuse. Starting in 1972, Australia has continued to increase mandated reporting laws for child abuse and neglect for professionals who come into contact with children (Mathews and Kenny, 2008). Canada also introduced reporting legislation in the 1960s, and in the US, beginning with the passage of the 1974 Child Abuse Prevention and Treatment Act (CAPTA), a number of laws regarding mandatory reporting have been enacted. New Zealand and the UK, on the other hand, do not have mandatory reporting laws because of concerns about over-reporting (Mathews and Kenny, 2008).

Assessment and interventions of child abuse cases

- Culturally grounded assessment of the quality of the parent–child relationships
- Identification of cultural strengths of the family
- Sensitivity to cultural shame and stigma
- Psychoeducation with a focus on the family

There is very little data about the rates of reported child abuse cases among Asian immigrants in English-speaking countries. In the US, rates of reported child maltreatment cases among Asian immigrants are lower compared to African Americans, Caucasians, Hispanics, and Native Americans (Pelczarski and Kemp, 2006). However, the rates of reported physical abuse among Asian parents are higher compared to other groups. When Asian immigrant parents are referred to practitioners for alleged abuse, it is important first to assess if child abuse is indeed an issue or if there was a misunderstanding on the part of the reporting party. While there should be zero tolerance of physical abuse, practitioners need to be aware that many Asian parents still consider corporal punishment to be a part of education for their children. "Spare the rod, spoil the child" is a common belief among many Asian cultures. Thus, in the assessment process, practitioners need to evaluate if the children are able to develop a sense of trust and positive attachment ties with their parents rather than assume that parents were abusing or mistreating their children. Some Asian immigrant families choose to use traditional Eastern or homeopathic medicinal practices to treat ailments before seeking treatment from Western clinics or emergency rooms. Depending on the medical ailment, this delay in medical treatment in some cases constitutes medical neglect by American standards (Larsen *et al.*, 2008). Fong (1997) notes four issues that are especially important to consider during the assessment process:

1   the family's concept of child welfare;
2   the family as the unit of analysis and treatment;
3   family migration and location history, especially the values of the particular Asian society from which the family emigrates; and
4   cultural strengths that some Western-trained practitioners Americans might misinterpret as weaknesses.

   Prevention and treatment models need to incorporate belief systems, cultural variables of patriarchy, gender roles, shame, isolation, and normative values attributed to corporal punishment and physical abuse among these ethnic groups (Maker *et al.*, 2005). Professionals in the UK note that, against a background of disadvantage and racism against Asian families in the UK, professional intervention may compound or increase the sense of alienation and discrimination experienced by these families (Humphreys *et al.*, 1999). Asian immigrant families may be more likely to adhere to court-ordered assessment and treatment given their Asian respect for hierarchy and authority. Asian families may also cooperate out of fear of having the child removed from the family (Ho, 1994). However, compliance with court mandates does not guarantee that families will get the help they need to resolve the issues.

   Given the strong family orientation among Asian immigrants, it is crucial to involve the entire family in the prevention and intervention of child abuse. Child abuse should be approached as a problem of the entire family and framed as a problem, which reflects the major social and cultural transitions that they are experiencing as immigrants. The practitioner needs to be aware that the immigrant family may feel ashamed for having to deal with the issue of child abuse with a practitioner. However, if the family can be helped to realize that what they are doing in counseling is to restore the family's health and honor, they will be more cooperative in the process. It is important for clinicians to respect the traditional hierarchical structure of the family in therapy (e.g., begin the initial session addressing and listening to the parents first) (Larsen *et al.*, 2008), and establish rapport with the whole family. Practitioners can then emphasize how each member of the family can contribute to decreasing the family's social and cultural transitional predicament (ibid.). Again, given the strong family orientation among Asian immigrants, it is crucial to involve the entire family in prevention and intervention efforts. Once trust is established, the clinician can clarify how and why the alleged abuse has taken place (ibid.). It is also important to point out the family's strengths, and stressors.

   Practitioners can help Asian parents and children discuss their desires for success, especially in academic-related areas. The practitioner first tries to understand the extent to which the parents have sacrificed for their children and the level of their desire for their children to succeed academically (Larsen *et al.*, 2008). It is important to address what success means to them individually and what is acceptable for the whole family. If success means the same thing for the whole family and the child lacks certain skills or motivation, the practitioner can use the community's resources to help the child. On the other hand, if the child's meaning of success differs from that of the parents, then the practitioner continues to work with the family until a consensus is reached (ibid.). It is also important to explore the obstacles to the child's "success" such as an unsupportive teacher/learning environment. Taking a more systemic approach with the parents removes the onus of responsibility on the child.

Applying a psychoeducational approach is important when working with parents who have been referred for child abuse and neglect. In order to prevent future child abuse incidents, practitioners need to help Asian immigrant families understand the child abuse laws of the host country and promote practicing healthy parenting while being respectful of their native cultural beliefs and practices (Larsen *et al.*, 2008). When parents who are court-mandated to undergo therapy deny child abuse, it does not necessarily imply that they are unwilling to work for the safety of their children (Hiles and Luger, 2006). The work of the practitioner is to facilitate the healing and growth of the family as a whole, no matter how resistant the parents or the family may seem to the clinician (Larsen *et al.*, 2008).

Families with adolescents

In this section, we discuss relationships between Asian immigrant parents and their adolescent children. Building on issues discussed in Part I we will discuss 1) the interactions between adolescent development and parental expectations, 2) challenges that parents face as immigrants, and 3) challenges that adolescents face as children of immigrants. We will first provide a brief summary of adolescent development and culture- and immigrant-specific issues that can compound intergenerational conflicts between parents and adolescents, then present risk and protective factors, and ways to work with Asian immigrant families and adolescents that are based on a relational framework.

Psychological well-being of Asian immigrant adolescents: risk and protective factors

Cultural beliefs and practice in regard to adolescence

In Western cultures, adolescence is conceptualized as a period in the life cycle where an individual achieves a sense of identity and autonomy as an individual. Failure to achieve a secure identity is believed to lead to low self-esteem and a poor self-concept (Erikson, 1980). Identity development includes gender identity, and in the case of minority adolescents, an ethnic identity.

In the United States, among White and upper to middle-class communities, turning 13 is considered to be the beginning of adolescence with more freedom from parental control (Garcia-Preto, 2010). However, many adolescents of minority groups, including immigrants, are called upon to assume adult responsibilities such as taking care of their younger siblings or helping with their family-owned businesses (Garcia-Preto, 2010). In many Asian families, adolescents are still expected to be obedient and respect their parents despite their additional responsibilities. Furthermore, while becoming independent and autonomous is an important goal for Western adolescents, this is not the case for Asian youth. Asian cultures tend not to view adolescence as a separate life stage since maturation is considered as a lifelong process. Thus, Asian parents with a traditional value orientation tend to not encourage autonomy for their children, and this increases the risk of intergenerational conflicts.

Physical development

Physical changes during adolescence include growth spurts and hormonal changes. Neuroscientists also note that changes in adolescent brains can lead to erratic behavior and poor judgment among adolescents (Yurgelun-Todd and Killgore, 2006). Researchers find that many Asian American adolescents grow up with a less positive body image and self-image compared to their European American cohorts (Yee *et al.*, 1998). There is evidence that some Asian youth are less satisfied with their physical characteristics than their White cohorts (Pang *et al.*, 1985). Sexual and physical development is a topic that is not discussed in most Asian American families. This can be problematic for adolescents who are in the midst of developing their own sexual identity. Boys, in particular, are confronted with "emasculated images" of Asian American males in the media, which can affect the development of a healthy sexual self-image (Leong, 1994).

Ethnic identity development

In addition to normative issues of adolescent development that are associated with cognitive, psychological, and social development, immigrant adolescents face stressors because of their minority status and challenges related to acculturation and identity development (Eyou *et al.*, 2000; Yeh *et al.*, 2008). In addition to gender identity development, adolescents among minority groups including Asians need to form an ethnic identity. Ethnic identity includes a sense of belonging, attitudes and beliefs, knowledge, and ethnic values, and membership in a particular group (Phinney and Ong, 2007). Developing an ethnic identity can be challenging since adolescents also have to respond to the way in which society defines them and often discriminates against them. Forming a positive ethnic identity is crucial, yet this can be challenging. The development of ethnic identity can be viewed as a dynamic process that changes over time according to the context of peoples' lives and different challenges that people face (Phinney, 2003).

Research demonstrates that a strong ethnic identity is linked to a variety of positive psychosocial outcomes among Asian immigrant adolescents, and serves to protect individuals from the negative consequences of racism and discrimination (Chae and Foley, 2010; Yip *et al.*, 2008).

Asian adolescents, regardless of whether they are first or second generation (children of immigrants), also need to negotiate between their own culture and the culture of the dominant society. The following is a model that is suggested by Phinney and colleagues on the four different ways that adolescents negotiate their family culture and the host culture (Phinney *et al.*, 1990). Some adolescents become alienated from their own culture as well as the majority culture (1). Very few adolescents become alienated or marginalized to the point of being alienated from either culture (Schwartz *et al.*, 2010), but many deny their own culture (assimilation) (2), or the host culture (withdrawal) (3). Research indicates that feeling positive about both their own culture and the host culture (i.e., integrate both cultures) (4) is associated with positive well-being among adolescents. For example, a study of 427 immigrant Chinese between 12 and 19 years of age in New Zealand reports that students who were integrated into the mainstream culture had higher self-esteem (Eyou *et al.*, 2000). Integrating both cultures accompanies cognitive flexibility, an awareness and willingness to consider ways to adapt or make changes without getting stuck in a narrow view of responding to challenges and conflicts, especially with their parents (Ahn *et al.*, 2008). Immigrant parents generally expect children to maintain some aspects of their own culture, and immigrant youth have to adopt to different social roles and obligations by "shifting selves" (Yeh *et al.*, 2008).

(1) **Alienation/Marginalization** Own Culture (-) Negative self-image Estrangement from own culture Fail to adapt to majority culture	(2) **Assimilation** Majority Culture (+)/ Own Culture (-) Assimilate into majority culture Exclusion of ties with own culture
(3) **Withdrawal/Separation** Own Culture (+)/Majority Culture (-) Withdraw from contact with majority group	(4) **Integration/Biculturalism** Own Culture (+)/Dominant Culture (+) Retain ethnic culture and adapt to majority culture

Figure 5.1 Immigrant youth and cultural identities. Source: (Phinney, *et al.*, 1990)

Intergenerational relationships between Asian immigrant parents and adolescents

- Differences in language, values, and lifestyle
- Asian parenting style and the adolescents' social world

In Western cultures, when children reach adolescence, family relationships are expected to change from a system that protects children to a system that prepares adolescents to achieve independence and prepare to enter adulthood (Garcia-Preto, 2010). Most families have to undergo changes as they change the rules for their children (Yang, 2009). Family therapists note that intergenerational conflicts are common during this transitional phase (Garcia-Preto, 2010). The turmoil that families experience as their children enter adolescence is complicated among immigrant families because of differences in acculturation between parents and their children. Most Asian immigrant parents did not go through similar stages as adolescents while they were growing up. As children grow into adolescence and seek greater autonomy, tensions may grow around issues of dating, role expectations, career choices, and family obligations (Ahn *et al.*, 2008). Many of these issues are not unique to immigrant families. However, family conflicts may be more amplified by differences in acculturation levels or language barriers between parents and adolescents.

As Asian adolescents explore and negotiate their goals, peer group affiliations, and identity development, they can experience conflict between the collectivistic values of their family and Western culture that values individualism and autonomy. Many are not able to seek guidance and support from their parents because of the differences in worldviews (Qin, 2008). Language barriers between immigrant parents and their English-speaking children can also deter parent–child communication. The role reversal between parents and their children because of the parent's lack of English proficiency can contribute to the unstable parent–child relationships, making family dynamics increasingly complex (Rhee *et al.*, 2003)

Hwang (2006), in studying Asian immigrant families in the US, proposed a concept called Acculturative Family Distancing (AFD), which has two dimensions: (1) a breakdown in family communication which is caused by different rates of language acculturation, and (2) cultural values that are incongruent between parents and children. The breakdown in communication and incongruent cultural values is thought to increase over time, and cause greater emotional, cognitive, and behavioral distance between parents and their adolescent children, which in turn leads to family conflict (Hwang, 2006). A study of Acculturative Family Distancing among Chinese high school students and their mothers in the US indicates that larger cultural gaps increase depression for both adolescents and their mothers (Hwang *et al.*, 2010)

Conflicts between values of independence and autonomy versus interdependence and conformity are common among parents and adolescents. Doing daily chores and homework, engaging in social activities with friends, dating, attending college, and making career choices can precipitate conflicts. While these conflicts can be understood as developmental issues that are common to all families, they are often amplified by the perceptions and responses of both parents and children in the family that are influenced by different sets of cultural values and norms and immigrant-specific circumstances (Chung, 2006; Qin, 2008).

Asian immigrant parents tend to focus on how their adolescents should solve their problems in concrete ways rather than discuss the experiences that their children are going through. This may deter adolescents from sharing their concerns and emotional distress. The parents' lifestyle tends to revolve around work and socialization within their kinship network and ethnic enclave, which may create disconnection with the social world of their children. As mentioned previously, as children grow older and enter adolescence, they are often expected to take on more responsibilities at home and this can also exacerbate emotional distance among members in the Asian immigrant families.

As noted earlier, the "authoritarian" style of parenting within a hierarchical and collectivistic culture does not undermine the mental health of adolescents as it does within Western liberal societies (Chao, 2001). However, it is the inconsistency between parenting styles and the culture that the adolescent is immersed in outside of the home that creates the conflicts and emotional distress for adolescents (Dwalry, 2008). In the case of Asian immigrant families, many parents are often not able to provide guidance or serve as role models because of language barriers, long hours of employment, and changes in roles within the immigrant families (Chung, 2012).

According to research, traditional values of family obligation have been transmitted to younger generations in Asian immigrant families. For example, a study of Chinese and Filipino adolescents in Northern California demonstrates that they have a strong sense of family obligation and tend to seek advice from their parents and siblings (Fuligini *et al.*, 1999). Overall, compared to their White counterparts, Asian adolescents in the study, had stronger cultural values and greater expectations about their duty to assist, respond to, and support families. At the same time, a recent study of Korean and Vietnamese college students indicates that children of immigrants tend to idealize the "normal American family." The students' image of the American family is one where parents:

1   are democratic;
2   respect the autonomy and individual well-being of their children;
3   encourage emotional expressiveness;
4   are intimate and emotionally nurturing; and
5   are supportive, understanding, and forgiving of their children.

(Pyke, 2000)

These students viewed their own families in a negative light compared to their idealized image of the American family. They saw their own parents as:

1   having high expectations for duty and responsibility;
2   emphasizing the importance of family over the individual;

3 being overly strict; and
4 being emotionally distant.

Consequences of intergenerational conflicts

- Mental health issues among adolescents
- Gang membership

Intergenerational conflicts in Asian immigrant families are a concern because of the negative impact on adolescent mental health and the frustrations of immigrant parents who feel inadequate in supporting their adolescent children. According to recent statistics in the United States, Asian female adolescents in the United States aged 14–24 have the highest rates of suicide among their peer group (Office of Minority Health, 2007). Another US national survey indicates that 30 percent of Asian American girls in grades 5–12 reported suffering from depressive symptoms, ranking highest among Caucasian, African American, and Latino girls in the same cohort (The Commonwealth Fund, 1998). Young Asian female adolescents also report more self-harmful behaviors than males (Nguyen *et al.*, 2004). Studies of Asian female adolescents in Australia also report that the struggles around role conflict lead to depression (Woelz-Stirling *et al.*, 2001).

While many Asian adolescents perform well academically, many internalize the pressure from their families to succeed and have difficulties coping with disappointments and setbacks in academic performance as well as in relationships with peers. Asian adolescents are often targets of racial discrimination and bullying at school, and the lack of support from their environment, especially their parents, poses major risk factors for depression and even suicidal ideations (Fong, 2002; Rosenbloom and Way, 2004). When adolescents are depressed, the symptoms of lethargy and inability to concentrate are usually perceived as personal weaknesses by those parents who are not familiar with mental health issues. Instead of trying to understand factors that are troubling their children, many parents exert more pressure because they believe that self-discipline and motivation will resolve the problems. Adolescents who perceive greater cultural conflicts with parents are at higher risk for symptoms of depression. For example, a longitudinal study of South East Asian adolescents reports that perceived intergenerational conflict in early adolescence is associated with depressive symptomatology in late adolescence (Ying and Han, 2007). Among Asian Indian adolescents, low self-esteem, anxiety, and increased family conflict were observed among adolescents whose parents were not acculturated and were unsupportive of their Western values and lifestyle (Farver *et al.*, 2002).

Cultural dissonance between parents and children weakens parent–child attachment, and this in turn increases the likelihood of delinquent behavior and gang membership (Bui, 2009; Choi *et al.*, 2008). There is a lack of research on youth violence/gang activities among children of Asian immigrants. One notable exception is the cluster of studies among Southeast Asian youth. Data indicates that gang involvement is related to poverty, alienation (Hong, 2010), lack of integration into their own ethnic community (Hong, 2010), exposure to stressful life events (Ngo and Le, 2007), and difficulties in schools (Choi, 2007). Intergenerational relationships are also associated with gang involvement (Hong, 2010). Harsh punishment and child maltreatment are predisposing risk factors for delinquency and gang-related activities as are lack of parental supervision and cultural dissonance between parent and child. Southeast Asian youth who experience intergenerational conflicts perceive parental attachment as excessive control. On the other hand, youth who are attached to their parents have less risk of delinquent behavior (Chang and Le, 2005) while low levels of parental support because of process of migration predicts violence among youth (Spencer and Le, 2006). Vietnamese and Asian American youth who have more opportunity to spend time with parents are less likely to engage in delinquency and gang-related activities because they wish to avoid parental disapproval and shaming (Le *et al.*, 2005).

Working with intergenerational conflicts in Asian immigrant families

In working with Asian immigrant children, adolescents, and parents, it is important for practitioners to appreciate the values associated with the traditional parenting style from a historical, cultural, and psychological perspective so that they can effectively engage the family and assess its strengths and vulnerabilities (Chao, 1994; Stewart *et al.*, 2002).

Practitioners need to pay attention to intergenerational dynamics and consider the impact of immigration and acculturation. With some families, it is important to consider the positive aspects of extended families and include them as important resources in the helping process (Sonuga-Barke and Mistry, 2000). For practitioners with Westernized training it is important to understand the ways that families show affection through actions, not words (Rastogi, 2007). Because most Asian parents have an indirect communication style, it is important for the practitioner to be active in finding and validating positive emotions in the family and to convey to the children how the parents care for them. Parents also need to feel understood and supported, and this can be done by validating their hard work, disappointment, and frustration when their children do not understand the sacrifices they have made. Having the practitioner validate family strengths and feelings is often a new experience for the family and one that models a new way of processing the intergenerational conflicts. Parents come to appreciate practitioners for their support and advice and practitioners can act as an important bridge to also help parents understand and accept their children's problems.

Voices of practitioners

In the following section, we will discuss how practitioners work with children, adolescents, and their families in Asian immigrant communities, specifically on the nuances of the major issues discussed in the literature review section, which include:

- intergenerational issues in Asian immigrant families;
- the importance of developing a holistic view of the dynamics underlying these intergenerational issues;
- practice challenges in working with Asian immigrant families;
- use of relational approaches to enhance engagement and intervention.

The practitioners whom we talked with work in a variety of settings including child welfare protective agencies, social service organizations, and mental health clinics. Some families that the practitioners work with are self-referred or referred by schools and hospitals; others are mandated for treatment by the New York City Administration for Children Services (ACS), and school officials in New York City. The client population is primarily of low socioeconomic background and represents diverse Asian ethnic groups including Chinese, Korean, Filipino, South Asian, and Vietnamese. The presenting problems vary depending on the referral sources. Those referred by ACS generally involve reports of children with unexplained bruises and injuries, or reports by children themselves who claim that their parents are using excessive physical discipline with them. Families referred by the school generally involve serious academic and behavioral problems of the child or adolescent as well as signs of depression and suicide. The self-referred cases present similar behavioral and mental health problems, generally parents in these cases are at a juncture where they feel they have not been successful in resolving the issues and want professional intervention. We will discuss how the varied nature and circumstances of the presenting problem create different challenges in engagement and intervention.

The scope of intergenerational issues

The practitioners agree that problems among Asian immigrant families have become far more complex in recent years. In the past, communication problems and conflicts over career and marriage choices used to be the major issues of contention between parents and adolescents or young adults. However, there has been a significant increase in the range of presenting problems. School phobia, absenteeism, poor time management, and delinquent behavior at school and at home are major complaints reported by frustrated parents about their school-aged children. In the case of families with adolescents, parents are distraught over their children's apathetic behavior, such as leaving home, withdrawing from family activities, and persuing activities on the Internet, and their lack of control and influence over them. The parents also express shock and helplessness that their children threaten to report them to child protection services as a leverage when they try to discipline them.

Parents who cannot keep up their communication with the school system because of language barriers and hectic work schedules are not able to detect any mental health and substance abuse issues until their children exhibit serious symptoms such as eating disorders, panic attacks, self injurious behavior, and suicide attempts. Indeed, the practitioners agree that an increasing number of

Asian children and adolescents no longer fit the "model minority" stereotype of the compliant, well-disciplined, and academically successful student.

A multi-dimensional and empathic view of intergenerational issues

- Different sociocultural realities between parents and children: values, stressors, and coping mechanisms
- Dissonance in the use of traditional Asian parenting practice with children in Western societies: corporal punishment; communication style; concept of emotional support.

According to practitioners, it is important to understand the interplay of psychodynamic, cultural, and environmental issues impacting the interactions between the parents and the children and the circular dynamics within each Asian immigrant family system. Depending on client populations, stressors related to the clients' low socioeconomic background such as financial difficulties, poor working conditions, and lack of knowledge on child development issues, are a pervasive factor that adversely magnify the interactive dynamics.

From the practitioners' perspective, intergenerational conflicts in immigrant families are often rooted in the daily interactions between parents and children. As indicated in the literature review section, Asian immigrant parents often experience a loss of control and mastery in their lives because of underemployment and acculturation difficulties. Practitioners with a psychodynamic orientation observe that the parents' feelings of loss and helplessness are often played out in their focus on their children's compliance with daily routines and chores because of their need to gain a sense of gratification from ensuring order and cooperation in the family. Such a focus is also reinforced by the traditional Asian cultural emphasis on the parents' role in instilling a sense of discipline and responsibility among their children. The parents' identity and pride are, therefore, closely linked to their ability to get their children to do chores and follow directions. It is difficult for children and adolescents living in a world of technology, social media, and a culture that emphasizes instant gratification and innovation to appreciate the values of their parents. Many adolescents do acknowledge to their practitioners that they know that their parents care about them and that they do want their parents' approval. However, they experience their parents' behaviors as "nagging" and "overly critical." As a result, they ignore their parents or become belligerent and respond with typical Westernized adolescent responses such as "I don't care," "shut up," or "leave me alone," which in the eyes of their parents are highly disrespectful. These frequent squabbles certainly undermine the communication and quality of the relationship between parents and children. It is common for parents and children to be at odds with each other. Among low-income Asian immigrant families, there is also a lack of social and recreational opportunities for them to bond and repair relationships. Acculturation difficulties exacerbate daily skirmishes and lead to the escalation of acrimonious interactions. When practitioners ask parents to reflect on their reactions toward their children, the parents often state:

I am stressed and I have no time, and she never listens to me; so I yell. What else can I do?

When I can't get him to do what he's supposed to do, I have no choice but to hit him to teach him a lesson.

An adolescent's account of an argument she had with her parent reflected similar dynamics:

My father flipped out at dinner tonight. I dropped rice on the table and he said "look what you did." I intentionally made him angrier by putting more rice on the table. He slammed the table and started yelling at me, "I paid money for that rice." So I put the rice back on the plate and didn't eat it. When I came downstairs again, my father was still angry. He sat me down and asked why I was "so bad" because I didn't always "do what he tells me."

Underlying the frustration of these remarks and exchanges are the parents' association with their own childhood experiences in their home country where there were taught to obey their parents and do what they were told. These immigrant parents also belong to a generation that condoned the use of corporal punishment when children were oppositional, dishonest, and involved in any immoral behavior. These parents believe that they should have absolute authority over their children to make sure that they attain high moral standards and proper behavior. The parents grew up in an era where there was lack of knowledge of child development, and little attention was paid to issues underlying children's aberrant behavior, such as sense of insecurity, learned aggression in a hostile environment, and jealousy among siblings. The traditional approach emphasized the inculcation of "right" and "wrong" behavior through the parents' delineation of expectations for their children and the use of corporal punishment as a deterrent of unacceptable behavior. The Asian practitioners, in reflecting on their own childhood experiences, indicate that they are less inclined than the current generation to interpret the traditional parental practice as harsh or unreasonable because the sociocultural context of their generation is very different. Their witnessing and knowledge of their parents' hardships in a politically unstable and impoverished environment in their home countries and their parents' sacrifices after immigration often motivated them to be compliant and disciplined in the family. Growing up in an era when racial discrimination was much more prevalent in the host countries, they were more aware of their ethnic heritage and values as a minority group. There were also less materialistic lures and social media distractions to compete for their time, and they were able to fulfill their obligations at home, which in turn diminished their parents' concerns in monitoring their behavior.

The following case vignette illustrates the interplay of cultural conflicts, environmental stressors and influences, socioeconomic background as well as personality clashes that culminated in estranged relationships in Asian immigrant families and unresolved behavioral issues of the children as they struggled with developmental issues and stressors at school and at home.

Case vignette: Mr. and Mrs. Li

Mr. and Mrs. Li, immigrants from China, had two sons, Tom, aged 12, and John, aged eight. Both sons were born in the United States, but sent to their paternal aunt to be taken care of in China until they reached school age. Tom was diagnosed with Attention Deficit and Hyperactive Disorder and had been prescribed medication and placed in Special Ed class. At home, Tom was often defiant, negligent in his self-care, and fighting with his brother, who was compared favorably to Tom. It seemed that Tom had a lot of anger toward his mother who continued to work and left him with neighbors until his younger brother returned to the US.

Mr. and Mrs. Li were referred by the Administration for Children Services to seek family counseling because Tom had told school officials that his parents hit him. Apparently Mrs. Li hit Tom when he was acting out at home and would not listen to her when she intervened. When his dad heard about the incident, he demanded an explanation of his behavior from Tom. Tom ignored him and continued to play games on his computer. Mr. Li became very angry and scratched Tom's hands when he physically forced him to move away from the computer. After the initial investigation, ACS decided to close the case. But Tom continued to claim that his mother was physically abusive toward him.

When the family arrived for their first session, they held different perceptions as to the causes of the problem.

Mrs. Li had learned something about ADHD from other Chinese parents but felt that the medication should have been sufficient for Tom to behave himself. She blamed her husband's aunt for spoiling Tom and not teaching him good values and behavior when he was in China. She was still very angry with Tom and wanted to vent her frustration in regard to his defiant behavior toward her. Every so often, she would ask the practitioner, "Do you have any suggestions for me when Tom does not listen to me? I have tried everything." Underlying Mrs. Li's frustration was also a sense of insecurity about her ability as a mother in the US. Mrs. Li came from a village in China, had little education, and did not speak English.

Mr. Li was also angry but focused on the fact that Tom did not seem to show remorse that he had done something "wrong," especially the audacious act to report the case to ACS. He kept saying to Tom that he needed to "*jiang dao li*," a Chinese idiom that translated to the importance of reflecting on his behavior based on fairness and the principles of right and wrong.

Tom was quiet because apparently he was a little afraid of his father, who had been in the US for a longer time and spoke some English.

However, when he spoke with the practitioner privately, he insisted that his parents were picking on him. Apparently, he also felt insecure of himself because of his diagnosis and being in a Special Ed class. He seemed to be having some issues with making friends at school, and felt he was ridiculed because of his Chinese accent and lack of fashionable attire. However, he did not think his parents would understand these issues. His words were, "They only care about my grades and how I behave at home."

In a subsequent family session attended by Mrs. Li and her sons, the practitioner engaged them in playing some games to observe and facilitate their interaction.

The first game was an electronic game that involved each family member taking turns to score. Since Tom was familiar with this game, he was eager to play the game and verbalized his desire to beat his brother and his mother. Mrs. Li was silent after Tom scored high points. She looked visibly upset when Tom assumed an authoritative role and tried to show her what to do, and said to her several times, "You can't do this!"

The second game involved each member drawing and telling a story to be finished by another person. At one point, Tom drew two snakes, and claimed that one was him and the other was his mother, and his snake wanted to attack and devour his mother's snake. Mrs. Li became emotional, and said, "Why did you want to eat me? I gave birth to you!" Tom looked surprised by his mother's reaction. He was silent for a while, and then said matter-of-factly, "Why can't you just draw a lion to help your snake?"

The case vignette highlights the collectivistic and hierarchical values implicit in the Asian parenting practice, i.e., the importance of teaching children to be deferential to the parents and fulfill their obligations and responsibilities. While Mr. and Mrs. Li focused on Tom's challenging behavior and did not seem to understand his underlying emotional needs, they also perceived the behavior as an indication of their own failed parenting practice. The use of physical punishment apparently was the only resort they knew to discipline their defiant son. The dynamics in the game playing was revealing in terms of the differences in cultural values between the two generations. Tom's competitiveness and creativity in winning the games with little consideration that his "opponent" was his mother was typical individualistic behavior among Western children and adolescents, and deemed acceptable in school and other social settings. However, Mrs. Li, who was raised under the Confucian practice of filial piety, perceived his aggressive behavior as inappropriate and disrespectful.

The following case vignette illustrates another dimension of the intergenerational issue that is compounded by cultural norms of communication, as well as the lack of knowledge and acceptance in regard to mental illness in the Asian immigrant community.

Case vignette: Mr. and Mrs. Phan

Mr. and Mrs. Phan, immigrants from Vietnam, were referred for family counseling to support the recovery of their 15-year-old daughter, Lily, who suffered from selective mutism, school phobia, and depressive symptoms. Lily had been hospitalized twice in the past year for aggressive behavior at home toward her parents and siblings and making suicide threats and gestures.

Mr. and Mrs. Phan had little education when they grew up in a rural area in Vietnam. Both held menial jobs that required them to work long hours. They currently lived with Mr. Phan's mother who was the primary caretaker for Lily and her two other siblings when they were young. They had a difficult time accepting that Lily required psychiatric treatment, and could not identify any stressors that might have triggered the mutism and the aggressive behavior. Lily's grandmother suggested that Lily might have been "scared" by some evil spirits, which was a common belief in regard to abrupt changes in children's behavior in her village. Mr. and Mrs. Phan did acknowledge that Lily always needed more supervision to finish her daily chores and homework, and would throw tantrums when she became frustrated. But they attributed her behavior to the lack of parental supervision. After Lily's first hospitalization, Mrs. Phan quit her job and stayed home while Lily received home instruction from the Department of Education. But Mrs. Phan was inconsistent in helping Lily adhere to her treatment regimen.

In the first family session shortly after Lily's second hospitalization, Mr. and Mrs. Phan came with Lily and her grandmother. They appeared to be upset about being questioned by the social worker, and stated repeatedly that Lily needed to pull herself together, just like her siblings. At that point, Lily spoke in broken Vietnamese that her parents didn't understand her. Mr. Phan said defensively that Lily should know that her parents spent all their time working and did not have a chance to learn English. He suggested that she should take some Vietnamese classes in the community or ask her siblings who spoke fluent Vietnamese to translate for her. Lily got visibly upset and shot back with "You don't care about me. You only care about my sister and brother." Mr. and Mrs. Phan got angry as well, and said, "You don't think we care about you? We provide for you and let you do everything you want to do." A long silence ensued. Grandma then stood up and acted like she was looking at the pictures on the wall while she wiped her eyes. Mr. Phan also walked away and stood by the window. Mrs. Phan lowered her head. Clearly everyone in the family was affected but no words were exchanged and no gesture was made to reach out to each other.

The family session of this case vignette captures some poignant emotions that were not articulated by any of the family members. While it is easy to empathize with Lily, who seemed to have failed to win her parents' approval and acceptance due to family dynamics and personality issues, one can also detect the parents' guilt and worries underlying their authoritarian stance and stoic presentation. Their non-acceptance of Lily's mental health issues can be partly a defense against shame and cultural stigma, and the idea that they failed to ensure the well-being of their daughter. The exchanges between Mr. and Mrs. Phan and Lily also highlighted the cultural and generational differences in communication of thoughts and feelings. Mr. and Mrs. Phan stayed with concrete issues and responses, even though Lily was trying to express her feelings of being rejected by her parents and they were clearly affected by her emotional outbursts. While personality traits, childhood experiences, and perhaps the low socioeconomic background of Mr. and Mrs. Phan had shaped their communication style, their reticence about their inner thoughts and feelings is not uncommon among Asian immigrant parents. One might also question if Mr. and Mrs. Phan provided sufficient emotional support to Lily. In the Asian culture, emotional support for family members is communicated implicitly through care-taking behavior provided in the context of patience and intuitive sensing of the family member's needs. It was likely that the combination of Mr. and Mrs. Phan's poor parenting role model in their own upbringing, Lily's sensitivity and aggressive responses to her parent's lack of attunement to her needs, and the differences in cultural communication style had fostered a vicious cycle of deterioration in their relationship.

The third case vignette, which involves a young Asian woman struggling to define a sense of autonomy for herself, illuminates the complexities of this developmental task when she is caught between a collectivistic-oriented Asian immigrant family and the individualistic mores of Western society.

Case vignette: Kim

Kim was a 19-year-old who emigrated from Korea with her older brother to reunite with their parents at age nine. Kim had a history of panic attacks and had recently been hospitalized for the severity of her symptoms. Kim's recent episodes of panic attacks seemed to be precipitated by her parents' strong opposition to her dating a young man of Latino descent and her ambivalence in regard to going to college. Kim had attempted to register for college classes previously, but each time she experienced physiological symptoms as well as fears of going outside of her home.

Kim did not complete high school but was able to obtain her high school equivalency diploma to qualify for college admission. She had gotten herself a job as a store cashier. Her parents, however, had been pressuring her to go back to school. They alternated between offering to pay for all her personal expenses and threatening to throw her out of the house. Kim felt resentful that her parents gave her older brother much more latitude in going to college at his pace and dating women of his choice. Her parents, who were devout Christians, also seemed to talk about her circumstances more freely with their fellow Korean parishioners, and Kim felt patronized and humiliated when she was often asked about her future plans and offered well wishes by these parishioners.

In her sessions with her social worker, Kim acknowledged that she was conflicted about going to college. On one level, she knew her parents were right that she should complete college: "I can't be a cashier for the rest of my life." On the other hand, she did not want to be perceived as following the footpaths defined by her parents, especially after she had to comply with her parents' wishes to stop seeing her boyfriend. In reflecting over her relationship with her parents, Kim felt that she was never given a voice on major decisions about her life, including when her parents left her and her brother in the care of their grandmother for two years while they tried to settle down in the United States. Kim still recalled feeling anxious and abandoned when her parents "disappeared" with no explanation or good-bye. On occasions when she tried to tell them about this traumatic experience, her parents would become defensive and said, "Why do you always have to bring this up? Why can't you just forget about this? We had to plead with your grandmother to accept this imposition. We couldn't just say good-bye and let your grandmother deal with the two of you crying."

Kim's emotional struggles seemed to stem from her inability to reconcile value differences rooted in Asian and Western cultures that she had internalized as a bicultural adolescent. While her Asian self did not wish to move out of her parents' house or confront her parents in regard to her anger, her Western self felt that she had to be able to make some major decisions for herself, such as dating and career options, as a step to gain a sense of independence. However, Kim tended to agree with her parents that attaining a college education was important for her future and dating the Latino young man could be a distraction. It was likely that she had also internalized some of her parents' values. So the conflicts became an issue of how she could agree and disagree with her parents without losing her voice and feeling she was being submissive. From her parents' perspective, they also had the dilemma of balancing support with guidance for Kim. Her panic attacks and hospitalization were an indication that they might have placed too much pressure on her, but as parents, they also felt they needed to supervise her around her decision-making. As indicated by the practitioner who shared this case vignette, both Kim and her parents essentially were looking for better ways to communicate their distress and support each other during this challenging period in Kim's life.

In all of the preceding vignettes, the Asian traditional concept of parental support, which revolves around attunement to the children's concrete needs and dispensation of advice, seemed to have become a major cultural divide between the parents and their children. While the parents felt frustrated that their children did not appreciate and benefit from the sacrifices they made in providing a secure future for the family, which included leaving their children in the care of extended family members, the children tended to interpret their parents' focus and action as excessively practical and lacking sensitivity to their emotional needs. This is an intergenerational issue that needs to be understood in the context of the socio-economic times and needs of each generation. The parents, who generally experienced poverty and loss of family ties during an era of war and/or political and economic instability in Asian countries, did not have the luxury to consider their emotional needs other than the comfort of having their daily and basic needs met. One can speculate that the parent generation tends to repress their emotional needs as a survival strategy. Their children, on the other hand, were raised in a stable home environment in an affluent Western society, where they have been encouraged to be in touch with their emotional needs and express their thoughts and feelings.

Challenges in working with Asian immigrant families

- Containment of the family's reactive emotions and management of counter-transferential feelings
- Building empathic connections with the family's underlying feelings and emotional needs
- Brokering of cultural values between generations: perceptions of problems and solutions
- Building trust and motivation to seek changes.

The complexities of the case vignettes that are presented in the previous section illuminate the challenges in engaging the families and developing strategies in interventions. Underlying each presenting problem are layers of biological, psychological, social, and cultural issues that shape the different perceptions and responses of the family members. Parents who are mandated to seek counseling by child welfare administration tend to be angry and defensive about the alleged complaints of child abuse, and focused on their children's aberrant behavior as the cause of the problem. They can be resentful that their parental rights were violated by outsiders who "intruded on the privacy of their family issues." They are less willing to divulge relevant information and discuss family dynamics and underlying issues, and perceive the counseling sessions as an imposition on their hectic work schedule and another financial burden. These parents naturally harbor a lot of fear that their children would be taken away from them. Among those who are undocumented immigrants, they also fear that they will be reported for deportation. The primary concern of these parents is to comply with the counseling mandate and secure a satisfactory dissolution of the complaint. It is not uncommon for these parents to feel hostility and distrust toward practitioners who are viewed by them as "outsiders," or "one of us who do not have our best interests in mind."

Parents who are referred by school officials or self-referred tend to focus on the presenting problems, such as absenteeism, delinquent behavior, and substance abuse, and expect the practitioners to address the behavioral problem directly with their children with measurable outcomes. They view the practitioners as experts who can take over their responsibility of teaching their children to become more disciplined and motivated to make positive changes. The practitioners acknowledge that they generally feel a great deal of pressure from the parents' remarks such as, "We have tried everything. Tell us how you can help us," "Nothing's changed since we last saw you. He [child] is still the same," or "Have you ever had success with kids like ours?"

The initial responses of the children and adolescents who attend individual and family sessions tend to be a mix of fear, resentment, defiance, and resignation. There are varying degrees of resentment in reaction to being told to seek counseling, and their anticipation that the family sessions would be just another opportunity for their parents to berate them on their problems. Their silence, curt answers, emotional outbursts, avoidance of eye contact, and strained body language certainly add more tension to the dynamics in the sessions.

The practitioners agree that immersing in Asian family dynamics invariably brought back memories of their own relationship dynamics with their parents and siblings. Listening to some parents who expressed their anger toward their children in familiar cultural idioms, such as comparing them with their siblings, or threatening to disown them, can trigger strong negative countertransference. In order to maintain an empathic and objective stance, the practitioners indicate that listening for the subtle feelings of anxiety and shame underlying the parents' harsh words is helpful in getting in touch with the parents' vulnerabilities and emotional needs. However, it is also difficult for practitioners not to feel the burden of responsibility to effect some changes in the children's behavioral problem when parents want to entrust their hopes to the practitioners. Practitioners caution against the risk of alienating the children when they focused on behavioral markers for fear of disappointing or antagonizing the parents. Thus the biggest challenge is to engage *both* parents and children in the change process as a family. To do that, it is important to gain a sense of the common grounds between the emotional needs of both the parents and the children. In the three case vignettes that were presented, the parents were essentially looking for validation that they fulfilled their obligations as parents and a sense of gratification that their children were on a promising academic and career path in a country in which they had made tremendous sacrifices to build a better life for their family. The children were looking for validation of their parents' unconditional love and acceptance of their identity and emotional development in a Western society. Somehow these needs were overshadowed by the interplay of personality issues, immigrant-specific stressors, and dissonance between Asian and Western parenting practice. Practitioners agree that finding ways to address these needs can provide a break in the impasse between the parents and the children and pave the way for more constructive conversation in the family session. In the following section, we will discuss the practitioners' use of relational approaches in engaging the family and enhancing their communication of thoughts and feelings in a culturally relevant context.

Use of relational approaches

- Showing acceptance of parenting practice and respect for parents' values
- Facilitating intergenerational communication and bonding in a culturally relevant context
- Providing education on parenting practice that is congruent with the family's norms and values
- Immersing fully in family dynamics: sharing the anger, pain, and anxiety of each family member in the helping process.

From a relational model perspective, clients are more motivated to reflect on issues and make changes in their lives when they feel unconditional regard and acceptance by others. The practitioners find that Asian immigrant parents generally are aware of issues of cultural dissonance in their parenting practice, and that they are more inclined to examine their role in the estranged family dynamics and accept suggestions to modify their ways of disciplining and relating to their children if they do not feel criticized. Validation of their sacrifices and resilience as immigrants as well as their challenges as parents straddling two cultures are effective empathic approaches that provided a non-judgmental and strength-based context to begin a dialog on parenting practice. Some practitioners disclose discreetly about their knowledge and family experience of intergenerational issues when they sense that parents harbored some feelings of shame and guilt. We will illustrate these approaches using the previous case vignettes.

In the case of Lily who was hospitalized for selective mutism and depression, her parents and grandmother tried to hide their tears and presented a very stoic and at times, defensive stance. Instead of acknowledging or probing their affective state, the practitioner made a comment to normalize the parenting challenges of immigrant parents. Lily's parents nodded appreciatively. Mr. Phan then remarked that the hospital social worker, who spoke through an interpreter, had asked him for his input to help his daughter. He seemed to be insulted and shamed by his interpretation of the remark, *"Why did she ask me? I'm not the expert. I don't even speak English. Or did she think I did not do enough? My daughter is Americanized. She doesn't want to listen to me. What can I do?"* While the social worker's good intentions to involve the parents might have been lost in translation, the parents' sensitivity to criticism was evident.

In the case involving Kim who suffered from panic attacks, the social worker met privately with the parents, listened to their immigration stories and empathized with the hardships they endured. As they talked about the parents' experience as children and compared that to Kim's generation, the father said, *"We know this is not Korea. Children in America want a lot of freedom."* The social worker, however, did not pressure the parents in regard to modifying their parenting practice with Kim. Instead, she expressed appreciation for their insights. Later on, when the social worker suggested a family session with Kim, the father seemed reluctant and cancelled the session a couple of times. While the social worker sensed some resistance, she did not raise it with the parents. Shortly after that, the father told Kim that she could see her Latino boyfriend under the condition that they would meet in the house when he and her mother were around. This idea was the parents' gesture of concession without relinquishing their authority. The social worker realized that it was important for the parents to maintain a sense of pride and control in a hierarchical family, which they feared would be undermined by confrontation and accusations by Kim at the family session. By not pursuing the issue of a family session, the social worker communicated her sense of respect for the parents' wishes and created a safe space for them to initiate changes at a pace they were comfortable with, which was a major step toward mitigating the conflicts experienced by Kim.

In engaging Tom and his mother presented in the first case vignette, the social worker assumed the role of a cultural broker by contextualizing the mother's anger and Tom's aggressive behavior toward his mother. Instead of pointing out the cyclical repercussions of their acrimonious exchanges toward each other, the social worker validated the mother's feelings of being disrespected and Tom's need for attention and approval, and framed the situation as a family overwhelmed by transitions and not able to hear each other's needs. Sensing that the mother felt some shame about having sent her children back to China, the social worker did not delve into how attachment issues could have affected Tom's behavior in the initial session. Instead she focused on making interpretations of their positive feelings toward each other when they were playing games, i.e., Tom's desire to help his mother to win the game, and the mother's wish to be a partner of Tom's team and not his opponent. This paved the way for more bonding between mother and son in future sessions.

The practitioners agree that they often have to play an active role in facilitating the exchange of positive emotions between parents and their children in Asian immigrant families. They observe that it is often easier for parents to verbally express approval and encouragement than affection, which is a common communication norm in the Asian culture. While there are words that express emotions in the Asian languages, they are mostly found in literary works and not used in informal conversations. However, as one practitioner put it, "Such practice goes beyond the language barrier between generations." Many immigrant parents apparently still adhere to the traditional belief that when their children made some trespasses, it would be inappropriate to show verbal or physical affection until they are able to make amends or a commitment to change their behavior. While some children are able to accept that their parents are "strict" and "traditional," those who do not have secure ties with their parents and are looking for attention and validation can perceive such a response as punitive and rejecting. Some practitioners view this as another issue of cultural dissonance whereby the parents follow the principles of discipline and fairness and the children act out of their emotional needs. In the following case vignette, the practitioner was able to facilitate communication of positive emotions between the parent and her child while showing acceptance of the parent's belief system.

Case vignette: Mrs. Santos

Mrs. Santos was referred by school officials to seek family counseling with Maria, her six-year-old daughter who had been hitting other children at school. Mrs. Santos and her husband were immigrants from the Philippines. Mr. Santos had been working long hours and on weekends since Mrs. Santos gave birth to a son two years ago and had to stay home to take care of their children. Mr. Santos also supported his parents who lived in the Philippines by sending money back on a regular basis.

In the first session, Mrs. Santos told the family counselor that she was very embarrassed and distraught by being called into school about Maria's behavior. A couple of times she was humiliated when she had to apologize to the other parents. She had tried to reprimand Maria who always acted compliant in front of her, but somehow was not able to stop her aggressive behavior at school. Mrs. Santos became increasingly angry in the session as she characterized Maria's behavior as having no regard for others and respect for authority. The family counselor noticed that Maria looked frightened and glanced at her mother several times, but Mrs. Santos would not make any eye contact with her.

In the second session, the family counselor asked mother and daughter to play a game, which required each one of them to take turns to look for a cotton ball that the other person had hidden inside her clothes. Maria at first would circle and walk around mom who looked very serious. At the family counselor's encouragement, Maria moved closer and used her fingertips to poke lightly at her mother's shirt. As the family counselor cheered her on, Maria finally grabbed her mother's shirt and found the cotton ball. Maria smiled broadly and rested her head contentedly on her mother's lap. When it was Mrs. Santos's turn, Maria became giggly with her mother's touch and Mrs. Santos started to smile and became playful with Maria. The game apparently renewed the bonds between mother and daughter. Mrs. Santos acknowledged that she had not seen Maria looking so happy for a long time. Maria nodded her head emphatically when the family counselor asked if she enjoyed playing with her mother. However, she added, "But mommy has no time for me. She is busy all the time." The family counselor suggested a trial period of Maria and her mother spending some quality time together on the condition that Maria would work on not hitting other children at school.

By providing an opportunity for Mrs. Santos to witness her daughter's yearning for closeness and affection, the family counselor was able to help Mrs. Santos understand her daughter's emotional needs underlying her behavioral problems without challenging her parenting practice. When Mrs. Santos's maternal instincts overcame her anger and she was able to respond spontaneously with affection toward Maria, she communicated her availability for Maria to learn new skills in problem solving and regulation of emotions from her.

After the practitioners engage the families and enhance their motivation to make some changes, they may provide education about parenting practice that addresses the underlying issues of the children's behavioral and mental health problems. In doing so, they emphasize the importance of reframing issues that resonate with the family's values and strengths, as well as eliciting input from the parents. For example, the practitioner might acknowledge the use of corporal punishment as a culturally time-honored tradition in disciplining children, but would point out that it has its "side effects," such as, children might learn to use physical force with other children, or parents might have to step up on the punishment when the children became less fearful of it. Or when parents minimize the signs of suicide of their children that school officials brought to their attention, some practitioners would characterize a child harboring suicide ideation as analogous to having a seed planted in his head, which would flourish given the proper exposure to risk factors such as academic failure, being the target of bullying at school, and parental disapproval. The practitioners would ask the parents for input in identifying any recent behavioral issues of their child and help them make the connection to stressors that the child might be struggling with. In cases where parents reassured their child that he could share any concerns with them, but might add a typical cultural and immigrant perspective that talking about dying would be alarming to other people and get the family in trouble, the practitioner would normalize the parents' fear of being stigmatized and engulfed in the bureaucratic protocol of the school and child welfare system. She would point out how children who are loyal to their family may want to protect their parents and not want to burden them with their stress. This approach resonates with the cultural emphasis of filial piety, and tends to be effective in motivating the parents to reflect on how they can provide more open and supportive responses.

Overall, the practitioners indicate that it is important to infuse a sense of hope and empowerment in providing parenting education. Parents need to be reassured that their role as parents will not be undermined by Western values and norms, and that they still have "the power" to make their children feel better. When practitioners offer a Western perspective of child development issues, they generally preface by stating that the objective of their discussion is to elicit input from the parents to make the best of Asian and Western parenting approaches so that their children will benefit from the wisdom of their ethnic heritage and the resources of their Western society. This approach is evident in the previous case vignettes whereby parents were encouraged to communicate more support to address their children's underlying issues but in a way that was relevant to their personal experience, socioeconomic background, values, and family history.

The practitioners also note that adherence to the relational model helps them stretch their professional boundaries to be more compatible with the collectivistic orientation of the Asian culture. In their experience, Asian immigrant families generally prefer the practitioner be the individual who works with different members of the family separately once a trusting relationship has been established. From these families' perspective, trust entails the practitioner's understanding and acceptance of immigrant-specific stressors and Asian parenting values. The practitioner will then be considered an "insider" of the family who is privy to secrets, shameful behavior, and feelings between family members. The practitioner, therefore, has the burden of maintaining an objective stance and distilling information and emotions that need to be shared with the family. At the same time, the practitioner also has to be genuine in showing empathy and engaging specific family members in the change process.

In the following case vignettes, we will examine how practitioners assume multiple roles with family members by immersing themselves strategically in family dynamics to initiate changes.

Case vignette: Annie

Annie, a 12-year-old girl of an immigrant family from China, was referred for counseling at the local children and family service center for her history of defiant behavior and her recent episode of hitting an assistant principal at school. Annie lived with her parents, Mr. and Mrs. Wong, her six-year-old brother, and her grandparents. Mrs. Wong worked part time as a home health aide, often leaving Annie and her brother under the supervision and care of her grandparents. Mr. Wong worked as a restaurant worker out-of-state and only came home once a week.

Joan, the family counselor, initially reached out to Mrs. Wong, and they had a long conversation on the phone. Mrs. Wong did not sound hopeful that Annie's behavior would change, but wished to comply with the school's request so that Annie would not be suspended. She claimed that Annie was angry and difficult at home as well, particularly toward her and her brother. She had tried to use corporal punishment to discipline Annie, but stopped when Annie started to fight back. Mrs. Wong was reticent about her husband and her in-laws' role in the family, and claimed that her erratic job schedule did not allow her to meet with Joan in the near future. She did, however, agree to make arrangements for Annie to seek counseling on an individual basis.

In working with Annie, Joan initially spent time listening to her complaints about school and family life. It appeared that Annie felt very alone, especially at home, and deep down wanted her mother's attention. Joan decided to make a home visit to observe and engage the family. When Joan arrived on a day that Mr. Wong was off from work, she noticed that Mrs. Wong tried to talk to Mr. Wong about their children's recent behavioral problems, but Mr. Wong barely responded. At one point, the grandmother interrupted with some harsh criticisms of Mrs. Wong, claiming that she should have supervised the children more closely. Joan engaged the grandmother in conversations about her life and how she managed to care for her own husband as well as the grandchildren. Then she validated Mrs. Wong's frustration in supervising her children and invited Mrs. Wong to meet with her privately to discuss parenting practice. Mrs. Wong finally took up her offer and seemed to like the opportunity to get some attention and support. As Mrs. Wong confided details about her husband's passivity and her mother-in-law's hostility toward her, Joan gained a clearer picture of the generational dynamics of attention-seeking and displacement of frustration among the female members in the family. When Joan shared her observation with Mrs. Wong, she looked surprised that Annie might be looking for attention from her, "We are always fighting. And she speaks more English now. What does she want from me?" Mrs. Wong, however, did agree to talk with Annie if Joan would be present.

When Joan broached the issue with Annie, she was ambivalent, but finally agreed when Joan promised to help her verbalize her feelings and mediate if the discussion became too tense. They "rehearsed" in Chinese what Annie wanted to say to her mother. Annie settled with a culturally endearing phrase between parents and child that loosely translated to "I want my mom to dote on me (*shek sai ngoh*)."

At the beginning of the session, Joan spoke about her impressions of the strengths of both Annie and Mrs. Wong, and their similar traits of being observant, sensitive, vocal, and strong-willed. Joan asked Mrs. Wong to share some fond memories of Annie when she was a young child. This strength-based approach helped to set a positive tone for bonding between mother and daughter. When Annie was asked to talk, she became emotional in mid-sentence and started to cry. Mrs. Wong seemed touched as Annie revealed her vulnerability, and also became teary-eyed. Then she took out a tissue and wiped Annie's tears. At the end, Mrs. Wong thanked Joan and said, "I understand what I have to do."

After this session, Joan made a couple more visits to the family while continuing to meet with Annie individually. Mr. Wong appeared to be more interactive as he noticed that Mrs. Wong and Annie were on better terms. Joan continued to make small conversations with the grandmother despite her temperamental moods and harsh remarks. Joan's interactions with the grandmother appeared to be helpful to Mrs. Wong who remarked at one point that "I guess grandma just needs an outlet for her frustrations."

From an Asian cultural perspective, Joan was successful in facilitating positive changes in family dynamics via her empathic interactions with and role modeling for different family members. She did not push for direct expression of positive or negative feelings between family members, but facilitated their subtle shifts of attention and perceptions toward each other in a culturally relevant context.

Case vignette: Ahmed

Ahmed, a 15-year-old adolescent from a Pakistani immigrant family, was referred to a mental health clinic for counseling due to a brief psychotic episode. During his hospitalization, he revealed that he had been troubled by some violent sexual fantasies about a female student in his class.

Ahmed grew up in a very strict family. Ahmed's father had a college degree in accounting from Pakistan, but felt he was not able to advance his career due to his heavy accent. Ahmed's mother had not worked for a couple of years and seemed to suffer from depression symptoms. Ahmed had an older brother who was rebellious and had left home since dropping out of school. Subsequently, both parents had high expectations for Ahmed to adhere to a restrictive social role commonly prescribed in their Punjabi and Muslim community, and to be successful in his academic pursuits.

When Ahmed first met with Nikita, the mental health counselor, he was reluctant to talk. His parents, Mr. and Mrs. Talib, requested to meet with Nikita separately to discuss their expectations and their perception of Ahmed's problems. They believed that Ahmed was under the bad influence of his older brother who had refused to practice the Muslim faith. Nikita asked the parents to help her understand the major tenets of the Islamic religion. Mr. and Mrs. Talib, in turn, asked Nikita to clarify the purpose and parameters of counseling. As they seemed to establish a rapport with Nikita, Mrs. Talib asked if she could also meet with Nikita periodically to get an update of Ahmed's progress. Nikita reassured both parents that she would welcome their input.

As Ahmed became comfortable with Nikita, he started asking her a lot of personal questions about her marital status, history of dating, and her opinion of pre-marital sex. Nikita decided that it was important for her to self disclose discreetly in order to normalize his interest in sex and the ideological struggles for young Asians growing up in a Western society, and at the same time, model for him in managing these conflicts without feeling guilty and anxious. Eventually the discussion progressed to how Ahmed could handle the pressure from his parents. Ahmed indicated that he would like to do well in school so his parents would be proud of him. He would also like to continue to follow the Islamic faith, which was part of the identity he grew up with. However, he felt overwhelmed by the expectation of his parents and the teachings of Islam that he could not harbor any sexual thoughts. Nikita suggested that he read up on Islamic literature to see if there was a difference between having sexual desires and acting them out. The following week Ahmed returned and said with a smile, "It seems like Allah will not punish us for thoughts that we do not act on." Nikita added, "And neither will your parents. I think they just wanted to make sure you can exercise self restraint." By reframing the intentions of Ahmed's parents and supporting Ahmed's ties with his family and his Islamic faith, Nikita was able to co-construct with Ahmed a non-threatening perspective in "toning down" some of the harsh voices he had internalized. At the same time, Mrs. Talib also began to see Nikita regularly, and the focus of her discussion gradually shifted from telling Nikita what she thought Ahmed would be talking about in his session and giving advice to Nikita, to sharing her own marital distress and worries. It appeared that it was important for Mrs. Talib to project her hopes and sense of control onto Ahmed's behavior. After listening to Mrs. Talib's fear that her husband might be having an affair, Nikita asked Mrs. Talib if she would like to invite her husband to join her in the session. Mrs. Talib indicated that she actually would like Nikita to speak with her husband separately and ask if there was another woman in his life. Mrs. Talib's suggestion put Nikita in a delicate position that would jeopardize the balance of her objective yet empathic "immersion" in the family dynamics. But she knew that Mrs. Talib would not fully appreciate her using the rationale of professionalism and client confidentiality in declining the suggestion. So Nikita asked Mrs. Talib if she expected her husband to inquire about what she and Ahmed had been discussing in their sessions. Mrs. Talib thought he might leave it to Nikita's discretion because the family regarded her as a "fair" and "honorable" person who could be the "keeper of family secrets". Nikita nodded and said she felt honored by the family's trust in her. Then she said, "What it means is that I can't tell anyone anything. But what I can do is to ask everyone to share information that is important in a family session." Nikita also offered to encourage Mr. Talib to discuss how he and Mrs. Talib could work together to better support Ahmed in his recovery – a premise that was culturally relevant and uncontroversial – and would foster closer ties in their relationship. Mrs. Talib seemed hopeful with this prospect.

Mr. Talib didn't meet with Nikita until a few months later. Ahmed had been doing better at school, and Mr. Talib came under the pretext of showing his appreciation for Nikita's help. Mr. Talib spent most of the session venting about job-related stress. Toward the end, when Nikita asked if he felt he could get more support from his family as a subtle inquiry about his marital relationship, Mr. Talib nodded and said, "I need to work harder at that."

Nikita terminated counseling with the family shortly after her session with Mr. Talib and Ahmed's satisfactory completion of his school year. While she never held a family session with all three members in the same room, she was able to provide timely and individualized support to each one of them as a strategic approach to enhance the strengths of the family in addressing the crisis of the presenting problem.

In both case vignettes, the practitioners used themselves differentially in supporting reciprocal changes between parents and child, couples, and extended family members. From a relational model perspective, both practitioners stretched their professional roles and boundaries to become a trusted and supportive "confidante" of the family. Their focus on strategic interactions with the family members versus direct expression and interpretation of thoughts and feelings between family members was a departure from the traditional Western model, but appeared to be effective and culturally relevant in these cases.

In the next and final case vignette, the practitioner faced the challenge of working with a parent who had anger management issues and difficulties regulating her emotions when she disciplined her child. Her use of relational approaches in being a close ally who walked the parent through an emotionally difficult journey in making positive changes is discussed in the following section.

Case vignette: Mrs. Hu

Mrs. Hu, who emigrated from Taiwan with her husband to the US, sought counseling for herself and her eight-year-old daughter, Linda. Mrs. Hu was concerned about Linda who seemed to have become angry and agitated easily, and showed little interest in her schoolwork and friends. When Mrs. Hu met with Fong, a psychologist, she acknowledged that Linda's change of behavior had something to do with their estranged relationship. She had been staying home to take care of Linda while her husband traveled back and forth to Taiwan to take care of a small business he owned. Since Linda started school a couple of years ago, she had become more outspoken and would challenge Mrs. Hu when she used corporal punishment to discipline her for any wrong doings. Mrs. Hu would become enraged at what she perceived as Linda's provocative behavior, and would hit Linda until she cried and went hiding in her room. Mrs. Hu looked remorseful and ashamed as she recounted the circumstances. She realized that Linda had gotten to be like her as a child when her parents disciplined her harshly, but somehow she could not stop herself from hitting Linda when she felt the anger swelling inside her. When Linda came into the session, Mrs. Hu cried and apologized to her, and indicated her interest in working with Fong on managing her anger. Fong asked Mrs. Hu if she would promise not to use physical punishment with Linda so mother and daughter could take some time to bond again. Mrs. Hu agreed to bring any problems she might have with disciplining Linda into the session.

In Mrs. Hu's subsequent session, Fong encouraged Mrs. Hu to share her own childhood history of being disciplined by her parents. Apparently Mrs. Hu's parents were extremely strict and at times physically abusive toward her. Mrs. Hu recalled how she could tell which shoe her father was using to hit her even when she closed her eyes because the hitting happened so often. After sharing some of the stories, Mrs. Hu stopped, stating that it was too painful for her to continue. A couple of days after the session, Mrs. Hu called Fong to say that she wanted to quit counseling. She had never told anyone about the abusive details, and she had doubts if she should revisit those traumatic times. Fong disclosed that Mrs. Hu's stories had brought up memories of her own upbringing and stories of other parents, and it had been difficult for her as well. Fong told Mrs. Hu gently but firmly that she did not want to give up on her and Linda because she felt that they had already embarked on this arduous journey together. This empathic, genuine, and collaborative approach re-engaged Mrs. Hu, who agreed to continue her sessions.

Another crisis emerged shortly thereafter when Mrs. Hu came in very distraught and reported that she had badly bruised Linda during another altercation. Fong felt she had no choice but to report the incident to the Administration for Children Services. Mrs. Hu was extremely upset with Fong, and threatened to quit again. Fong validated her anger, "I am here to listen. It is important that you let me know how you feel about me, because we are in this together." Fong also promised to advocate for Mrs. Hu to ensure that Linda would not be removed from the home. Fong's communication that she could accept Mrs. Hu's anger and was not afraid of it was an important corrective experience for Mrs. Hu. Looking back, Mrs. Hu's willingness to stay in counseling was a turning point in the therapeutic process. Evidently she had learned from Fong that there were other options in handling angry feelings.

In subsequent sessions, Fong externalized Mrs. Hu's anger as something she acquired from her childhood history that had gone out of control. She also began working with Mrs. Hu on developing some skills to practice mindfulness as a means to regulate her anger. Mrs. Hu felt hopeful and empowered, and was eager to learn. Fong and Mrs. Hu spent several sessions practicing how to observe, describe, and accept her thoughts and feelings from moment to moment while toning down her reactive emotions. Fong encouraged Mrs. Hu to express her angry feelings toward Linda and herself without using words that were laden with emotions. She role modeled to Mrs. Hu by stating that she herself was angry at "the fact that Mrs. Hu had hurt Linda physically and emotionally." Mrs. Hu indicated that the approach of being mindful of her angry thoughts without reacting to the associated emotions and history made good sense, but it was not easy to put it into practice, especially when she was home alone with Linda. Fong offered to be her "lifeline" if she would like to call her anytime she felt she could not control her anger. Mrs. Hu was touched by Fong's genuine desire to help her, and vouched to try her best to manage her emotions. In the following session, Mrs. Hu told Fong that she had slipped once, but stopped short of hitting Linda. In the middle of her anger outburst, she thought of Fong, but was too ashamed to make the call. However, it did seem that the idea that Fong would be there for her helped break up her anger.

Mrs. Hu had a couple more episodes of similar anger outbursts. Fong was patient and supportive throughout the process. Then one day, Mrs. Hu called Fong, telling her excitedly that she finally was able to observe her thoughts and stop the anger from escalating.

This case vignette highlights the importance of using relational approaches in working with emotionally charged issues between parent and child as well as the practitioner. From a psychodynamic perspective, Mrs. Hu had been strongly defended against her anger toward her parents' abusive behavior, but her daughter's defiant behavior had threatened those repressed feelings, and she had responded by acting like her own parents toward Linda. Through the strong therapeutic alliance and corrective experiences with Fong, Mrs. Hu was able to get in touch with some of her rageful feelings as a helpless child, and at the same time, let go of them as she felt empowered and supported by Fong. Ultimately Mrs. Hu was ready and able to learn new skills in regulating her emotions, again with the support of Fong as her coach and ally.

The cases vignettes presented by the practitioners offer a glimpse of the complexities of intergenerational issues in Asian immigrant families, and the challenges of working with parents who hold different perceptions of the nature of their problems and the helping process. Oftentimes the practitioners had to take risks in being part of the family dynamics to elicit trust and broker changes among family members who have different needs. Their use of self in expanding professional boundaries and communicating empathic understanding of the family's stressors exemplifies the core tenets of the relational model.

Discussion highlights

Traditional Asian parenting style

The applicability of the concept of "authoritative" and "authoritarian" parenting styles, however, has been questioned for Asian families, because they do not fully describe Asian styles of parenting. (p. 95)

Once children reach school age, instead of expressing physical affection, parents communicate their love for each other and their children through fulfilling their obligations to the family, and sacrificing their own needs for their children. (p. 95)

While there should be zero tolerance of physical abuse, practitioners need to be aware that many Asian parents still consider corporal punishment to be a part of education for their children. (p. 100)

Intergenerational issues in immigrant families

The turmoil that families experience as their children enter adolescence is complicated among immigrant families because of differences in acculturation between parents and their children. (p. 105)

Working with Asian immigrant families

It is important to understand the interplay of psychodynamic, cultural, and environmental issues impacting the interactions between the parents and the children and the circular dynamics within each Asian immigrant family system. (p. 110)

It is important to gain a sense of the common grounds between the emotional needs of both the parents and the children. (p. 118)

Practitioners emphasize the importance of reframing issues that resonate with the family's values and strengths, as well as eliciting input from the parents. (p. 122)

Asian immigrant families generally prefer the practitioner be the individual who works with different members of the family. (p. 122)

6 Working with survivors of intimate partner violence

Irene W. Chung and Tazuko Shibusawa

Intimate partner violence, behavior by a partner that results in physical, psychological, or sexual harm to the other partner, is a problem that affects women worldwide (Garcia-Moreno *et al.*, 2006). Although it is difficult to estimate the prevalence of partner violence because of discrepancies in data collection methods, studies compiled by the World Health Organization (WHO) indicate that 10 to 69 percent of women report experiencing physical abuse by an intimate male partner (World Health Organization, 2002). The paucity of population-based studies does not allow us to determine if rates of domestic violence are higher in Asian countries than in Western countries. However, there are reports that suggest that rates of partner abuse in Asian countries are higher than those in Western countries. In the United States the incident rates are 20 percent of the population (Tjaden and Thoennes, 2000). The WHO reports that 3 percent or fewer women reported partner abuse in the previous 12 months in Australia and Canada while the rate reported by currently married women in Korea was 38 percent (World Health Organization, 2002). Non-population-based studies in China indicate that 21 percent of married women in Beijing and 90 percent of married women in rural China report having been physically abused by their husbands (Hicks, 2006). According to a government study in Japan, 25 percent of women reported experiencing physical battering by their husbands or male partners (Cabinet Office Japan, 2009).

Worldwide, intimate partner violence can lead to murder. According to the WHO, 40 to 70 percent of female murder victims are killed by their husbands or boyfriends (WHO, 2002). A significant proportion of homicides occur when women try to leave their partners. In some Asian cultures, women who are thought to have brought dishonor to their families are murdered in the name of honor (Papp, 2010).

Asian immigrant women are particularly vulnerable to intimate partner violence because most Asian cultures are patriarchal and hierarchical and men have power over women. Some immigrant communities condone violence toward women (Bhuyan *et al.*, 2005; Bui and Morash, 1999; Yoshioka *et al.*, 2001). The purpose of this chapter is to discuss clinical practice with women who are survivors of intimate partner abuse in Asian immigrant communities. We first provide an overview of intimate partner violence, present issues that are unique to Asian immigrant women, and discuss how relational approaches can be used in providing assistance to these women. In this chapter, we use the terms *intimate partner violence* and *domestic violence* interchangeably.

Intimate partner violence

- Range of abusive behavior
- A systemic view of the precipitants of intimate partner violence

Intimate partner violence includes physical, psychological, and sexual abuse. Physical abuse includes slapping, hitting, kicking, choking, burning, beating, and using of weapons against a partner (Jordan *et al.*, 2010). Psychological abuse includes acts such as threatening and intimidating partners, and denying emotional or financial support (Jordan *et al.*, 2010). Controlling behaviors that isolate women from family and friends and that monitor and restrict access to others is also a form of psychological abuse. Sexual abuse includes forced sexual intercourse and other forms of coercion (World Health Organization, 2002). Physical abuse in intimate relationships is often accompanied by psychological abuse and sexual abuse (ibid.). Most women who are abused by their male partners experience multiple acts of aggression over time. Violence is often triggered when women do not comply with the wishes of their male partners.

Intimate partner violence was first brought to public attention by feminists in the US in the 1970s (Johnson and Ferraro, 2000), and was initially understood as a result of the patriarchal family structure that gave men license to abuse their partners (ibid.). In recent years, there has been increasing recognition of the need to examine abuse from different system levels including larger contextual factors such as poverty, discrimination, and social policy (Sokoloff and Dupont, 2005) as well as couple interaction patterns, and individual batterer characteristics. Poverty is a risk factor for violence because of increased stress levels, which in turn can precipitate violence (Goodman *et al.*, 2009).

Studies of male batterers indicate that substance abuse (Cunradi *et al.*, 2002) and psychological pathology such as borderline personality organization (Dutton, 1994) are strongly associated with intimate partner violence. Exposure to violence in childhood often predicts both perpetration and victimization of violence in adult life (Cavanaugh and Gelles, 2005). In general, there are two patterns of violence: severe violence that escalates with multiple forms of abuse and in which the male partner becomes increasingly possessive and controlling, and a more mild form of violence known as "common couple violence" in which frustration and anger erupt into occasional physical aggression (Johnson, 1995). Researchers note that in the case of "common couple violence," women also engage in violence. However, women do not inflict the same type of severe or escalating violence on their male partners (Hamel, 2007). Women are also more likely to get injured by their male partners and use violence as a form of self-defense (Johnson, 1995).

Intimate partner violence in Asian immigrant communities

- Increasing mental health concern
- Nature of abuse

Survivors of intimate partner violence among Asian immigrant women are diverse in terms of country of origin, religious background, socioeconomic background, age, length of stay in the host country, and immigration status (documented versus undocumented). Although intimate partner violence is increasingly recognized as a problem in Asia and in Asian immigrant communities, there is still a paucity of research on this topic (Yick and Oomen-Early, 2008). Studies in Australia and New Zealand report that immigrant women including Asians tend not to report abuse because they are dependent on their husbands for their legal status (Saroca, 2007; Tse, 2007). Asian communities in Australia and New Zealand also tend to hide domestic violence to protect the community reputation so as not to foster negative public perceptions of their countries of origin (Tse, 2007).

Studies of prevalence of intimate partner violence among Asian immigrant women in the US ranges from 24 to 60 percent (Lee and Hadeed, 2009). There is no conclusive evidence that Asian immigrant women in the US have higher rates of victimization than non-Hispanic White women (Cho, 2012). However, data do indicate that intimate partner violence is a serious problem in Asian immigrant communities. In a study using the 2003 National Survey of Children's Health Study of Violent Disagreement, Wang and colleagues found that Asian respondents reported more violent disagreements (13.7 percent) than Whites (9.9 percent). Furthermore, Asian immigrants were more likely to report heated arguments than native-born Asians. Parenting stress increased the likelihood of violent disagreements (Wang *et al.*, 2011). A community study of Chinese immigrant women living in Boston reports that lifetime prevalence was 17 percent among women who were ever married, 8 percent for severe violence in the lifetime.

Forced marriages have also been identified as a form of intimate partner violence in the UK, which has a large number of South Asian immigrants. Some Asian immigrant women are abused by extended family members such as their in-laws (Dasgupta, 2000). A study conducted among South Asian women in Boston reports physical as well as emotional abuse by both parents-in-law (Raj *et al.*, 2008), including isolation, economic control, verbal abuse and degradation, criticism of the woman's own family, complaints about dowry, controlling intake or access to food, and not being allowed to eat with other family members (ibid.). Severe exploitation of household work by in-laws has also been reported in the UK (EACH, 2009). Conflict with in-laws is also a risk factor for intimate partner violence among Chinese immigrants in the US (Lee, 2000).

Factors that contribute to intimate partner violence in Asian immigrant communities

Intimate partner violence and culture

Although many researchers caution against using culture as an explanatory variable for violence, studies indicate that in some Asian cultures, patriarchal norms are used to justify abuse by Asian societies (Lee and Hadeed, 2009). For example, among Vietnamese immigrants, husbands who believed in traditional gender norms were more likely to inflict violence (Bui and Morash, 1999). Likewise, studies among Korean immigrants in the US indicate that women with more traditional Korean values experienced more abuse by their husbands than those who were less traditional (Y. I. Song, 1996), and that women in male-dominant marriages reported higher levels of violence in the relationship (Kim and Sung, 2000). In China violence is commonly used as a way to make women obey (Xu *et al.*, 2001). Indian women face abuse when they do not live up to the expectations of *sewa* (selfless service), expectations to be submissive, docile, and dependent in the context of patriarchal family structures (Shirwadakar, 2004). In countries including Bangladesh, Cambodia, India, and Pakistan, wife-beating is regarded as a consequence of a man's right to inflict physical punishment on his wife (World Health Organization, 2002). In such countries women also agree with the idea that men have the right to inflict violence on women as discipline (ibid.). In a community survey among Chinese, Korean, Cambodian, and Vietnamese adults in the US, Yoshioka and colleagues found that 24 percent to 36 percent of the sample agreed that violence was justified in some instances depending on the women's behavior (Yoshioka *et al.*, 2001). It is important to note that there are differences based on nationality. In Yoshioka's study, Vietnamese and Cambodian respondents were more likely to endorse the use of violence compared to Chinese and Koreans.

Immigration-related issues

- Changes in gender roles and family dynamics
- Lack of support from family of origin
- Untreated symptoms from pre-migration traumas
- Immigrant status

There is no consensus regarding the association between immigration-related stressors and intimate partner violence. Some studies show no relationship while other studies indicate that multiple stressors from immigration do contribute to intimate partner violence (Lee and Hadeed, 2009). Studies in the Korean American community report that women whose husbands were under higher levels of stress reported higher rates of physical violence (Kim and Sung, 2000). Immigration can bring about changes in gender roles and power dynamics among Asian immigrant couples because of changes in employment and acculturation levels. Women may find employment faster than men or may desire the more egalitarian relationships that they observe in the host culture. Shifts in relationships can challenge traditional patriarchal structures, triggering men to maintain their power by inflicting violence (Lee and Hadeed, 2009). A study of Chinese immigrant male batterers in the US found that compared to non-violent husbands, men who were abusive experienced loss of decision-making power as well as loss in income after immigration (Jin and Keat, 2010). Difficulty with anger control and avoidance of attachment has been associated with partner abuse among Korean American batterers (Kim and Zane, 2004).

Immigrant women often leave their family behind in their home countries and are not able to talk to them about their struggles because they do not want to worry their family. Research among South Asian women in the US indicates that women with no family in the US were three times more likely to be physically abused than those who had family in the country (Raj and Silverman, 2003). This is because these women tend to be isolated and do not have a source of family support to protect them. Tse, in his study of Asian survivors of abuse in New Zealand, notes that Asian women who married native-born New Zealanders are not able to seek support from their families in their homeland because their families believe that all White men are good and give women all the freedom they want, and that there is no violence in Western society (Tse, 2007).

Intimate partner violence is also found in immigrant communities where people have experienced trauma prior to or during the immigration process. The consequences of trauma from war, torture, re-education camps, and being forced to leave one's country for survival can contribute to domestic violence (Bhuyan *et al.*, 2005). In one study of Vietnamese women, abusive husbands had been political prisoners (Shiu-Thornton *et al.*, 2005). Research among Cambodians indicates that experiences with genocide may increase the likelihood of domestic violence (Yoshioka and Dang, 2000). The exact connection between exposure to genocide and battering is not clear; however, research indicates that exposure to previous violence does predict male-to-female violence (Bell and Naugle, 2008). One study among Southeast Asian women reports that two out five have experienced intimate partner violence (Wong *et al.*, 2011). It is likely that men who suffer from severe depression due to PTSD might not be able to modulate their emotions and impulse control.

Studies in Australia, Canada, the UK, and US document that Asian women who immigrate through arranged marriages are especially vulnerable to abuse because of their visa status. These women fear the possibility of deportation because their legal status in their host country is dependent on their partner's status. The fear of losing legal status is also found in Asian women who immigrate through arranged marriages to Asian men as well as women who marry native-born men (Anitha, 2010; Saroca, 2007; Tse, 2007). Most Asian immigrant women in Canada immigrate with their husbands, which makes them vulnerable since they are dependent on them for their legal status. If a woman has not yet obtained permanent residency status, she cannot stay in Canada if she loses the sponsorship of her husband. In the UK, immigrant women who are abused can apply for Indefinite Leave to Remain if they are able to provide evidence that domestic violence was the cause of the break-up, but not all women are aware of this policy or are too fearful of seeking help lest they anger their husbands (Anitha, 2010).

Consequences of intimate partner violence

Intimate partner violence has serious health and mental health consequences. Being a victim of violence has been linked to fractures, chronic pain syndromes, gastrointestinal disorders, irritable bowel syndrome, lacerations and abrasions, ocular damage, respiratory disorders, and reduced physical function (WHO, 2002). Some women also suffer from gynecological and sexual disorders including infertility, pregnancy complications, miscarriages, and sexually transmitted diseases. Other consequences are unwanted pregnancies and unsafe abortions.

Psychological and behavioral consequences of abuse include depression and anxiety, eating and sleep disorders, panic disorders, psychosomatic disorders, feelings of shame and guilt, poor self-esteem, PTSD, suicidal behaviors, and self-harm. Intimate partner violence is associated with increase in depression among Chinese immigrant women in Boston (Hicks, 2006) and Southeast Asian women in the Washington DC area (Wong *et al.*, 2011). Psychological distress is also expressed in the form of physical symptoms among Asian immigrant women. South Asian women who have been abused report night fevers, chest pains, and swooning (Kaliivayalil, 2010).

Domestic violence has long-term negative health consequences for survivors, even after the abuse has ended (Zlotnick *et al.*, 2006). Women who have experienced intimate partner violence are also more prone to substance abuse (Bonomi *et al.*, 2009). For example, a study among Southeast Asian survivors in the Washington area reports that they were more likely to report smoking and drinking beer and other alcohol than women who were not abused (Wong *et al.*, 2011).

Help-seeking and service utilization

- Variety of help-seeking behaviors
- Obstacles due to cultural stigma and lack of culturally competent services

Asian immigrant women in English-speaking countries are less likely to report incidents of abuse or to seek help (EACH, 2009; Lee and Hadeed, 2009). In general, Asian immigrants have low rates of utilizing services for personal problems (Abe-Kim *et al.*, 2002) because of:

1 lack of service awareness;
2 lack of culturally sensitive services;
3 stigma about having problems;
4 a sense of shame; and
5 a need to maintain family unity.

Traditional cultural values also serve as barriers preventing Asian immigrant survivors from seeking help. Many Asian immigrant women are socialized to accept male dominance and do not view abuse as something they can avoid (Hicks, 2006; Song, 1996). A strong belief in the woman's role in the family also hinders women from seeking escape from the abuser (Shirwadakar, 2004). As studies of South Asian women in New Zealand indicate, many immigrant women are not educated about legal rights as a wife (Pillai, 2001), and do not know that they have the right not to be abused. Some women call the crisis hotline because they are not sure if what they are experiencing is abuse (H. Wang, personal communication, 9 May 2012).

Shame and embarrassment can deter women from seeking help. Studies of South Asian immigrant women report that they are not able to leave abusive relationships because of the need to maintain family honor (*izzat*) and to avoid bringing shame (*sharam*) to the family (Gill, 2004; Shirwadakar, 2004). Women who are involved in interracial marriages also might not seek help because of fear of discrimination from their own ethnic community (Bui, 2003).

Fear of retribution from their husbands also deters women from seeking help (Preisser, 1999). This fear is not unfounded since women who try to leave their male partners are at risk for re-victimization including murder (Ahmad *et al.*, 2009; Bybee and Sullivan, 2005). For other immigrant women, seeking help can be an admission that their marriage has failed (Shirwadakar, 2004), and they continue to hope that their partners will change. Coping mechanisms that include minimization, and denial of the trauma can also deter women from seeking help (Hattendorf and Tollerud, 1997).

Some women do seek help from the criminal justice system by calling the police or having neighbors or children do so (Bui, 2003). A study of Vietnamese immigrant women in the US indicates that even when they call the police, they want the police to help stop the violence but not have their husbands arrested (Bui, 2003). In the US, non-citizens who are charged with domestic violence can be deported, which is another reason why some immigrant women are reluctant to call the police.

At the same time, it is important to combat stereotypes of Asian immigrant women as victims and identify their strengths. While some women accept violence as a part of life, many are not passive victims. They try to adopt strategies to maximize their safety and that of their children. Some women resist, others flee, while others attempt to maintain family harmony by giving in to their husband's demands. Some women try to protect themselves and their children by keeping silent to avoid conflict. Others talk back, hit back, and challenge their partner. South Asian survivors in one study found that women did not fit the stereotype of the passive female – instead they challenged their partners (Abraham, 2000). Another study of South Asian women in the UK also indicated that women do try to seek help from their friends and contact domestic violence services (Anitha, 2010). It is also important to note that many community activists and social service workers in Asian immigrant communities have worked hard to provide culturally and linguistically specific services for Asian women in Canada, UK, and the US (Asian & Pacific Islander Institute on Domestic Violence, 2012; EACH, 2009).

Services and interventions

Most domestic violence programs in the US include:

1 a crisis hotline;
2 an emergency shelter;

3   advocacy;
4   counseling; and
5   case management.

(Bennett *et al.*, 2004; Bybee and Sullivan, 2002)

Similar services are also available in Australia, New Zealand, Canada, and the UK (Australian Domestic & Family Violence Clearinghouse; Resolve Alberta, 2010; Women's Aid, 2011). Hotlines serve as a point of entry for most women who seek help. Telephone counselors provide information and referral services as well as crisis intervention assistance. Shelters offer a place of refuge and a place for survivors to think about their options. Shelters try to help women attain independence by linking them to economic and educational resources and housing. They also provide advocacy for services and resources for women after they leave the shelter. Support groups are common at shelters (Sullivan, 2006). In the US, support groups commonly run for ten to 12 weeks closed groups and have been found to improve women's self-esteem, sense of belonging, sense of control, and reduce stress (Sullivan, 2006). Shelter use is associated with increase in self-esteem, decrease in depression, increase in help-seeking behaviors, increase in personal empowerment and access to professional services. Among women who experienced severe violence, women who used shelters left the abusive relationship sooner than those who were not in the shelters (Panchandadeswaran and McCloskey, 2007).

Interventions for Asian immigrant women must be tailored in culturally appropriate ways. This is because of:

1   cultural expectations regarding Asian women about their obligations to the family;
2   cultural values that stigmatize separation and divorce;
3   lack of resources for women to survive on their own and to become financially independent; and
4   as with women of other ethnicities, most Asian immigrant women's roles and identities are embedded in their relationships with their families.

As with all survivors of domestic violence, it is important to not focus solely on physical abuse, but psychological, sexual, and financial abuse as well. Ongoing violence is associated with self-blame and decrease in self-worth, which contributes to depression (Kim and Kahng, 2011). Many also develop PTSD as a result of the abuse. It is important to keep in mind the sense of shame that many Asian immigrant women experience for having to 1) admit that they are in an abusive relationship, and 2) talk about the issue with a non-family member.

Initial assessment

Assessment of lethality is primary when working with survivors of intimate partner violence, and it is important to work with the woman in developing a safety plan. The Asian & Pacific Islander Institute on Domestic Violence compiles documents including Safety Plans in many Asian languages (www.apiidv.org/resources/translated-materials.php, accessed 25 February 2012).

In addition to issues of safety, other areas of assessment include:

- individual factors – social support, sense of self, sense of control of the environment, self-esteem, social support;
- personal resources – awareness of own emotional needs, self-reflection, ability to accept aloneness, ability to be self-protective, ability to foresee consequences, willingness to seek help;
- mental health status and trauma history – traumatic memories, current mental health state;
- perception of abuse – how they perceive the abuse (e.g., whether they perceive that the abuse is wrong);
- perception of available resources.

Counseling

Counseling services are offered individually and in support groups in shelters as well as social service agencies. Because clients do not necessarily remain in therapy, it is important to determine priorities such as safety planning and referral for social and legal services early on in the helping process. Most counseling services include treatment modalities that are informed by feminist theories, which seek to empower women (Hattendorf and Tollerud, 1997). Counseling programs usually focus on addressing the impact of violence and helping survivors recover from trauma and build self-esteem and self-efficacy. Specific modalities include supportive therapy, cognitive therapy, problem-solving therapy, self-esteem building, trauma therapy, and grief counseling. A common thread in most domestic violence counseling programs is exploring battering from the perspective of power, control, and gender inequality (Bennett *et al.*, 2004).

Studies of counseling for survivors of domestic violence indicate that psychoeducational and supportive counseling that is based on a strengths perspective for battered women is effective in empowering survivors and in improving self-esteem, anxiety, and depression, and in enhancing a sense of control and coping abilities (Bennett *et al.*, 2004). A report from Taiwan using the strengths perspective in shelters illustrates the way they placed emphasis on rebuilding the client's informal support system (Song and Shih, 2010). The authors found that the strengths perspective led to a decrease in self-blame, an increase in self-acceptance, ability to express oneself, self-care, self-capacity and potential, enhanced stress-coping ability, and a decrease in frequency of violence (Song and Shih, 2010).

Countertransference issues

People who work with victims must listen attentively to their stories, provide emotional and informational resources, and help survivors realize that they have choices (Dunn and Powell-Williams, 2007). Most women who seek help are in crisis situations and are overwhelmed by the time that they seek help from service providers. Some women are in life-threatening situations with their partners and the high-pressured situation can provoke countertransference reactions in practitioners (Babin *et al.*, 2012). Crisis hotline workers may have only have one opportunity to assist callers, which results in a lot of pressure on the hotline worker. Shelter workers experience stress over the nature of domestic violence and can become frustrated and discouraged when women return home to an abusive partner (Brown and O'Brien, 1998). They experience a reduced sense of personal accomplishment when their clients refuse help or return to their abuser (Babin *et al.*, 2012).

Exposure to victim stories can also be traumatizing. Such exposure can threaten emotional well-being (Jenkins and Baird, 2002). Secondary exposure is known as vicarious traumatization (McCann and Pearlman, 1990) and indicates how practitioners' own worldview changes (viewing the world as less safe) and they start to experience similar symptoms as the survivors such as intrusive thoughts and nightmares. This can lead to burnout (Babin *et al.*, 2012). Working with victims of abuse can arouse feelings of helplessness, guilt, and responsibility in clinicians (Gibbons *et al.*, 1994). Hence, it is important for clinicians to be aware of their own reactions so that they can remain empathic without becoming disaffected or overly sympathetic (Gibbons *et al.*, 1994).

Voices of practitioners

Our literature review section outlined several interrelated areas of foci for practitioners working with survivors of intimate partners in Asian immigrant communities:

- the enhancement of the survivors' motivations to seek a better quality of life that is meaningful to them;
- the nurturance of the strengths and sense of self of these women;
- the restoration and enhancement of the women's level of functioning, for example, their judgment, perception, modulation of affect and impulses, problem-solving capability, and coping mechanisms.

In this section, we will present culturally specific practice issues when working with Asian immigrant women who experience interpersonal violence, and the way in which relational approaches enhance the practitioners' work with this client population. The practitioners who contributed to our discussion worked in three major urban agency settings in the United States: 1) telephone hotlines, 2) shelters for women and their children, and 3) counseling programs. Although the services offered by each setting differ in focus, all the practitioners played multiple roles in providing concrete and emotional support to their clients. The practitioners concurred with the literature discussion that the healing process for this client population had to be viewed as a multi-stage progression, and the outcome of the contacts with practitioners in different settings could not be gauged separately. Their experience indicated that therapeutic changes for Asian immigrant women, who also had to overcome cultural expectations and immigrant-specific circumstances, are often a lengthy and individual process marked by setbacks and compromises. Our discussion of the practitioners' work needs to be considered in this context. We do, however, believe that the therapeutic experience, shaped by the practitioners' relational approaches, renewed and sustained their clients' sense of hope in seeking a better quality of life.

Domestic violence hotlines

Domestic violence hotlines in Asian immigrant communities provide information and referral services to women with diverse needs, and respond to women who are in crisis situations. The problems that women present are as diverse as their age range, socioeconomic background, and immigration history. Some women are ready to leave their homes and ask specifically for assistance to move into a shelter. On the other end of the spectrum, are women who are not sure if their spouses' behavior could be considered "abusive." There are also a substantial number of women who are not ready to make any decisions, but call because they just need to talk with someone about their circumstances. Many women call several times before they are ready to make any specific requests, while others have limited choice in the face of escalating violence in the family and ask for resources such as legal consultation and emergency funds, or information about order of protection.

Most of the practitioners who answer telephone hotlines in various Asian languages do not have the opportunity to meet their clients with whom they share conversations about their intimate personal lives. Most clients seem to appreciate the physical distance that telephone calls offer because of the greater sense of anonymity and control in regard to the nature and amount of information that they share. This implicit incentive for women contemplating seeking help, however, presents tremendous challenges for practitioners who have to engage clients in a single telephone conversation, and where assessment and intervention have to be initiated as a seamless process.

Developing a genuine and empathic relationship over the phone

Underlying the problems presented by women who contact hotlines is psychological suffering that includes fear, helplessness, shame, and anxiety. For many of these women, making the first call for help is the outcome of a long contemplative process and a gesture that signifies a major change in their lives. As one practitioner aptly put it, "it's not just about ending the violence for many Asian immigrant women; it's about ending their identity growing up in a patriarchal culture, and a life that has defined their being for a long time." At the same time, contact with an empathic individual in her native language after a long period of suffering in silence and isolation can be an overwhelming yet comforting experience that evokes the caller's longings for family support and the desire to be taken care of. It is common for the practitioner to have to respond to clients who are hyperventilating, crying uncontrollably, or remaining silent. In these situations, practitioners need to forego the screening protocol and offer emotional support and engage the women in conversation, making supportive remarks such as "Are you alright?" "Take your time, I can wait" or "It's not easy to talk about your personal business, I understand." There are also crisis situations where the practitioner has to give instructions to women who call under difficult circumstances such as the following example.

Vignette #1

A practitioner received a call from a recent immigrant from Korea. She was married to a Caucasian man and relocated with him from an urban area to the suburbs where she was totally isolated, and was not allowed to leave the house by herself. The woman was extremely nervous on the phone because she was calling the hotline by hiding behind some bushes in her garden. Upon realizing that she did not have any paper and pen with her to take down the phone numbers she needed, the practitioner quickly came up with the idea that she should look for a twig to scribble the information on the ground, and she followed his suggestion. By staying with this caller through these emotional moments, the practitioner made a genuine connection with her and was able to initiate a therapeutic relationship so that the woman could make follow-up calls or connect with other practitioners once she entered the domestic violence service system.

Working with the limited cues of the callers' thoughts and reactions on the other end of the phone, practitioners have to be very mindful of any subtle changes in their callers' tone and pace of speech, the pauses and focus in their narratives. While many callers begin the conversation with complaints about their spouse and the abuse to which they were subjected, some also feel ashamed for revealing a dark family secret to an outsider, or displaying negative emotions and disloyalty toward their intimate partner. Some callers rationalize the abuse with comments such as – "I married him for the green card." Practitioners' intuitive sensing of these feelings from a psychological and cultural perspective helps them craft responses that provide a sense of acceptance for these callers' mixed emotions. Practitioners generally do not probe the callers' feelings or interpret their ambivalence in their conversation. Instead they talk about the general cycle of domestic violence behavior and offer some thoughts for the callers' reflection. They focus on concrete issues such as safety and the well-being of the callers and their children, which usually elicits appreciative responses.

Vignette #2

One Chinese caller, who appeared initially to be uncomfortable with discussing her abusive experience, started to share that she had lost a lot of hair. She also complained that she had lost her appetite and could barely finish a bowl of noodles. The specifics of how she had been affected captured her mental anguish as a victim even though she did not delve into her emotions. The practitioner responded softly with a Chinese affective expression "*Aiyah*" that denoted her exasperation and empathy with the caller's suffering. The brief but powerful communication and connection prompted the caller to start crying, and share more about her circumstances.

Another common engagement approach used by practitioners is to talk about the general hardships and struggles of other Asian immigrant women who are domestic violence survivors, and ask the caller if she can relate to some of these experiences. One may question if this approach deviates from the Western practice model that emphasizes the therapeutic value of the client's direct verbalization of her narratives. From the perspective of the relational model, the universalization of these women's experiences offers important therapeutic benefits. Hearing that she is not alone in her predicament alleviates some of the cultural stigma that inhibits the caller from sharing her experience, and rekindles a sense of hope that, just like others who sought help, her life can improve. Knowing that the practitioner has worked with other Asian immigrant survivors helps the caller feel understood and assured that she will not be judged. At the same time, the practitioner's elicitation of her input conveys a sense of empowerment and respect for her choice of participation.

Forging a sense of partnership over the phone

For many of the callers, their contact with the hotline practitioner is the first genuine conversation about themselves since their lives of abuse and social isolation started. It is important for the callers to feel supported in any small steps that they are ready to take to improve their lives. Over the course of the phone conversation, the practitioner utilizes different opportunities to create a sense of partnership and active collaboration with the caller. For example, the practitioner might summarize the narratives of the caller and suggest: "Let's think of a way for us to move away from this situation," and gently guide the caller to consider the next step of action. For those who are not ready to leave their homes, the practitioner might review with callers the pros and cons of different options such as getting an order of protection and the risk of antagonizing the abuser and escalating the violence. The practitioner will ask detailed questions of the caller's safety plan and make sure the caller learns how to ask for an interpreter in English if she has to call the police. The practitioner's thorough assessment and anticipation of the needs of the caller forges a bond that possibly stays with the caller after the phone conversation. One caller poignantly expressed her appreciation as, "It's good to know that someone looks out for me."

Domestic violence shelters

Practitioners who work in the shelters are in the unique situation of having extensive contact with their clients on a daily basis over a period of several weeks. Their primary role is to help the women become self-sufficient and start a new life in the community, and the scope of their work revolves around providing case management and some supportive counseling services. However, achieving independence is an objective that goes beyond the procurement of employment, financial benefits, housing, and other concrete services. For women who have endured years of abuse and internalized their spouses' domination over them, the psychological healing process is another major task in the arduous journey to their independence, such as the development of a positive sense of self, trust in relationships with others, and mental acuity in problem-solving and daily living tasks. From a relational model perspective, the practitioners' supportive and egalitarian relationship with their clients is the therapeutic tool that will strengthen the clients' sense of trust in themselves and others, and restore a sense of control over their lives. However, there are challenges inherent in the shelter setting where women are transitioning into a new environment and new roles, and where being with other survivors of domestic violence can be a stark reminder of their victimization and the fact that they no longer have a home, and possibly the support of their family and community. For Asian immigrant women whose sense of self is built around familial obligations and interdependence within their kinship network, their initial relief of being in a safe place is often replaced by feelings of ambivalence, self-blame, and fear of the uncertainty of the future that are amplified by the loss of that identity. For those who move into the shelter with their children, their complaints of missing home and a familiar environment can evoke feelings of guilt and further self-doubt. For those who have to leave on their own, they may also have to cope with similar emotions. These complex feelings are often displaced onto the practitioners and other clients over issues of communal living – abiding by the rules and regulations, sharing of facilities, and so forth – and the systemic obstacles of securing concrete services.

Creation of an egalitarian and emotionally supportive relationship

The practitioners at the shelter have to be very mindful of their interactions with their clients individually as well as on a group basis. On one hand, their dedication and willingness to go out of their way to help their clients settle into the shelter – accompanying them to apply for benefits, shop for clothing, checking in on them when they have physical complaints, etc. – generally elicits trust and appreciation from the clients. On the other hand, practitioners can also be the target of scrutiny for being partial to specific clients, making unsupportive comments or being the authority figures who have privileges over the clients. These are inevitable familial dynamics when practitioners are the major source of compassion, nurturance, and resources at the shelter. For practitioners, it is important to manage the negative countertransference that is being triggered and channel the induced feelings into a corrective experience. To minimize the power differential inherent in the relationship and reinforce the clients' negative experience with conflicts, many of the practitioners acknowledge the clients' challenging comments that they were dismissive or impatient with the clients, and thank them for the feedback. Practitioners may share that they are also feeling the stressors and pressure at the shelter, and their own susceptibility to stress gives them a sense of the experience and struggles of their clients. This empowering approach pre-empts acrimonious feelings and power struggles between the practitioner and the client, and most importantly, offers an opportunity for the client to assert her voice and her needs. Over time, both the practitioner and the client become more adept at reading each other's emotional cues, and sometimes eye contact with a brief nod or gentle pat on the shoulder in a group setting is sufficient to repair any ill feelings.

Providing a sense of acceptance and empowerment in support groups

Some practitioners also utilize group meetings as a format to raise issues of conflicts and estranged relationships among clients in a supportive and culturally relevant manner. They frame the issues in the context of the demands of sharing living quarters and its adverse effect on everyone's tolerance of stress. For example, the issue of children fighting with each other is reframed as stemming from the lack of private space and the attention from their mothers who are preoccupied with utilizing the kitchen and laundry facilities in their allotted time; or the issue of not tidying public facilities is attributed to the pressure to rush to work or job interviews. Thus issues are generally brought to the attention of everyone without placing the blame on any individuals. Some practitioners also remind clients of their resilience as survivors, and ask everyone to identify each other's strengths. The tone of acceptance and the implicit exchange of good will among the clients in the group setting have proven to be effective in alleviating conflicts and reinforcing their obligations at the shelter.

Counseling services

Practitioners in counseling agency settings also work with a vast array of clients with a wide spectrum of presenting problems and circumstances. Among those who receive counseling are women who went through the hotline and shelter systems and seek further support; those who were referred by the police or child welfare agencies, but are not ready to take a stance against their spouses' abuse; and others who are not able to leave their homes because of the lack of resources and do not want the stigma associated with going to a shelter. In working with these women, practitioners need to be mindful of the complexities of the situation that the women are in and the importance of respecting their choices and the pathway they choose to pursue what is important to them. One practitioner poignantly pointed out that "It is presumptuous to think that an Asian immigrant woman will want to leave her husband just because she is being abused." Thus the therapeutic goal in the helping process is really about empowering the client to make decisions for herself – one small step at a time.

Creation of a safe space for reflection and empowerment

The women who seek help display a variety of help-seeking behaviors that include cooperation, compliance, advice-seeking from the practitioners, ambivalence, and resignation that the abuse was "destiny" or as "something that husbands do in our culture." Although these behaviors might be shaped by clients' circumstances, such as the urgency of the presenting problem, the inadequate problem-solving skills and resources of the clients, and the needs of their young children, there is often a re-enactment of an internalized fragile sense of self that is palpable in their interactions with the practitioners. Remarks such as "Tell me what I should do?" "What do you think is good for me?" "How can I do this to my children?" are layered with feelings that the women do not trust their abilities and right to do the best for themselves. From a psychodynamic perspective, many of them are also defended against the pain and shame of being controlled and mistreated by their loved ones and try to make sense of their tolerance of the abuse by using their familial roles and obligations defined by the cultural values of inter-dependence and self-sacrifice. Some women also become demanding and angry over time, accusing the practitioner of not being able to do more for them or give them directives. These behaviors seem to indicate that clients perceived practitioners as benign authority figures who should resolve their inner conflicts and the associated feelings of guilt and anxiety by taking over the responsibility of decision-making over issues that were stigmatized in their culture. From a relational perspective, they are also indications of the clients' developing trust in the practitioners' expertise and commitment to help them, and that they are engaged in the helping process.

The practitioners' understanding of the issues and emotions underlying the varied help-seeking behavior of their clients is essential in maintaining their empathy and crafting therapeutic responses. They convey a sense of acceptance by validating the clients' remarks and behavior in the context of cultural expectations and immigrant-specific circumstances. Some of the practitioners apologize for not being able to make decisions *for* the clients but offer to review the options *with* them. Others extend their boundaries whenever possible and accompany their clients to court or other entitlement offices. This approach was important in strengthening the sense of partnership that the clients look for from a cultural and psychological perspective. It also provides a corrective experience that the practitioner genuinely cares about the client despite the times she caused disappointments and doubts in the helping process.

In the following section, we will present case vignettes to illustrate the different relational approaches used by the practitioners in meeting the myriad needs and help-seeking behavior of their clients.

Case vignette: Mrs. Wong

Mrs. Wong, an immigrant from China, was referred to the community mental health clinic for counseling after the neighbors called the police about a suspected episode of domestic violence. Mrs. Wong had been married for 15 years. She was unable to work due to a chronic back problem, and often depended on her husband to help out in the household. Mr. Wong worked long hours in a fish market in Chinatown, and barely made enough money to support the family. Mrs. Wong suffered from debilitating pain and sometimes had to spend her day in bed. Mrs. Wong and her husband seemed to be under a lot of stress and there had been constant arguments leading to Mrs. Wong being hit by her husband. Their ten-year-old daughter would often sleep in the middle of her parents' bed to mitigate the conflicts and protect Mrs. Wong.

When Mrs. Wong came to her first session, she told Jasmine, her psychologist at the clinic, that the incidents of her husband hitting her were not "domestic violence" because "there was no blood shed." Mrs. Wong also said that even though her husband was "wrong" in hitting her, this was a "private" matter that should stay in the family. Jasmine said she respected Mrs. Wong's opinion, and that her primary concern was to ensure that Mrs. Wong and her daughter would not get hurt. Jasmine also reassured Mrs. Wong of the confidentiality of the sessions, and did not pursue the issue of domestic violence right away. She spent the new few sessions encouraging Mrs. Wong to talk about her back pain and her frustrations for not being able to do more chores around the house. As Mrs. Wong described how she creatively managed to do some chores and care for her daughter on the days that she was in a lot of pain, Jasmine was able to validate her strengths and resilience. Eventually Jasmine inquired about Mrs. Wong's relationship with her husband, and Mrs. Wong wistfully said, "Sometimes I want to leave him, but part of me feels indebted to him; he has done a lot for the family." Jasmine validated Mrs. Wong's ambivalence, and asked if she would consider doing some role-play to minimize the escalation of conflict when her husband was home. As Mrs. Wong described a typical heated conversation with her husband preceding the hitting, Jasmine was able to identify inflammatory remarks such as, "Yes, I know I am useless. Why don't you hit me already?" or "Kill me then, if you dare." In pointing out how Mrs. Wong needed to refrain from making these remarks, Jasmine was able to validate her anger toward her husband and at the same time emphasize the priority of safety for herself and her daughter.

As Mrs. Wong felt supported and learned to manage her anger and frustration, she also agreed for Jasmine to reach out to her husband and invite him for a joint session. Apparently she was feeling stronger, less resentful, and also more hopeful about having a better family life. Jasmine framed the invitation to Mr. Wong as an opportunity to build on the strengths of the family, and Mr. Wong agreed to attend a session. At the beginning of the session, Jasmine engaged Mr. Wong by asking him about his work, and validated the pressure and hardship of being the sole breadwinner of the family. Jasmine also pointed out that despite their conflicts both Mr. and Mrs. Wong worked hard to raise their daughter and wanted the best for her. Mr. Wong lowered his head and Mrs. Wong looked tearful. With Mrs. Wong's permission, Jasmine shared that they had been working on how to handle conflicts without getting into physical fights because Mrs. Wong acknowledged that this issue had been undermining the integrity of the family and the development of their daughter. Without placing blame, Jasmine asked if Mr. Wong agreed that it would be important to stop the violence. After some silence, Mr. Wong said that keeping the family together was his top priority, and in his words, "As long as we can put rice on the table and share our meals together, that's what matters."

Mr. and Mrs. Wong subsequently had a couple more sessions together. With Jasmine's mediation, they were able to vent their frustrations but also focus on their contribution to the welfare of the family. Jasmine was able to secure some financial supplements for the family, which seemed to alleviate some of the conflicts. While Mr. and Mrs. Wong remained estranged to some extent, they were able to respect each other's boundaries, and there seemed to be no major incidents of domestic violence during the time Mrs. Wong was in treatment.

Case vignette: Mrs. Kim

Mrs. Kim, a Korean immigrant in her thirties, was referred by the women's shelter to seek counseling for her depressive symptoms. She had recently left her husband and moved into public housing with her adolescent son. Mrs. Kim came from a poor family and married her husband when he went back to Korea to look for a wife. Shortly after she arrived in the United States, her husband, who had a drinking problem, became abusive. Since her husband had put everything under his name, she left home with no resources. Mrs. Kim did not speak English and was illiterate in Korean as well. When Mrs. Kim first met Myung Hee, the social worker in the mental health clinic, she was reluctant to seek psychiatric treatment for her depressed moods, inability to focus, and flashbacks of the abuse. She told Myung Hee that she did not want to bring more stigma to her family, and that she just wanted to learn how to manage her symptoms and "move on" with her life. Myung Hee did not pressure her, but reframed her symptoms as her body taking on the stress that she had endured, which was a common experience of domestic violence survivors. Myung Hee suggested that Mrs. Kim wait and see if the symptoms would go away, and if not, she could consider taking medications from the clinic's psychiatrist for a short period of time.

Meanwhile Myung Hee focused on helping Mrs. Kim settle down in her new life. She accompanied Mrs. Kim to the Food Stamp and Medicaid Office for recertification interviews. At Mrs. Kim's suggestion, she helped Mrs. Kim enroll in English and job training classes. Eventually Mrs. Kim got a job assembling jewelry pieces at a small factory, and soon won the praise of her employer for her work ethic and performance. As Mrs. Kim gained more confidence in her ability, she became more spontaneous in her sessions with Myung Hee. She would revel in telling Myung Hee about her job and interactions with her coworkers. Other times she would be more reflective, and little by little, she would share the details of her abuse and cry in Myung Hee's presence. When Myung Hee went to Mrs. Kim's son's school, intervening on his behalf about a bullying incident, Mrs. Kim was grateful but also became emotional about how much pain she had caused her son. This was the first time Mrs. Kim articulated her feelings about her past. Mrs. Kim then asked for a consultation with the psychiatrist because she wanted "to be on her best on the job as well as for her son." Mrs. Kim was subsequently prescribed anti-depressants for a short period while she continued to share with Myung Hee her concerns and worries.

After a year of counseling with Myung Hee, Mrs. Kim decided that she was ready to take on another challenge, which was to take classes to prepare for naturalization. She came to see Myung Hee less often, because she "had learned how to take care of herself." A year later, she came to see Myung Hee, telling her proudly that she had passed her citizenship examination.

The following is a case where the client was referred for counseling because her husband was physically abusive toward their daughter. It was not until later that the practitioner found out that the client had also been abused. Although the client never sought help from the practitioner regarding the abuse, the practitioner was able to support the client in making positive changes in her life that eventually ended the abuse.

Case vignette: Mrs. Suri

Mrs. Suri, an immigrant from Punjab, India, was referred by the child welfare agency to receive counseling. Her 17-year-old daughter had filed charges against her father for physically assaulting her, and was placed in a relative's home. Mrs. Suri grew up in a rural area in Punjab and only had a few years of schooling. For many years, Mrs. Suri lived with her in-laws who mistreated her before her husband applied for her visa to immigrate to the United States. Mrs. Suri spoke little English and stayed home to raise her daughter and a son who had some learning disabilities.

When Mrs. Suri first met her social worker, Bhavi, a second generation South Asian whose family was from another region in India, she was skeptical that Bhavi could help her. Even though Bhavi could speak Hindi, Mrs. Suri commented that Bhavi looked "young" as a counselor. She asked if Bhavi was married and if her family was in the United States. Bhavi validated Mrs. Suri's doubts and disclosed her personal background growing up in an immigrant family, which seemed to help Mrs. Suri feel more at ease.

When Bhavi and Mrs. Suri talked about her daughter's alleged charges of physical abuse, Mrs. Suri said, "It's in our culture, don't you know? It's something that men do to their wives and daughters." Bhavi asked if Mrs. Suri's husband also hit her. Mrs. Suri initially said "Yes," and then recanted her statement. Bhavi did not press the issue further, and decided that it was more important to engage Mrs. Suri in the helping process.

In the next couple of months, Bhavi focused on developing a relationship that empowered Mrs. Suri, rather than talking about problems in her life. Mrs. Suri disclosed that she loved cooking, and her face always lit up when she talked about how she creatively prepared dishes that her husband and her children enjoyed. So Bhavi let Mrs. Suri take the lead and bring up whatever she wished to discuss in the session. At one point, Mrs. Suri asked Bhavi if she cooked for herself, and brought some food for her to take home for dinner. As the relationship evolved, Mrs. Suri seemed to take on the role of an older sister taking care of Bhavi, and relish the fact that Bhavi was appreciative of her skills and talents. Over time, Bhavi noticed that Mrs. Suri had taken time to groom herself, wear make up, and use more English words. Mrs. Suri also told Bhavi that she started taking yoga classes and going to a Punjabi temple where she could partake in meals and socialize with other people. Mrs. Suri was excited when she was accepted to cook in the kitchen of this temple.

Mrs. Suri surprised Bhavi when her husband completed anger management classes and her daughter had returned home. She voluntarily brought up the issue of her husband's abuse and disclosed some details to Bhavi. However, Mrs. Suri claimed that the physical violence had stopped since she learned how to avoid her husband and he seemed to be more mindful of the legal consequences. She also did not want Bhavi to bring up this issue in the family sessions with her husband and her daughter. It seemed that it was important for Mrs. Suri to share the abuse with someone she had come to trust, and after that, she could move on with her life.

The therapeutic experiences that the practitioners provided for their clients centered on a genuine relationship that was sensitive to their clients' concrete and emotional needs and an appreciation of their strengths in a culturally relevant context. The case vignettes illustrate how the clients felt empowered by their practitioners' involvement in their lives – as confidante, advisor, and a benign authority figure who mirrored their resilience and cheered them on in their quest to seek changes that were important to them. While there were different outcomes, the clients experienced positive change in how they viewed themselves and others. If we look at change as an evolving and ongoing process that is enhanced by an individual's sense of self, the practitioners across all settings played a significant role in supporting the survivors of intimate partner violence in seeking a better life.

Discussion highlights

Cultural and immigrant-specific factors that contribute to domestic violence

Patriarchal norms in Asian cultures are often used to justify abuse. (p. 133)

Shifts in familial roles can challenge traditional patriarchal structures, triggering some men to maintain their power by inflicting violence. (p. 134)

The consequences of trauma from war, torture, re-education camps, and being forced to leave one's country for survival can contribute to domestic violence. (p. 135)

Asian immigrant women in English-speaking countries are less likely to report incidents of abuse or to seek help. (p. 136)

Mental health consequences of being a victim of domestic violence

Psychological and behavioral consequences of abuse include depression and anxiety, eating and sleep disorders, panic disorders, psychosomatic disorders, feelings of shame and guilt, poor self-esteem, PTSD, suicidal behaviors, and self-harm. (p. 136)

Relational and culturally responsive approaches in working with Asian immigrant women who are victims of domestic violence

It is important to combat stereotypes of Asian immigrant women as victims and identify their strengths. While some women accept violence as part of life, many are not passive victims. (p. 137)

Practitioners generally do not probe the callers' feelings or interpret their ambivalence. (p. 142)

Practitioners' supportive and egalitarian relationship with their clients are therapeutic tools that will strengthen the clients' sense of trust in themselves and others, and restore a sense of control over their lives. (p. 144)

The therapeutic goal in the helping process is really about empowering the client to make decisions for herself – one small step at a time. (p. 146)

7 Working with Asian immigrant elders

Tazuko Shibusawa

The population of older Asian immigrants continues to grow in English-speaking countries. By 2026, Chinese and Vietnamese are expected to be the first and fourth most spoken languages spoken by older immigrants in Australia (Lee *et al.*, 2011). The number of older Asians in New Zealand is also growing and is expected to increase fivefold between 2001 and 2021 (Statistics New Zealand, 2006). The largest group of Asian elders in New Zealand is Chinese, and over 90 percent are foreign-born (Li and Chong, 2012). In the UK, approximately 11 percent of South Asians and 3 percent of Chinese are between 60 and 74 years of age (Evandrou, 2000). Asians are also the fastest-growing group among elders in the US, and are projected to increase from 3 percent in 2000 to 8 percent by 2050 (Federal Interagency Forum on Aging-related Statistics, 2012).

When working with older Asian immigrants, it is important to understand the aging process through a life course perspective and explore ways in which early life experiences shape late life. Different socio-historical periods provide different opportunity structures for individuals (Elder *et al.*, 2003). Access to health care, education, and employment in early life influence the life course. The majority of elders from rural areas of Asia had limited access to education, which reduced opportunities for employment in their new country. On the other hand, individuals who had access to education in their home countries were able to obtain well-paying jobs and prepare for a secure retirement in their host countries. Disadvantages in early life such as malnutrition can also result in chronic physical conditions in later life (Hertzman, 2004). A lifetime of adversity results in poor physical and mental health among Asian elders (Mui, 1993). For example, Bengali and Gujarati elders who held low-wage jobs in the UK report numerous health problems including poor eyesight, arthritis, rheumatism, and high rates of depressive symptoms (Lindbloom *et al.*, 2012).

The timing of immigration also influences subsequent life experiences. People who immigrate during young adulthood usually migrate at the beginning of their career and child-bearing years. Migrating in young adulthood enables people to settle down and grow roots in their new environment. Those who immigrate during mid-adulthood can find employment and receive a pension. In recent years, there has been an increase in older adults who immigrate in late life to be with their children. Although immigrants of all ages face stressors such as loss of a familiar environment, support systems, and identity and status, it is more difficult to adjust to a new environment in late adulthood than in young adulthood (Angel *et al.*, 1999; Kim *et al.*, 1991; Le, 1997; Phua *et al.*, 2001). Older immigrants are less capable of learning a new language and adapting to new surroundings than those who immigrate earlier in life.

Older adults, in general, have to cope with life cycle transitions such as finding new meaning in life after retirement, and coping with physical changes. Elders who immigrate in late life not only have to cope with the aging process, they also have to adapt to a new environment, face language barriers, and respond to changes in intergenerational relationships. These changes can have negative consequences on psychological well-being (Tsai and Lopez, 1997).

Financial security is a serious problem for many Asian elders in English-speaking countries. Elders who migrated in late life are not eligible to receive pensions. Although the Social Security system is designed as a safety net to protect elders in the US, close to half of Asian elders (53.7 percent) do not receive Social Security benefits because they immigrated late in life and have not paid into the Social Security system (AARP Public Policy Institute, 2004). Among the elders in the US, Bangladeshi (35 percent), Hmong (31 percent), Laotian (22 percent), Korean (22 percent), Cambodian (19 percent), Chinese (16 percent), Pakistani (15 percent), and Vietnamese (16 percent) elders also live under the poverty line. The percentage is smaller for Asian Indians (9 percent), Japanese (6 percent), and Filipino (8 percent) elders, because most Japanese elders are second and third generation, and a large number of Filipinos and Asian Indian elders immigrated to the United States in the 1970s and 1980s as professionals, enabling them to establish financial security for their retirement years. Asian immigrant elders, on the whole, are a vulnerable group with high rates of poverty, low educational attainment, limited English proficiency, and low levels of assimilation into mainstream society.

In this chapter, we will present an overview of aging and mental health, followed by issues that are specific to working with older Asian immigrants. We discuss ways in which practitioners can use relational perspectives to support the psychological well-being of Asian immigrant elders and their families.

Psychological well-being and older adults

Positive psychological well-being among elders is associated with good health, cognitive function, socioeconomic status, and advantages in early life such as education and access to health care. Social support and close relationships with family members are also important. Engagement in meaningful activities including volunteer work and spiritual activities also offer life-satisfaction, a sense of mastery, and self-efficacy for elders. Personality and outlook on life also influence psychological well-being.

Risk factors for psychological well-being in late life involve losses including decrease in physical health and cognitive functioning, loss of social status, and loss of loved ones (Blazer, 2002). Bereavement is a significant risk factor for depression among elders who lose a spouse (Turvey *et al.*, 1999). Financial difficulties, changes in living situation, interpersonal conflicts, and caring for ill family members can also result in depression and anxiety among elders. In the next section, we will discuss physical and mental health aspects of aging.

Chronic illness

Common chronic health conditions among older adults include heart disease, hypertension, chronic bronchitis, cancer, diabetes, and arthritis (Federal Interagency Forum on Aging-Related Statistics, 2012). In the United States, 90 percent of adults age 65 and over have at least one chronic condition and 77 percent have two or more conditions (Anderson and Hovarth, 2004). Studies in the US indicate that Asian women, especially those who immigrated in late life, are at risk for osteoporosis because of:

1   poor nutrition during childhood;
2   small body frame;
3   lack of exercise;
4   lack of knowledge about causes, preventions, and treatments; and
5   difficulty accessing medical care.

(Lauderdale *et al.*, 2003; Walker *et al.*, 2006)

Elders who immigrated early in life can develop chronic conditions because of the change in diet and lifestyle.

Disabilities

Physical function can also diminish with age, and hinder Activities of Daily Living (ADL) which include bathing, grooming, dressing, feeding, transferring, toileting, walking, and continence; and Instrumental Activities of Daily Living (IADL), which are cooking, cleaning, laundry, driving, using transportation, writing, reading, using the telephone, taking medicine, and managing money. In the general population, 23 percent of adults between the ages of 65 to 74, and 45 percent of adults 75 and older experience difficulties with ADL (Hooyman and Kiyak, 2002). According the 2000 Census, 35 percent of Asians aged 65 and over reported at least one disability, which was slightly higher than the rate among non-Hispanic White elders (Mutchler *et al.*, 2000). Compared to US-born Asian elders, foreign-born Asian elders reported higher rates of disabilities (Mutchler *et al.*, 2000). Among Asian elders in the US, South East Asian elders report the highest rates of physical disabilities.

Depression and anxiety

There are two types of older adults who experience depression: those who have struggled with depression throughout their lives (early onset), and others who experience depression for the first time in late life (late onset). In the United States, it is estimated that over 50 percent of elders have late onset depression while less than 50 percent have early onset depression (Fiske *et al.*, 2009). Older adults with early onset depression are more likely to have had a family history of depression and personality traits that are associated with depression (Brodaty *et al.*, 2001).

Onset of depression in late life is likely to be associated with structural changes in the brain, and may be related to vascular risk factors or cognitive deficits which may be an early phase of dementia (Fiske *et al.*, 2009). Depression can also interact with individual vulnerabilities that are due to cumulative adversity and stressful events such as physical illnesses and bereavement. These events can also trigger depression in individuals who have had a history of depression during their younger years.

Depressive symptoms among older adults

- sleep disturbance
- fatigue, psychomotor retardation
- loss of interest in living
- hopelessness about the future
- complaints about poor memory and concentration
- slower cognitive processing speed and executive function.

According to research worldwide, 1 to 5 percent of community-dwelling elders 65 years of age and older have major depressive disorder (Fiske *et al.*, 2009), and 14 percent have subsyndromal depression (VanItallie, 2005). The latter, also known as subthreshold or subclinical depression, does not meet the diagnostic criteria for major depressive disorder, but includes prolonged depressed mood, poor concentration, psychomotor retardation, and poor self-reported health (ibid.). Chronic pain, diminished physical mobility, and other changes in physical functioning can result in subclinical depressive symptoms. Unfortunately, depressive symptoms among Asian immigrant elders often go unnoticed by family and community members because people assume that the symptoms are a normal sign of aging.

Some studies report that older Asian immigrants have higher rates of depression compared to other elders in the host country, while other studies show lower rates of depression. There is no conclusive evidence about the rates of depression among Asian elders because of the paucity of research that is based on population-based samples. The inconsistent results among current research findings are due to:

1 different cultural conceptualizations of psychological distress and depression;
2 different measures that are used in research; and
3 different sampling methods.

(Sorkin *et al.*, 2011)

Measurements such as the Geriatric Depression Scale that is often used by researchers report findings on the number of depressive symptoms, but the number of symptoms do not necessarily equate with the diagnosis of depression.

Research based on community samples does indicate that depression is a problem among Asian elders (Bhatnagar and Frank, 1997; Diwan *et al.*, 2004; Dong *et al.*, 2011; Kim and Chen, 2011; Kuo, 2011; Kuo *et al.*, 2008; Lai, 2004; Lai and Surood, 2008; Ngo *et al.*, 2001; Pang, 1995; Silveira and Shah, 1998). Table 7.1 summarizes the contributing factors to depression that have been identified by research on Asian immigrant elders in Australia, New Zealand, Canada, UK, and the US.

Psychological and medical problems tend to co-exist more frequently among older adults than younger adults (Kogan *et al.*, 2000). Depression among older adults is associated with other diseases such as Alzheimer's and Parkinson's. In addition, depression is associated with higher risks of developing dementia or can co-exist with dementia (Lee *et al.*, 2011). Older adults also tend to take medications for various medical conditions that can cause depression (Goncalves *et al.*, 2009). Many Asian elders use traditional herbal medicine and it is important to find out

Table 7.1 Risk factors associated with depressive symptoms among Asian elders

Biomedical risk factors (all populations)	*Psychological and social risk factors (all populations)*
• Chronic physical illness and conditions • Chronic physical pain • Neurological or cognitive deficits • Poor nutrition	• Multiple losses • Adverse life events and stress • Social isolation and lack of social support • Interpersonal conflicts • Lack of socioeconomic resources and income (poverty) • Lack of education • Societal oppression and discrimination • Past history of depression or alcohol and other substance abuse • Exposure to unsafe environments

Risk factors among older Asian immigrants (in addition to above)

• Recency of immigration
• Limited English-speaking ability
• Gender (being female)
• Access to services
• Intergenerational cultural conflicts
• Lack of social support
• Traditional cultural values
• Poor housing conditions
• Living alone

if there is a negative interaction with Western medication, which may increase depression.

Medical conditions associated with depressive symptoms

- Dementia
- Parkinson's disease
- Rheumatoid arthritis
- Thyroid dysfunction
- Diseases of the adrenal glands
- Strokes
- Heart disease
- Hypothyroidism
- Vitamin deficiencies
- Chronic infection.

There is a common belief among the general public including the Asian immigrant community that depression is a part of late life and unavoidable. However, major depression can be treated effectively with medications such as selective serotonin re-uptake inhibitors, tricylic antidepressants, and monoamine oxidase inhibitors (Fiske *et al.*, 2009).

Psychological interventions are effective for dysthymia and minor depression (Pinquart *et al.*, 2006). Evidence-based psychological treatments for older adults with depressive symptoms include brief psychodynamic psychotherapy, interpersonal psychotherapy, cognitive behavioral treatments including behavioral activation, cognitive bibliotherapy, problem-solving therapy, and life review therapy (Fiske *et al.*, 2009; Gallagher-Thompson *et al.*, 2008; Lynch *et al.*, 2003). Preliminary research also indicates effectiveness of mindfulness-based cognitive behavioral therapy (Baer, 2006). Research also indicates that exercises including aerobic exercise and weight training are effective interventions for older adults with depression (Fiske *et al.*, 2009).

Anxiety

Anxiety, like depression, is prevalent among older adults and often co-exists with depression and physical illnesses (Byers *et al.*, 2010). While younger adults often experience anxiety on a cognitive level and express "feelings of guilt," older adults who have anxiety express being "worried," "fearful," "afraid," and "scared" (Kogan *et al.*, 2000). Anxiety is frequent in dementia, in the form of agitation, and it is difficult to differentiate them. In contrast to depression, very little research is available on anxiety among Asian elders (Iwamasa and Hilliard, 1999). As with depression, it is difficult to identify in elders because of the comorbidity with medical problems such as cardiovascular disease or Parkinson's disease.

Symptoms of anxiety among older adults

Cognitive
- Fearfulness
- Sense of dread

Physiological
- Headaches
- Intestinal distress
- Trembling
- Insomnia
- Heart palpitations
- Hyperventilation
- Dizziness
- Excessive sweating.

Symptoms commonly observed among older Asian immigrants

- Excessive worry
- Chronic concern
- Somatic complaints.

Demoralization

Demoralization is a concept that is used by some mental health professionals to describe the psychological distress that is experienced by individuals who are medically ill, especially those receiving palliative care or those who seek psychotherapy (Bellomo *et al.*, 2007; Cheuk *et al.*, 2009; Clarke *et al.*, 2006). Although there is insufficient research on demoralization to be included as a diagnostic category in the Diagnostic and Statistical Manual of Mental Disorders (DSM), the utility of this psychological construct has been recognized by a number of mental health researchers and practitioners (Cheuk *et al.*, 2009). Demoralization is viewed as a useful construct to understand and treat distress among elders, especially the despair that is associated with the loss of meaning and purpose in life. Individuals who are demoralized are not able to act assertively because of hopelessness, helplessness, and isolation. According to de Figueiredo (1993) demoralization starts with anger, resentment, sadness, anxiety, discouragement, and a feeling of incompetence which develops into a state where people give up. Demoralization is considered to increase rates of depression in elders (Kissane, 2001).

Trauma

Compared to research on children and adults, very little attention has focused on trauma and older adults (Busuttil, 2004). There are no epidemiological studies on the incidence or prevalence of PTSD in older adults, and very little is known about the negative interactions between unresolved distal and recent trauma, and stressors associated with aging such as diminished sensory capacities, decreased mobility, physical frailty, and multiple losses. Because of the lack of understanding about trauma and older adults, symptoms of trauma are often misinterpreted by professionals as mental illness or dementia (Allers *et al.*, 1992). Research on the long-term psychological effects of trauma have been conducted primarily among Holocaust survivors (Kellerman, 2001) and military veterans (Schnurr *et al.*, 2002). While these studies yield important information about the long-term effects of trauma, there is a dearth of information on the effects of early trauma on Asian elders. It is important to assess experiences of early trauma among elders because recent investigation indicates that symptoms that are highest after exposure decline for years and then increase in later life (Cook, 2001). Southeast Asian elders are at high risk for psychological distress, because of their prior exposure to war and experiences as refugees (Yee, 1997). Worries and sadness, described as a "sad heart," is experienced in one's heart, body, and spirit. Somatic symptoms related to PTSD that are expressed among Southeast Asian elders include headaches and dizziness. Cambodian elders talk about *pruiy chüt* which denotes bereavement over loss of country, community, and culture (Gerber *et al.*, 1999). Other Asian elders have also experienced traumatic events in their lives. For example, many Chinese elders lived through the Sino-Japanese war (1930–45), civil war (1945–9), and the Cultural Revolution (1966–76) before migrating to English-speaking countries (Mui and Shibusawa, 2008).

Suicide

The suicide rate among older adults in the US is 18 percent even though they comprise 13 percent of the population (Blazer, 2002). Depression is the major cause of suicide among older adults (VanItallie, 2005). Although older adults are less likely to verbalize suicidal thoughts they have higher rates of ideations of death than younger adults. They are also more likely than younger adults to visit a physician shortly before suicides. Physical illnesses, cancer, seizure disorder, pulmonary disorder, renal failure, vision and hearing impairment, and incontinence are associated with the risk of suicide in late life (Fiske *et al.*, 2009).

Older Asian immigrant women have higher rates of suicide among women of their age cohort in the United States. For women aged 75 and older, the suicide rate for Asian Americans and Pacific Islanders was 7.95 per 100,000, compared to the rates of 4.18 for Caucasian women and 1.18 for African American women (Centers of Disease Control and Prevention National Center for Injury Prevention and Control, 2004). A study in San Francisco, California reports that between 1987 and 1994, Asian women age 85 and older had the highest rates of suicide among their age group and gender group (Shiang *et al.*, 1997).

Dementia

Dementia is associated with the aging process. Symptoms of dementia include difficulties with short-term memory, orientation to time, space and person, concentration, and ability to perform complex tasks (McInnis-Dittrich, 2005). The most common form of dementia among older adults is Alzheimer's disease followed by vascular dementia. Alzheimer's disease is caused by neurofibrillary tangles and degenerative nerve endings, while vascular dementia is associated with cerebrovascular factors (Larson and Imai, 1996; McInnis-Dittrich, 2005). The rate of Alzheimer's disease among adults 65 to 74 is 1 percent and increases to 25 percent among adults 85 and older (McInnis-Dittrich, 2005). Diagnosing dementia in older adults is difficult because of comorbidity with other medical conditions (Lee *et al.*, 2011). Community outreach is key in getting Asian elders and their families to understand dementia and seek services (Chao *et al.*, 2011)

Studies on dementia among Asian immigrants in English-speaking countries indicate that they have less understanding of dementia compared to other populations. For example, many South Asians in the UK are not aware of the symptoms of dementia and those who recognize the symptoms do not seek help because of embarrassment (McGarry *et al.*, 2011; McInnis-Dittrich, 2005). Other Asians have never heard of the concept of dementia (Hasnain and Rana, 2010) or view it as a normal aging process (Gupta and Chaudhuri, 2008; Turner *et al.*, 2005) or as an "act of God" (Milne and Chryssanthopoulou, 2005). In Australia, literacy for dementia is also low in Chinese and Vietnamese communities (Lee *et al.*, 2011). When symptoms are recognized, they are interpreted as mental illness, which in turn is experienced as stigma. Asian family members also attribute symptoms to psychosocial stressors such as earlier traumatic experience, migration, and inter-generational conflicts (Liu *et al.*, 2008). As a result, many families do not seek help

Table 7.2 Stages of Alzheimer's disease

First stage	2–4 years	Loss of recent memory
		Mild personality changes
		Loss of spontaneity
		Social withdrawal
Second stage	2–12 years	Pronounced memory loss
		Inability to retain new information or learn new skills
		Disorientation and confusion
Final stage	1–3 years	Total physical dependency
		Unable to recognize family members
		Loss of ability to communicate

Source: Based on McInnis-Dittrich (2005).

when their elders show signs of dementia. Although Alzheimer's disease is a progressive disease, early detection and intervention can help facilitate quality of life of the elder and decrease caregiver burden and depression among family members (Mittelman *et al.*, 2004).

Family relationships and caregiving

The family plays a critical role in the lives of Asian elders. In the US, larger numbers of Asian Americans co-reside with their families compared to the overall elderly population. According to the US Census 2010, over 86 percent of older Asian men and 77 percent of older Asian women lived with their spouses and/or other family members (Federal Interagency Forum on Aging-Related Statistics, 2012). Conflict within families and lack of social support is associated with psychological distress among older Asian immigrants. Family relationships between older immigrants and their adult children are influenced by a number of factors. Culture gaps between elders and their adult children have a negative impact on psychological well-being (Mui and Shibusawa, 2008). Acculturation often results in shifts in power between generations, and the discrepancy between traditional roles and new cultural demands can be problematic for many older immigrants.

It is well known that traditional Asian culture stresses the importance of filial obligation, and that adult children are expected to care for their older parents. In the United States, almost a third of Asians in mid-life care for their elderly parents (American Association for Retired Persons, 2001). There is pressure not to seek help outside the family because to do so would imply that the adult children were not following the values of filial obligation (Arnsberger, 2005; McBride and Parreno, 1996). While many adult children face caregiver burden, the cultural values of filial obligation provide some caregivers with the sense of satisfaction that they are carrying out the families' responsibilities (Tang, 2011). For adult children who experience caregiver burden, it is sometimes difficult to feel comfortable to obtain outside assistance. For Muslim families, caring for families is considered a duty in life and one is not supposed to express any irritation when parents are difficult. Placing older parents in long-term care facilities is against the Qur'anic obligation (Hasnain and Rana, 2010).

Asian immigrant families tend to be smaller, and there are fewer family members who can care for the elderly. Most daughters-in-law, who are the designated caregivers of frail elders in Asian families, work outside the home. As a result, when Asian elders become frail, long-term care facilities are often the only option despite preferences for family care. However, the lack of culturally appropriate services poses difficulties for frail elders and their adult children.

It is important to note that changes in elder care are not only occurring in Asian immigrant communities in English-speaking countries, but also in Asian countries. There has been a decrease in families where three generations live together (Tam and Neysmith, 2006). Although placing elderly parents in long-term care facilities used to be unthinkable in traditional Asian societies, there has been an increase in the number of elders who reside in assisted living or skilled nursing facilities in many parts of Asia.

Help-seeking and service utilization

Like Asians in general, utilization rates of services among Asian immigrant elders and their families are low (Chen *et al.*, 2003; Chow *et al.*, 2003; Hu *et al.*, 1993). Service utilization is determined by both structural and cultural factors. For Asian immigrant elders who immigrated late in life, it is important to understand that not only cultural, but structural issues influence the ability for elders to receive services. Language barriers, low socioeconomic status, lack of health insurance, lack of mobility, and fragmented health care systems result in low utilization (Jang *et al.*, 1998). Lack of mobility and language are two other major barriers to access among elders (Pang *et al.*, 2003). The inability to communicate with physicians and pharmacists, to understand prescription instructions, and to deal with insurance policies severely restrict elders from seeking health care (ibid.). A study of Chinese immigrant elders in the US reports that elders did not use their Medicare or Medicaid benefits because they did not understand treatment and services that were covered (ibid.). Reluctance to seek services can also be related to past experiences of discrimination. For example, South Asians in the UK perceive poor services as racially motivated because of negative experiences in the past (Lindbloom *et al.*, 2012).

As indicated earlier, cultural factors that influence service utilization among Asian elders and their families include their beliefs about their problem (Saint Arnault, 2009), preferences for family care (Yamashiro and Matsuoka, 1997), resistance to have strangers provide services in the home (ibid.), and availability of culturally appropriate services including language, food, and activities (Worth *et al.*, 2009). Having same sex health care providers is important for some elders as in the case of Muslim elders (Hasnain and Rana, 2010).

Table 7.3 Barriers to service utilization

Structural factors	Cultural factors
Accessibility	Acceptability
Affordability	
Availability	
Asian immigrant elders	
Language barriers	Health beliefs
Lack of awareness	Preference for family care
Lack of health insurance	Distrust of non-family members
Lack of citizenship	Perception of Western medicine as
Inability to navigate within health care	being overly aggressive
system	Lack of familiar food and cultural
Lack of transportation	activities
	Sex specific staff
	Stigma

Cultural models of distress

According to Levkoff and colleagues, there are four stages that individuals go through to seek help for dementia. These stages apply to other health and mental health issues as well (Levkoff *et al.*, 1999):

1 symptom experience and recognition;
2 symptom appraisal;
3 decision to seek care; and
4 medical contact.

Symptoms of psychological distress are often experienced and expressed by Asian elders as somatic symptoms including headaches, backaches, pain in the neck, dizziness, diarrhea, and insomnia (Chung, 2002; Le, 1997; Silveira and Shah, 1998). Because Asian elders do not talk about depressed moods, it is important for practitioners to understand ways in which psychological distress is expressed through somatic complaints (Shibusawa and Chung, 2009).

Each culture has different models for explaining symptoms, illnesses, and their causes (Saint Arnault, 2009). These explanatory models also influence the way individuals decide to seek treatment (Hall *et al.*, 2011; Kleinman, 1988). Because Asians have a holistic view of health which emphasizes balance and harmony between mind and body, psychological functioning is not differentiated by physical functioning (Jenkins *et al.*, 1996; Lee *et al.*, 2000; Leung, 1998; Ma, 1999; Pang, 1991; Ranguram *et al.*, 1996).

According to Saint Arnault (2009), practitioners can use culturally specific symptoms as a starting point to explore how their clients perceive their distress. Asian clients often experience their symptoms of distress as signs of weak character or failure to carry out important social roles. As a result they will also "experience shame, humiliation, anxiety or fear" and will "avoid disclosing it out of fear of the social consequences" (2009, p. 264).

Implicit social support

A useful way to work with elders who do not want to talk about their distress is by providing *implicit social support*, where practitioners provide emotional support without having clients feel that they have to disclose personal problems (Kim *et al.*, 2008). According to Kim and colleagues (ibid.), when people from a European background are in distress, they seek *explicit social support* by reaching out to their social networks to seek advice or emotional comfort. In seeking *explicit support*, people need to talk about their distress or reasons for needing assistance. Asians, on the other hand, seek *implicit social support* by thinking about people they are close to, or by being with others without discussing their problems. *Implicit social support* enables Asians to seek comfort without losing face or worrying about being a burden on others. In the next session, we will illustrate how practitioners work with elders by providing implicit support.

Voices of practitioners

- Understanding individuals as family members
- Helping clients feel comfortable receiving services
- Collaboration with volunteers and service providers
- Implicit social support – addressing problems without talking about them.

Understanding clients as family members

Vignette #1

Joyce is a medical social worker who works for a health clinic in Chinatown in New York City. Joyce often facilitates workshops on health care proxy and advanced directives of older Chinese immigrants. Under New York law, individuals can appoint a family member or friend to make health care decisions on their behalf if they lose the ability to make decisions for themselves. Joyce gives the Chinese translation of the health care proxy and explains the decisions that their health care proxy must make about their treatment. Elders who have had relatives die all say that they do not want to be on life support. But elders who have never been exposed to end-of-life care immediately start to think about their children and wonder about their children's preference rather than their own.

When we approached Joyce to ask about her work and to discuss what she thought was unique about working with Asian clients, her immediate response was, "You can't see your clients as individuals. You have to think about the family members who are part of their lives. You have to think of them as members of a close network." When it comes to care, elders are not going to tell you what they want. They first think of what their children want. As a medical social worker, she has worked with elders who agree to go through painful treatments for the sake of their children, even though they would prefer to receive palliative care.

Service utilization

Case management is an important part of service delivery for older adults. Practitioners assess the needs of clients, and connect them to appropriate services. As mentioned previously, Asian clients often do not feel comfortable receiving services because of stigma. Not feeling or understanding that they are entitled to receive services also hinders Asian elders from accessing services.

Case vignette: Mr. Kato

Mr. Kato is an 85-year-old Japanese man who lives alone in a rent-controlled apartment. Mr. Kato came to the US after graduating from college in

Japan to pursue his dreams of becoming a professional artist. After attending a program in fine arts, Mr. Kato worked for a small printing company while continuing to paint in his free time. He retired when he was in his late sixties, and pursued his interest in photography. Mr. Kato's parents and sister passed away shortly thereafter. While Mr. Kato had some regrets about not having married and being with family in his retirement years, he was able to enjoy his independence until he suffered from a mild stroke a year ago. The stroke left Mr. Kato with a slight speech impediment and difficulties with walking. Since his stroke, Mr. Kato stopped socializing, and spends most of his day alone in his apartment. He was referred to a Japanese American social service agency through his neighbor. Keiko, the social worker at the agency did an intake by making a home visit. Sensing Mr. Kato's reluctance on the phone, Keiko emphasized that the home visit was a courtesy visit to Japanese elders in the community. When Keiko arrived, she made small talk and tried not to ask questions that might appear to be intrusive. At the end of the visit, Keiko offered to make arrangements for home health attendant services for Mr. Kato, and suggested that she find transportation services so that he could attend a monthly social group for elders at her agency. Mr. Kato rejected both suggestions, saying that he was doing fine on his own, and that he did not want a stranger to come to his home. Keiko could see that Mr. Kato was feeling demoralized, but sensing that Mr. Kato did not wish to be perceived as vulnerable and needy, did not press the issue. She then told Mr. Kato that there was a group of women who was looking for volunteer work and asked if he was willing to let one of them visit him and bring him Japanese food. She also told Mr. Kato that he would need to pay for the food. Mr. Kato thought about it and said, "Sure, if I can be of use." Since then the volunteer, who is part of the Friendly Visitor program at Keiko's agency, has been visiting Mr. Kato with food purchased at a Japanese market. Mr. Kato, in turn, prepares tea and they talk.

Keiko meets with this volunteer on a regular basis to get information about Mr. Kato and makes suggestions on ways to assess any physical and psychological changes. The volunteer reports that Mr. Kato seems to look forward to the visits and has her name and day of visit marked on his calendar on his wall. Keiko makes sure that the volunteer continues to structure her visits with Mr. Kato, visiting on prearranged days and that the duration of her visit is an hour and a half. Keiko also calls Mr. Kato twice a month to see how he is doing. On the phone, Keiko gently asks how Mr. Kato is doing and asks him to call if he ever needs assistance.

This is not the first time that Keiko has worked with a Japanese elder who lives alone and who refuses services. Keiko knows that elders who are home bound and socially isolated need to be connected to services. Many Asian elders, like Mr. Kato, do not feel comfortable receiving assistance because they fear that it would be a drain on their limited income. They also do not want to be a burden on others. Japanese elders, in particular, have a tendency to reject help because of the cultural value of "*enryo*," to restrain oneself from receiving favors from others. By using the concept of mutuality, Keiko created an opportunity for Mr. Kato to feel empowered and reciprocate the help. By connecting elders with volunteers, and monitoring their conditions and needs, Kato also created a support network for clients like Mr. Kato to maintain their cultural sense of dignity and interdependence.

Implicit social support

Case vignette: Mr. Park

Mr. Park is a 78-year-old Korean man who lost his wife from cancer a year ago. He has one son who is in his forties and two grandchildren. Mr. Park's son, who lives in the suburbs, wanted him to move in with his family after his wife's death. Mr. Park, however, wants to continue to live in the apartment that he used to share with his wife. Mr. Park also does not want to be a burden on his daughter-in-law, who works full-time while taking care of her young children.

Lynn, a Korean social worker, works for the hospice program where Mrs. Park passed away. The hospice program follows up with bereaved families for a year following the patient's death, and Lynn was assigned to work with Mr. Park. Shortly after Mr. Park lost his wife, Lynn contacted him by phone, and told Mr. Park that she was calling to see how he was doing after his wife's death. As she does with other clients, Lynn told Mr. Park that it was okay if he didn't want to talk about his wife, an approach that was respectful of the cultural belief that emotions are private and not to be intruded upon. Lynn always starts the conversation by asking how Mr. Park is doing physically, and asks questions about his daily life. Typical conversations include:

"How have you been sleeping?" "Has anyone been calling you?" "Who visited you?" "Have you been taking your medicine?" "Have you eaten today?" "You don't feel like eating? Oh, yes, it's hot today, isn't it? I can see why you don't feel like going out. Make sure that you drink a lot of water." These are caring conversations commonly exchanged between family members.

Mr. Park knows that Lynn works for the hospice program, and that she is calling to check up on him. As she does with other clients, when Lynn first called Mr. Park, she told him that she was calling to follow up to see how he was doing after the death of his wife, but that it was okay if he didn't want to talk about his wife, that she was calling just to let him know that she was available. Lynn knows that Mr. Park has her telephone number close to his phone because on one occasion she asked if he had her number, and she could hear him reach out and pick up a piece of paper with her number.

Lynn reflects on her approach,

> If my client says that he doesn't want to talk about his grief, I can't force him. But when I ask them about their daily routines, they feel cared for. They have my phone number, and they know they can call anytime. Ninety-five percent of the time, they don't call. But it's their knowing that I am there for them that counts.

Lynn continues, "Sometimes we talk about everything except the presenting problem. But that is how you support and work with Asian clients." Lynn used to wonder if she was being too overprotective of her clients by not discussing their bereavement process. But she now realizes that her clients appreciate her gentle approach and her sensitivity to their need to protect themselves from breaking down emotionally with someone outside of the family.

Lynn's statement is consistent with many other practitioners that we talked to. Many practitioners reported that when working with Asian elders, they talk around the presenting problem and do not probe or ask about their emotional reactions to the problem. They do not necessarily share their interpretation of the problems, but follow the clients' lead in the conversation. Sometimes, clients will volunteer private thoughts and positive changes that they have made in their lives. From a relational perspective, the sense of acceptance and implicit emotional support communicated to the clients are the therapeutic approaches that facilitated such changes.

Case vignette: Mrs. Lee

Mrs. Lee is a 79-year-old Chinese woman who was referred to Kathy, a mental health practitioner. Mrs. Lee had gone to her primary care physician because she was experiencing frequent heart palpitations and shortness of breath. Mrs. Lee also complained of neck pains, insomnia, and loss of energy. Mrs. Lee had lost weight and told her physician that she thought she had a serious digestion problem because she did not have an appetite. None of Mrs. Lee's physical exams or laboratory work identified medical problems. Mrs. Lee's physician referred her to a psychiatrist who diagnosed her with depression and referred her for counseling. Mrs. Lee was not familiar with mental health counseling, but was willing to give it a try as she had a long trusting relationship with her physician.

Kathy learned from Mrs. Lee's physician that Mrs. Lee was a widow and that her younger son had passed away a year ago from lung cancer. Mrs. Lee originally had three children, a daughter and two sons. But the eldest son had also passed away three years ago from a heart attack. Mrs. Lee associated Kathy as a colleague of her physician, and appeared comfortable with Kathy's knowledge about her past. She acknowledged during her intake session that she had stopped going out since her younger son's death, and she explained that she did not want to go to the senior center because she did not want to tell people about her son's death.

As Mrs. Lee talked about her immigration history and family life, she often spoke with regret that she and her husband left their two-year old younger son with her mother-in-law while they emigrated to the US to start a small business. She felt she had been a "bad" mother to her younger son, and wondered if she had caused the death of both her sons because of some wrong doings in her previous life.

Kathy realized that from a Western psychodynamic perspective, Mrs. Lee's depression and grief was related to her feelings of guilt for leaving her son behind when he was a child. But instead of focusing on discussing these feelings, which would have required Mrs. Lee to delve further into a painful past, Kathy focused on normalizing Mrs. Lee's reactions. Kathy reminded Mrs. Lee that the welfare of the family always takes precedence over individual members.

Kathy validated how Mrs. Lee had to make money for the family, and that Mrs. Lee had fulfilled her role as a parent for all her children by moving to the US.

Kathy's reframing and acceptance of Mrs. Lee's decision to leave her son behind actually helped Mrs. Lee to talk about her feelings of grief and guilt. Mrs. Lee talked about how her son never reaped the benefits of her hard work, and that it should have been her that died. Kathy responded by tapping into Mrs. Lee's beliefs about fate and reminded her about how lives are often predestined. Kathy normalized Mrs. Lee's feelings by stating that she was not the only Chinese parent who left their young children to be cared for by their grandparents. Kathy also told Mrs. Lee how she was being a good parent to her younger son by caring for his children.

From the perspective of the Cultural Model of Health (Saint Arnault, 2009), Mrs. Lee's depression can be understood as her feelings of failure to attend to her younger son when he was a child. Rather than conceptualizing Mrs. Lee's regret toward leaving her son as an expression of guilt, Kathy framed the feelings as shame that came from the regret of not having fulfilled her role as a mother. Kathy tried to empower Mrs. Lee by reframing how Mrs. Lee had been a good mother by moving to the US for the sake of the family.

The practitioners provided a supportive relationship for their older clients. They did not probe nor solicit clients to talk about their emotions. At the same time they conveyed empathy by attending to their clients' unspoken emotions by *being with* their clients. The practitioners also attended to the cultural meanings behind the clients' expressions. With Mr. Kato, the practitioner understood the cultural dimensions of his refusing to seek help, and did not force the issue. Instead, she found an indirect way of attending to Mr. Kato's needs by using a volunteer. For Mr. Park, the practitioner attended to his emotional needs the way a family or friend would, which is the basis of implicit support (Kim *et al.*, 2008).

Following up with clients on the phone, a common method used by practitioners who work with older adults and with people who are bereaved, is an effective way to offer implicit support to Asian elders.

Discussion highlights

Demographic characteristics of Asian immigrant elders

Asian immigrant elders, on the whole, are a vulnerable group with high rates of poverty, low educational attainment, limited English proficiency, and low levels of assimilation into mainstream society. (p. 153)

Psychological distress among Asian immigrant elders

Risk factors for psychological well-being in late life include decrease in physical health and cognitive functioning, loss of social status, and loss of loved ones. (p. 153)

Demoralization is viewed as a useful construct to understand and treat distress among elders, especially the despair that is associated with the loss of meaning and purpose in life. (p. 158)

It is important to assess experiences of early trauma among elders because recent investigation indicates that symptoms that are highest after exposure decline for years and then increase in later life. (p. 159)

Older Asian women in the US have higher rates of suicide among women in their age cohort. (p. 159)

Working with Asian immigrant elders

Because Asian elders do not talk about their depressed mood, it is important for practitioners to understand ways in which psychological distress is expressed through somatic complaints. (p. 163)

Sometimes we talk about everything except the presenting problem. "But that is how you support and work with Asian clients" [quote from a practitioner]. (p. 167)

8 Suicide assessment and intervention with Asian immigrants

Irene W. Chung

Introduction

Suicide is a worldwide public health concern. The loss of an individual's life to suicide leaves a devastating effect on families and communities across all cultures and societies. According to the World Health Organization (2008), which compiles data from 105 countries around the world, suicide ranks among the top three leading causes of death for those aged 15–44 years; in some countries, suicide rates have increased by 60 percent in the last 50 years. Globally, almost one million people die from suicide each year; it is estimated that by 2020, rates will rise to 1.53 million. These figures do not include suicide attempts, which are up to 20 times more frequent than completed suicide. They also are exclusive of countries that do not report on the prevalence of suicide.

The prevalence of suicide in Western and Asian countries

Due to cultural stigma, religious beliefs, and legal implications, there are variations in the methods used to report and classify the nature of deaths in different countries. So suicide rates may not reflect the true prevalence of the problem. Suicidologists recommend that comparisons of suicide rates and risks between countries should be made with caution, and that suicide rates should be examined from the perspective of fluctuations and changes in trends over a period of time and their relevance to social, political, and economic issues in a specific country (Goldney, 2010; Scowcroft, 2012; Varnik, 2012). Table 8.1 is a sample of suicide rates among the five English-speaking countries that host a substantial number of Asian immigrants. The World Health Organization has deemed these countries' methods of reporting as consistent with its standards, and considered their suicide rates to be in the mid-range among countries that submit reports on suicide rates (Hendin *et al.*, 2008).

Table 8.2 is a sample of suicide rates among Asian countries from which the majority of Asian immigrants migrated. With the exception of Japan, these countries tend to be less consistent and methodical in compiling and reporting their suicide data, which results in a paucity of information and issues of validity. Overall their suicide rates appeared to be in the high range. Yet some researchers

Table 8.1 Suicide rates 2004–11, English-speaking countries

Suicide rates 2004–11 (per 100,000)					
Country	Year	Male	Female	Total suicide rate	Record low	Record high
England	2009	10.9	3.0	6.9	6.7 (2005)	10.7 (1955–60)
United States	2007	18.45	4.68	11.27	7.6 (1950)	12.7 (1975)
Canada	2004	17.3	5.4	11.3	7.1 (1955)	14.0 (1980)
Australia	2006	12.8	3.6	8.2	8.2 (2006)	14.9 (1965)
New Zealand	2011	19.36	6.2	12.65	9.1 (1965)	15.3 (1995)

Table 8.2 Suicide rates, Asian countries

Suicide rates 1993–2009 (per 100,000)					
Country	Year	Male	Female	Total suicide rate	Record low	Record high
Japan	2009	36.2	13.2	24.4	14.7 (1965)	25.1 (1955)
Philippines**	1993	2.5	1.7	2.1	0.7 (1960/70)	2.1 (1993)
India	2009	13.0	7.8	13.0	8.47 (1989)	11.4 (2010)
China*	1999	13.0	14.8	13.9	13.9 (1999)	17.6 (1987)
South Korea	2009	39.9	22.1	31.0	7.4 (1990)	31.0 (2009)

*Limited validity found in statistics for China – results were based on select sample sizes and locations. No real composite data for the country as a whole was found. Next to the Philippines, statistics for China were the most outdated of all countries.

** Limited availability for rates in the Philippines. However, there are indications that suicide trends in the Philippines are in keeping with the increases seen in a number of Asian countries – most notably Thailand, South Korea, Japan, and Hong Kong. In contrast, many Western countries have experienced reductions in rates since the 1980s (Redaniel *et al.*, 2011).

believe that these rates are still likely underestimates of suicide in many of the Asian countries, especially China and India whose populations make up more than one-third of the world's population, and regional studies have indicated high incidents of suicide in rural settings where there are greater administrative difficulties in collecting data on suicides (Beautrais, 2006; Hendin *et al.*, 2008; Li *et al.*, 2012; Vijayakumar, 2004). According to World Health Organization estimates (2008), China, India, and Japan may account for 40 percent of the world's suicides, and along with other Asian countries, for as high as 60 percent of the total number of suicides.

From a historical perspective, the predominance of suicide mortality has shifted from countries in Western Europe to Eastern Europe within the past 60 years, with recent trends indicating that it is moving to several countries in Asia. China is currently the only country in the world whose female suicide rate exceeds that of males. South Korea, with the highest female suicide rate in the world and extremely high male suicide rate, is projected to be the country with the top suicide rate worldwide (Varnik, 2012). While economic downturn, and social and political instability are generally the contextual issues that precipitate the increase of suicide trends in any given country, cultural values and norms in shaping how individuals react and adapt to these changes are equally important influences (De Leo, 2002; Beautrais, 2006; McKenzie *et al.*, 2002). As practitioners, we need to understand that suicide is rarely an impulsive act. It is a cumulative outcome from the interplay of various dimensions of an individual's life. In the following section, we will utilize an integrative approach in discussing the major theories that examine the complex phenomenon of suicide.

The complexities of suicidal behavior

- Social context
- Psychological struggles
- Personal proclivities and coping mechanisms
- Cultural influences.

Historically, the study of suicide began with the work of Durkheim (1897) who postulated that the failure of social institutions, i.e., government, church, and family, to provide a sense of integration and purpose was the root cause of suicidal behavior prompted by feelings of isolation, alienation, and hopelessness. Freud (1916) and other psychodynamic-oriented theorists, on the other hand, focus on the individual's intrapsychic dynamics of coping with psychological pain and losses, and the conscious and unconscious communication of distress and conflicted emotions toward loved ones through the suicidal behavior, which can symbolize retaliation, self-punishment, or longings for reunion or a mix of all these emotions (Hendin, 1978; Menninger, 1938; Schneidman, 1993).

With the advance of neuroscience, recent studies on suicide have focused on physiological and genetic factors impacting impulse control, emotional and mood regulation, as well as substance abuse that may present impairments in judgment and coping mechanisms in times of stress (Bartels *et al.*, 2002; De Leo, 2002; Joiner, 2002; Mann, 1998; Oquendo *et al.*, 2000). At the same time, the increasing prominence of cognitive therapy in the last two decades also produced findings that show a robust correlation between suicide and cognitive vulnerabilities such as dichotomous thinking, cognitive rigidity, and deficient problem-solving capacity, particularly among adolescents (Ellis and Rutherford, 2008). Aaron Beck, a pioneer of cognitive therapy, identified hopelessness in his studies as a key psychological factor that is independent of depression in suicide ideations, attempts, and completion (Beck *et al.*, 1990; Beck *et al.*, 1999).

There is an increasing consensus among suicidologists that suicides and attempted suicides are complex phenomena that cannot be explained by or attributed to a single trigger or direct cause. The aforementioned cognitive vulnerabilities, for example, can be perceived as both genetic predisposition and learned perceptions due to environmental influences. Hopelessness is subjectively experienced by the individual and influenced by cultural values of purpose and meaning in his life and the quality of external support he receives. The varying rates and patterns of suicide as characterized by age groups, gender, and geographical settings in different countries are strong indications that sociocultural issues such as gender roles, help-seeking values and norms, support systems, and resources can amplify the aforementioned biological and psychological risk factors. As mentioned earlier, studies have indicated that there are high rates of suicide among young women in China and India in rural settings, citing interpersonal problems exacerbated by their traditional low socioeconomic status, lack of mental health services, and poor support systems as major suicide risk factors (Bhugra and Desai, 2002; Ji, 2000; Kamal and Loewenthal, 2002; Phillips *et al.*, 2002; Qin and Mortensen, 2001; Yip *et al.*, 2000; Zhang *et al.*, 2004). However, none of these factors could stand alone as the sole cause of the young women's suicide. It is the culmination of the reciprocal and circular dynamics of the psychological, biological, social, and cultural factors in these young women's life that needs to be examined as a cohesive narrative. This inclusive and interactive perspective provides a more process-oriented and contextualized approach in understanding the complexities of suicidal behavior (Bhugra, 2002; Chung, 2011; De Leo, 2002; Leenaars, 2008; McKenzie *et al.*, 2003).

In this chapter, we will utilize this multi-dimensional and systemic approach in discussing assessment and intervention of suicidal behaviors among Asian immigrants. We will focus on individuals with serious intention to end their lives underlying their suicidal thoughts, plans, and attempts. We will first discuss study findings in regard to these suicidal behaviors among Asian immigrants in English-speaking countries and their implications of risk and protective factors relevant to this population as well as practice challenges. In the last section of the chapter, we will present experiences and reflections from practitioners in the various Asian communities as well as their use of relational approaches that are integrated into assessment and interventions.

Suicidal behavior in the Asian immigrant communities

- Paucity of data and research challenges
- Inconsistent outcomes between national data and small sample studies.

There is a dearth of literature and studies on suicide and suicidal behavior in the Asian immigrant communities in the US and other English-speaking countries (Bhugra and Desai, 2002; Cheng *et al.*, 2010; Kennedy *et al.*, 2005; Leong *et al.*, 2008). With the exception of studies in the United Kingdom where young South Asian women were the target of inquiry, the existing literature tends to address Asian ethnic and immigrant groups as one singular population without reference to the specific sociocultural differences of each group and the within-group differences between immigrant and second generation Asians in the host country (Cheng *et al.*, 2010; Duldulao *et al.*, 2009; Ineichen, 2008).

In terms of suicide rates among Asians in the English-speaking countries, the only information available pertains to the US and New Zealand, which appear to be within mid-range or even lower compared to other racial groups (see Table 8.3). Apparently, ethnicity is not reported on death certificates in the United Kingdom, Canada, and Australia (Bird, 2011; Canadian Vital Statistics System 2010; Scowcroft, 2012), thus making it difficult to compile accurate data of suicide rates among its ethnic groups.

In Australia, a study that examined the patterns of suicide rates among immigrant groups from 1974 to 2006 shows an unusual trend between Asian female and male immigrants (Ide *et al.*, 2012). Asian women, especially those from India, had the lowest suicide rate compared to all immigrant groups during that period. Older women from Korea, China, Hong Kong, and Japan also showed lower suicide rates compared to other female groups in Australia as well as those in their home countries. On the other hand, Asian males showed comparable suicide rates with those in their home countries. Suicide rates of Asian males from Korea ranked high along with other immigrant males from several European countries. The study, however, did not offer any insights into the low suicide rates among Asian immigrant women.

Findings from small national and local study samples with Asians and Asian immigrants in the United States and the United Kingdom seemed to indicate that suicidal behavior might be a regional concern:

- A study on help-seeking behavior among Asian Americans indicated that suicidality was listed as the second most frequently reported clinical issue (after

Table 8.3 Suicide rates, Asian populations

Suicide rates: Asian population (per 100,000)			
Country	Year	Asians	General population
New Zealand	2011	5.36	6.2
United States	2007	11.27	6.18

Note: The lifetime estimate of suicide attempts and suicide ideation among Asian Americans representative of four major subgroups from a recent national study of 2095 participants was 8.8 percent and 2.5 percent respectively – a moderate rate compared to other racial groups (Cheng *et al.*, 2010).

depression) by a sample of 1,783 individuals from seven Asian ethnic groups – Cambodian, Chinese, Filipino, lu Mien, Japanese, Korean, and Vietnamese (Akutsu and Chu, 2006).

• A data report from the New York City Department of Health and Mental Hygiene (2012) indicated that suicide rates among Asians in New York City increased by 67 percent between 2000 and 2008, mostly due to the huge increase of suicides among Asian women.

• Older Asian women between the ages of 65 and 84 had the highest suicide rate among females from different racial backgrounds in the US in 2007 (Bartels *et al.*, 2002; Heron, 2011; Xu *et al.*, 2010). The fact that their suicide rate increased with aging was a sharp contrast from the general suicide rate among older females. Given the short history of immigration among Asian women in the United States, there is a good possibility that the majority of these older Asian women were immigrants.

• A similar trend was found among older Chinese immigrant women aged 65– 85 in England and Wales during the period 2001–5 (Shah *et al.*, 2011). Their suicide rate was also higher than that of older males worldwide which generally increases with aging.

• In the past three decades, young South Asian women from the various coun- tries in the Indian subcontinent, predominantly those in the 18–24 age group, have shown higher rates of suicide and suicide attempts compared to South Asian males and other racial groups in the United Kingdom (Bhugra, 2002; Bhugra and Desai, 2002; Burr, 2002; Glover *et al.*, 1989; Hicks and Bhugra, 2003; Ineichen, 2008; McKenzie *et al.*, 2003; Neeleman and Wessely, 1999; Soni Raleigh and Balarajan, 1992). Conflicts with family, violence by spouse, and depression were cited as the major risk factors for these women. Their circumstances and stressors were similar to those faced by South Asian women in the Indian subcontinent who also showed a high suicide rate and whose deaths by burning are often dismissed as "kitchen accidents" (Kamal and Loewenthal, 2002). Apparently the female submissive roles in the hierarchical familial and social structure in India remain a major stressor for these women after their immigration to the UK.

The varying rates of Asian immigrant groups in different countries need to be examined more closely from the perspective of the interplay of cultural beliefs and the social environment of the host countries. Some researchers believe that there is a strong correlation between suicide rates of immigrants and those in their countries of origin because of their identification with culturally defined help-seeking behavior, coping mechanisms, and perception of stressors (Ide *et al.*, 2012; Mullen and Smyth, 2004; Kennedy *et al.*, 2005). However, it is also important to consider the response of the host culture to the specific ethnic immigrant group (McKenzie *et al.*, 2003). It is not uncommon that Asian immigrants encounter racism and discriminatory policies as additional stressors (Cheng *et al.*, 2010). On the other hand, the host country's embracement of racial diversities and offering of opportunities for personal gains and enriched quality of life will ameliorate some of the acculturation difficulties faced by immigrants.

Overall, it is difficult to ascertain the prevalence and severity of suicidal behavior among Asian immigrants based on the limited findings of studies that are available. Many researchers believe that suicides and attempted suicides among Asians are generally underreported due to personal and familial shame associated with cultural stigma and the substantial number of Asians who are not consumers of the mental health system (Akutsu and Chu, 2006; Cheng *et al.*, 2010; Kahn and Reza, 2000).

Suicide risk and protective factors in the Asian immigrant communities

- Common suicide risk and protective factors
- The interplay of acculturation difficulties, mental illness, and help-seeking behavior in the context of the sociocultural realities of Asian immigrants

Suicide risk factors are characteristics of an individual or a group of individuals from a similar sociocultural environment as well as negative events that may heighten the possibility of contemplating and attempting suicide (Rudd *et al.*, 2006). Conversely, suicide protective factors are individual and group assets as well as circumstances that provide motivation for living, sustain hope, and support coping mechanisms in times of setbacks and distress.

Based on research findings, a history of suicide attempts is one of the highest suicide risk factors for individuals (Chandrasekaran and Gnanaselane, 2008; Skogman *et al.*, 2004; Wang and Mortensen, 2006). Researchers attributed the risk to heightened sensitivity to suicidal ideations and diminishing fear and pain associated with exposure to self-harm behavior (Ellis and Rutherford, 2008; Joiner, 2002). Psychiatric and personality disorders, family history of suicide, and conflicts with family are also significant individual risk factors that contribute to impairment of judgment, impulse control, problem-solving, as well a sense of loss and isolation.

On a societal and community level, cultural values, which ascribe meanings to circumstances and behavior, can become both suicide risk and protective factors (Lester, 2008). For example, the ending of one's life to preserve the honor of an individual or group is acceptable in some societies, whereas abandoning one's responsibilities and obligations to the family is frowned upon. In a hierarchical and patriarchal society, women's roles and self-worth are built around subordination to their spouses and elders in the family. The implication to some of these women who may not be able to change a tradition that is deeply ingrained in the fabric of society can lead to a sense of helplessness and an internalization of their anger, all of which are psychological precursors to suicidal ideations. On the other hand, their attachment ties to their children or the sense of gratification gained from raising their children may mitigate their suicidal risk.

Suicide risk factors cannot stand alone as predictors of an individual's suicidal behavior. They should be examined in the context of the individual's subjective experience and his or her current protective factors. They are cautionary markers for practitioners as they work with clients who may exhibit signs of suicide or struggling with multiple stressors.

As individuals, Asian immigrants have to cope with life stressors that are universal in all societies such as unemployment, marital problems, chronic illness, and loss of loved ones. However, their migration to a different environment where they are challenged by acculturation issues, such as language barriers, incompatible job skills, loss of supportive networks, changes in lifestyle and identity, etc., can severely undermine their coping mechanisms and sense of well-being. Studies have shown that acculturation stress can culminate in depression and increase the risk of schizophrenia among immigrant groups (Kuo and Tsai, 1986; Silveira and Ebrahim, 1998; Eaton and Harrison, 2000). In addition, the negative meanings they attribute to these stressors as shaped by cultural and immigrant values such as personal failures in the pursuit of immigrant dreams, and the lack of support and resources they receive in alleviating the stressors can become another source of distress. So acculturation difficulties and the sociocultural realities of immigrants can become significant correlates of suicide risk factors (Chung, 2011; Hjern and Allebeck, 2002; Leong *et al.*, 2008; Sundaram *et al.*, 2006).

The interplay of psychiatric illness and sociocultural issues can be another factor that poses additional suicide risk to the Asian immigrant populations. Findings of studies in the US and European countries indicate that pervasive feelings of hopelessness caused by depression, impulsivity and poor judgment aggravated by labile moods, and psychotic symptoms such as auditory delusions severely impaired the mental acuity of individuals and put them at great risk of harming themselves in times of distress (Blair-West *et al.*, 1999; Kreyenbuhl *et al.*, 2002; Oquendo *et al.*, 2000). In addition to depression and the spectrum of schizophrenia disorders, Asian and other ethnic immigrants who came as refugees or undocumented immigrants are at risk of suffering from post traumatic stress disorder (Fazel *et al.*, 2005). Studies have shown that individuals tend to recover from transient emotional and physical symptoms after exposure to traumatic events, but their risk for PTSD increased with life stressors (Brewin *et al.*, 2000).

In the United States, studies have shown that 90 percent of individuals who die from suicide carry a diagnosis of psychiatric illness, but less than one-third of them have sought treatment (Cavanagh *et al.*, 2003; Conwell *et al.*, 1996). While most people who suffer from mental illness do not attempt suicide, this is a strong indication that undiagnosed and untreated mental illness is a serious suicide risk. For Asian immigrants, their perception of mental illness and willingness to seek treatment is very much influenced by cultural beliefs and immigrant-specific circumstances. Findings of studies among Asians in their home and host countries indicate that there is a general lack of recognition and acceptance of mental illness, which is oftentimes attributed to character weakness and personal failure (Jang *et al.*, 2009; Thompson *et al.*, 2002; Zane and Mak, 2003). In addition, there is also the obstacle of the lack of bilingual and culturally responsive mental health services for those who wish to seek treatment (Chu and Sue, 2011). In the US, studies have found that the lower use of mental health services is inclusive of all Asian subgroups and differences in age, gender, education, and geographic location (Abe-Kim *et al.*, 2007; Meyer *et al.*, 2009). Among Asian Americans with a probable mental illness, only 28 percent utilized mental health services, in contrast to 54 percent of the general population (Wang *et al.*, 2005). The under-utilization of mental health services has also been found among Asian immigrants in Canada (Chan-Yip and Kirmayer, 1998; Chen and Kazanjian, 2005), Australia (Stuart *et al.*, 1996; Thompson *et al.*, 2002) and the United Kingdom (Gupta, 1991; Pilkington *et al.*, 2011). Findings of these studies indicate that cultural stigma and shame associated with mental illness and the lack of culturally relevant services are major deterrents to the utilization of services. A qualitative study of Chinese immigrants from low socioeconomic backgrounds who suffered from psychiatric disorders and attempted suicides in New York City showed that more than two-thirds of the 31 participants were not knowledgeable of mental health services in the community until their mental illness symptoms became severe or *after* their suicide attempts (Chung, 2011). Prior to their suicide attempts, their lack of knowledge of mental health symptoms and lack of support from their families to seek psychiatric treatment had left them in a vicious cycle of seeking indigenous or medical treatment, resuming employment and/or family responsibilities, and experiencing more severe symptoms that undermined their level of functioning. Their suicide attempts were generally made in a state of hopelessness with feelings of failure and helplessness as well as intolerable physiological symptoms from the untreated mental illness.

The aforementioned study also offered a nuanced view of another aspect of help-seeking behavior that can be a suicide risk factor for Asian immigrants. In the Asian culture, familial approval and support is a major protective factor in times of distress (Leong *et al.*, 2008). However, the stressors experienced by the suicide attempters – marital conflicts among the women, difficulties with main-taining unemployment among the men, and inability to pay back family debt for smuggling fees among the undocumented immigrants – were issues deemed as personal failures in the fulfillment of cultural obligations and responsibilities. In the study, half of the women did not disclose their marital problems to their families; two-thirds of the men did not disclose their employment issues to their families. The small number of men and women who shared their distress with their families in their home country were advised to endure their hardships. The social realities of these immigrants – lack of financial and social resources to start a new life also created more obstacles in help-seeking and amplified their suicidal behavior (Chung, 2010).

Suicide assessment and intervention

The suicide assessment process

- Common signs of suicide
- Agency protocol for suicide assessment
- Challenges for practitioners.

Warning Signs (Affective and behavioral)		**Risk Factors**
• Writing/remarks suggestive of suicide, death, hopelessness • Impulsive, risk-taking behavior • Preoccupation with death or violence • Sudden changes in personality, daily routine • Withdrawal from friends/activities • Giving away property or disregard for one's belongings	**vs**	• Persistent relationship problems (family, friends, partner) • Social isolation • History of previous suicide attempts • Substance use/abuse • History of depression • Significant loss (death of loved one, employment) • Recurrent feelings of hopelessness and helplessness due to prolonged perceived, unmanageable stress or pressure • Setbacks in academic, career or personal pursuits

Figure 8.1 Suicide warning signs vs. risk factors

Signs of suicide are different from suicide risk factors that we discussed earlier (see Figure 8.1). Warning signs are affective and behavioral indications that an individual may be at imminent risk of suicide. They include remarks or writings that hint at a sense of hopelessness toward life, impulsive and risk-taking behavior, preoccupation with death or violence, and changes in personality or daily routine (Rudd *et al.*, 2006).

In agency settings, a practitioner generally meets with the client immediately to explore his/her suicidal ideation and plan when warning signs of suicide are observed. The practitioner will then consult with supervisory staff to further assess the client's risk and protective factors and determine if the client requires hospitalization or referral to outpatient mental health services.

There are a host of suicide risk assessment instruments developed to measure psychosocial variables that correlate with the severity of suicidal ideation among adult and adolescent populations. The most common ones are the Scale for Suicide Ideation (Beck *et al.*, 1997), the Reasons for Living Inventory (Linehan *et al.*, 1983). However, suicide risk assessment instruments tend to be lengthy and impersonal, and are used more for research rather than at agency settings (Jobes, 2000). The suicide assessment protocol of most agencies generally focuses on the development of an appropriate referral plan based on the client's suicidal thoughts and plans and her internal states such as psychotic symptoms and sense of reality, and specific risk factors such as living alone and access to lethal means.

Unfortunately there are no assessment approaches that can accurately predict if and when an individual will kill herself. The complexities of suicidal behavior as impacted by the individual's internal and external forces present tremendous challenges in suicide assessment. Suicidal feelings wax and wane (Daigle, 2005;

Freedenthal, 2007). Life events and circumstances also change over time. Thus ongoing suicide assessment and timely intervention as a proactive measure is important for individuals deemed as having high suicide risk (Granello and Granello, 2007).

The suicide assessment process is often a daunting task for practitioners (Ellis and Patel, 2012; Jobes and Drozd, 2004). Exploring details of suicidality can often evoke the practitioner's instinctive fears of human mortality and conflicts with personal values. Some practitioners who are not experienced in suicide assessment may harbor the fear that exploring and validating the client's reasons for having suicidal thoughts will be perceived as a sanction for their suicidal behavior. The issue of professional liability and malpractice charges in the event of the client's acting out his suicidal ideation is always a looming burden for the practitioner. Thus the practitioner's reactions and feelings of discomfort in a client's suicidal crisis can hamper her ability to be supportive toward the client.

Suicide intervention and treatment

- Psychopharmocology and psychiatric hospitalization
- Treating suicidal behavior as a central issue and not symptoms of mental illness
- Integration of approaches: cognitive and behavioral, psychodynamic and relational theories
- Providing assessment and intervention as a seamless approach.

Studies have shown that the traditional treatment trajectory of psychopharmocology and psychiatric hospitalization for suicidal patients have not been substantially effective in reducing their suicidal risks (Baldessarini *et al.*, 2006; Cipriani *et al.*, 2005; Jobes, 2000; Meltzer *et al.*, 2003). Other studies also indicated that a client's non-adherence to medication regimen and short periods of hospitalization as mandated by managed care are serious impediments to this treatment modality (Gipson and King, 2012; Jobes and Drozd, 2004).

On the other hand, there are only a small number of clinical trials focusing on effective interventions and treatment for the reduction of suicidal behavior, due to the concern with liability and logistical issues of research with suicide high-risk individuals (Linehan *et al.*, 2012). Thus far, outcome evidence on cognitive and behavioral approaches has shown some measures of effectiveness (Ellis and Goldston, 2012). These approaches focus on helping clients enhance their self-awareness and coping skills in regard to identified "cognitive vulnerabilities" such as low threshold of affect distress· tolerance, constriction of thought process, and problem-solving capabilities during a suicidal crisis triggered by specific events. Other approaches that showed promising outcomes focus on mitigating the sense of hopelessness and the lack of interpersonal connection commonly experienced by suicidal clients (Daniel and Goldston, 2012; Joiner, 2005). Overall, there is consensus among suicidologists that it is important to offer an integration of approaches that address the individualized needs of the suicidal client (Ellis and Goldston, 2012).

In the following section, we will present some contemporary models that integrate assessment and intervention approaches from cognitive behavioral therapy, psychodynamic and relational theories.

Use of safety plans as a short-term intervention

In recent years, practitioners in both acute and non-acute clinical settings have increasingly utilized the safety plan as an intervention when the suicidal risks of a client seem to be less imminent. This is a transition from the traditional approach of using a written contract with the patient whereby she agrees not to harm herself and that she will contact resources listed on the contract if she cannot manage her suicidal thoughts. Some suicidologists have expressed concern that the use of a contract is primarily a reassurance for the clinician and the institution without providing much help to the client in honoring the agreement (Kelly and Knudson, 2000; Kroll, 2000). The contemporary suicide plan intervention (SPI) adopts a cognitive behavioral approach that elicits the client's input in identifying triggers and warning signs of her suicidal thoughts, as well as her own strategies in alleviating these thoughts, i.e., venues of self-distraction such as watching TV, listening to music, or taking a walk. The plan is a collaborative effort that essentially provides an individualized intervention by empowering the client to develop adaptive coping strategies on an ongoing basis (Stanley and Brown, 2012). When the client is asked to think of family members and peers to contact, the clinician will explore with the client the nature of support she anticipates getting from these individuals. Finally, the client will be involved in planning for the removal of any lethal means to minimize the risk of impulsive acts.

Example of a safety plan

Step 1: Identify warning signs and triggers (in client's own words)
1   Suicidal thoughts: feelings of worthlessness or hopelessness
2   Hearing voices

Step 2: Internal coping strategies; things that can be done to distract self
1   Listen to music
2   Take a walk
3   Watch TV

Step 3: Social situations and people that can help to distract
1   Meet friend (name)
2   Go to a neighborhood coffee house

Step 4: People who I can ask for help
1   Family member (name), phone #
2   Friend (name), phone #

Step 5: Professionals or agencies I can contact during crisis
1   Psychiatrist (name), phone #
2   Clinician (name), phone #
3   Local hospital emergency department
    Address
    Phone #
4   Asian Mental Health Lifeline, phone #

Step 6: Making the environment safe
1   Keep only necessary, small amount of pills/medications in the home
2   Put scissors and knives in a locked, hard-to-reach place at home
(Adapted from Stanley and Brown, 2012)

Use of relational approaches in suicide assessment and intervention

There is increasing recognition among clinicians and researchers that suicidality needs to be treated as a central issue of the client and not just a symptom of mental illness that can be managed by psychiatric treatment (Jobes and Drozd, 2004; Joiner, 2005; Linehan *et al.*, 2012). The implication is that the client's experience of unbearable psychological pain as an underlying issue of suicide has to be addressed in the assessment and intervention process as well. This requires the practitioner to first understand and accept the client's perception of suicidal behavior as an "option" of coping with her stressors and resolving life dilemmas (Linehan *et al.*, 2012). Showing acceptance of the client's perception and being there with the client are key relational approaches that create therapeutic bonding with the client. Many suicidologists believe that a suicidal client's willingness to disclose his suicidal thoughts directly or indirectly is actually an indication that he is seeking human connection that may mitigate his desire to die. In other words, there are always feelings of ambivalence underlying every individual's suicide plan and act. Most people look for reasons to live as they ponder over their reasons to die (Daigle, 2005; Freedenthal, 2007). Jobes (2000, p. 12) aptly indicates that a practitioner who is willing to "offer a real *relationship*" to the client and "truly joins (her) in the depths of suicidal behavior" while maintaining clinical judgment and wisdom creates for the client a powerful and viable option to suicide. On the other hand, the traditional neutral stance of the practitioner can be perceived as a rejection and reinforces the client's suicidal ideation that life is not worth living.

The therapeutic relationship in a suicidal crisis also emphasizes the importance for the practitioner to listen empathically to the client's narratives and understand what it means for the client to be suicidal. Studies have found that the opportunity for the client to discuss her suicidal ideations and ventilate her distress with an empathic practitioner can diffuse the suicidal crisis (Apter *et al.*, 2001; Callahan, 1994; Ruddell and Curwen, 2002; Westefeld *et al.*, 2000).

The use of a strong therapeutic alliance based on acceptance of and empathy for the client's suicidal ideations has been adopted with success in several suicide assessment and intervention protocols such as the Dialectical Behavior Therapy (DBT) and the Comprehensive Assessment and Management of Suicidality (CAMS) in outpatient settings (Jobes, 2000; Jobes and Drozd, 2004). As a major component of the collaborative process, the practitioner helps the client organize his feelings, impulses, and perceptions into a cohesive narrative that lends insights into the client's psychological pain, the sources of his stress, his perception of hopelessness, the negative aspects of his self-worth, and the specifics of his arousal symptoms. A comprehensive and individualized treatment plan that may include psychoeducation, cognitive and behavioral approaches, psychotherapy, family therapy, and group therapy is developed to address the range of issues identified in the assessment process.

Voices of practitioners

There was a general consensus among the practitioners who shared their experiences with us that suicidal ideation and attempts are common among the Asian immigrant client population that they serve in New York City. A coordinator of a multi-lingual mental health hotline for Asians in New York City estimated that 70 percent of their phone callers expressed suicidal ideation (T. Luo, personal communication, 30 July 2012). A social worker of an inpatient psychiatric unit estimated that 80 percent of the Korean patients admitted were due to suicidal behavior (J. Lim, personal communication, 15 August 2012). A recent report released by the New York City Department of Health and Mental Hygiene (2012) indicated that there was a 67 percent increase of suicides among Asians from 2000 to 2008 due to a substantial increase in suicides by Asian women.

The demographic and psychosocial profiles of the Asian clients served by these practitioners are similar in many ways to those discussed in our literature review of the suicide-risk immigrant population in other Asian communities. They are generally of low socioeconomic background, and appear to struggle with acculturation stressors, depression or other mental illness, as well as a multitude of negative life events such as employment issues, family conflicts, and social isolation. While it is likely that the interplay of their background, life stressors, help-seeking behavior, and their environment may not be totally representative of other Asian immigrant communities, the voices of the practitioners presented in the following sections do offer us a glimpse of the challenges of working with suicidal Asian immigrant clients and how their use of relational approaches helped to engage these clients in diffusing their suicidal crisis.

Practice challenges

Suicide assessment and intervention is an integral part of intake and ongoing work with Asian immigrant clients in all mental health settings. In other settings, practitioners are trained to explore their clients' suicidal ideations when they observe signs of suicide among their clients. These agency protocols are important as a "start", as one practitioner put it, but posing suicide assessment questions to clients, especially Asian clients who are disinclined to answer sensitive questions and disclose their emotions directly, may not be sufficient. There is generally a great deal of shame associated with having to disclose one's past and/or current suicidal behavior. Unlike altruistic suicides that are sanctioned by some Asian cultures as an honorable means to make a political or social statement, immigrant suicidal behavior is generally perceived by the individual and his family as an admission of personal failings and character weakness. In addition, those who are familiar with the mental health system are aware of the possibility of psychiatric hospitalization if they reveal their suicidal intent. This will create another layer of stigma and shame as well as disruption of their work and family responsibilities. Such negative feelings are palpable in the common remarks made by those who attempted suicide: "I did not really want to die"; "I just wanted to sleep"; "I heard voices telling me to jump"; "I don't belong here (hospital) ... It will really make me crazy if I stay."

Many practitioners acknowledged that the task of suicide assessment with Asian immigrant clients can be stressful and challenging. On one hand, they are charged by agency protocol to make a quick treatment recommendation that will protect the client as well as the liability of the institution. Hospitalization is a relatively direct disposition in the case of the client exhibiting psychotic symptoms and posing a threat to himself and/or others. However, the practitioners will have to exercise their clinical judgment judiciously when they are uncertain if their clients are being forthcoming in regard to the level of their distress and suicidal intention. While hospitalization can ultimately provide a safe environment for the client, the experience of being hospitalized, especially against one's will, and sometimes being taken away under restraints, can be very traumatic and humiliating for immigrant clients who speak little or no English. One practitioner recalled an undocumented immigrant client from China saying to her, "My family sent me off on a boat to America, and then you sent me off again to fend for myself." Thus the familial dynamics of ethnocultural transference and countertransference are inevitable when the practitioner becomes the client's major source of resource and support. It is difficult not to feel the tremendous sense of responsibility to make the appropriate assessment and plan for these clients.

A client's suicidal crisis certainly triggers a myriad of strong feelings between the practitioner and the client, and it can put a strain on the therapeutic alliance. The common practice wisdom in doing suicide assessment is to pose direct questions using words like "suicide" or "killing yourself" to avoid clients providing ambiguous and evasive responses. From an Asian cultural perspective, such a direct and personal question can be considered highly intrusive and offensive, and may easily alienate the client and induce feelings of failure and shame. However, the practitioners agree that Asian clients generally appreciate the direct inquiry on this important issue if it is communicated with concern and respect. In addition, the practitioners caution against the pitfall of assuming an authoritative position during such times. While literature has often suggested that talking with authority would be a culturally relevant approach to engage Asian clients, the practitioners felt strongly that telling the client that he should not kill himself or remind him of his obligations and responsibilities as "reasons for living" can come across as critical of the client at a time when the client needs unconditional acceptance and support.

Relational approaches in suicide assessment

In this section, we present a summary of the relational approaches that the practitioners used to create a more supportive and culturally relevant context in conducting suicide assessment:

Initiating the conversation

The practitioner starts with inquiring about specifics of the client's daily routines such as recent sleeping and eating patterns and then transitions to her emotional well-being. The practitioner listens to the client's narratives of her circumstances and stressors and makes empathic comments such as "It seems like you have gone through some very rough times. How have you been coping?" Some clients can be evasive in their response, and the practitioner may preface the question by saying, "Some people will think about ending their lives when life is so stressful." Other clients may make comments with death ideations: "Life is really tough. What's the purpose of living your life?" The practitioner will then pose the question using the client's words instead of making an interpretation of the nature of her emotional distress that she may not be ready to hear, "So if you feel that there is no purpose in life, are you thinking about killing yourself?" If the client answers "no" or minimizes the severity of her suicidal ideation, the practitioner will not persist and question the validity of the response even though the client's affect and tone of voice communicate hints of denial. From a relational theory perspective, it is important for the practitioner to view the client's behavior as a defense against her vulnerabilities or distrust of the practitioner. From an Asian cultural perspective, it is imperative that the practitioner does not turn it into an interrogation or investigation to "save face" for the client.

Exploring with new clients

If the practitioner does not know the client well and he is reticent about his life circumstances, she may take a respectful stance by asking for permission from him to talk about more "personal" issues. She will proceed cautiously starting with general questions about stressors and then checking periodically with the client in regard to his comfort level before posing more specific questions about suicide ideations. From a relational and cultural perspective, the practitioner alters the asymmetrical power dynamics inherent in the assessment process by letting the client take the lead in the discussion. While it appears that the client may decide to end the conversation, the feelings of empowerment and respect communicated to the client can often became an incentive for him to connect with someone who genuinely accepts him for who he is.

Probing for more information

In the event that a client denies his suicidal ideation or plan, some practitioners may pose questions to explore the client's protective factors such as "What stops you from killing yourself now?" But they will preface it with a personal remark such as "I am so glad to hear that you are not giving up on life." Other practitioners may inquire about the client's activity plans for the coming week to get a sense of the client's inner thoughts and preoccupation. Indeed, the practitioners often have to walk the fine line between accepting the Asian client's reluctance to disclose and creating or taking advantage of opportunities to engage the client in further discussion. The practitioner's own comfort level and attunement to the client's readiness are crucial in this process. A few practitioners recalled how their clients' responses to suicide assessment questions became more revealing as they intuitively picked up that their clients were communicating their distress tangentially and metaphorically and decided to stay in the conversation with the client. For example, a young South Asian female client who was screened in a hospital emergency room and assessed as "low suicide risk" with depression symptoms began to talk about her suicidal ideations in delusional terms when the practitioner accepted her remark that she saw someone standing behind him. As the practitioner engaged her in further conversation about that, she said "I hear that person telling me that he will be taking me away with him." Eventually her answers to suicidal thoughts also changed from "none" to "sometimes" to "often." The client also disclosed that her family often got upset when she talked about visions and voices, so she had tried to keep them to herself, which became increasingly difficult and triggered her suicidal thoughts.

The approaches presented by the practitioners illustrated some typical nuances in the suicide assessment process with Asian immigrant clients. The ideal scenario whereby the client will voluntarily disclose her suicidal thoughts and seek help rarely happens. The practitioners are in agreement that a client will only disclose information about his past and current suicidal behavior if he senses that "the practitioner is really trying to help and will not judge" him. The implication is that suicide assessment is only effective in the context of a trusting and supportive relationship with the practitioner. It is important to keep in mind that the purpose of suicide assessment is to pre-empt and prevent the tragedy of suicide, and it should include identifying the underlying issues of the client's suicide ideations to inform the treatment plan. Making a clinical judgment that a client is suicidal is not necessarily a therapeutic intervention. Even hospitalization of the client in the case of a suicidal crisis is not a guarantee that the client will not attempt suicide. Rather, the empathic connection between the practitioner and the client during the assessment process that helps the client regain his sense of hope in life and engage in treatment is the beginning of an effective intervention. Many practitioners recalled clients who volunteered information about their past suicidal behavior *after* they developed a trusting relationship with them. So suicide assessment is essentially a process that evolves with the relationship between the practitioner and the client.

The following case scenarios illustrate how the therapeutic relationship characterized by acceptance and empowerment of the clients provided a safe environment for them to disclose past suicidal behavior and offered opportunities for healing.

Case vignette: Ms. Kim

Mrs. Kim, an older widow who spoke little English, had been seeing Hae Na, her social worker at the outpatient mental health clinic for a couple of years. Mrs. Kim experienced panic attacks shortly after she emigrated to the US from Korea. She initially did not recognize the symptoms as panic attacks and began to have suicidal ideations when she felt she was a burden to her son and daughter who often had to come home from work to check in on her. During intake and subsequent assessment, Mrs. Kim minimized her suicidal ideations and claimed that they were just transient death wishes. Her panic symptoms subsided when she began taking medications and attending weekly individual and group therapy. Mrs. Kim became a grandmother recently and was pleased to be able to take care of her grandchild. Hae Na, in offering her congratulations, pointed out how Mrs. Kim had come a long way in her recovery. Mrs. Kim became emotional and started crying. She told Hae Na more details about how she struggled with her frequent suicidal ideations in the past and her specific plan of jumping off a bridge nearby at the early stage of her illness. She also revealed that her family had told her not to dwell on her suicidal thoughts, which made it more difficult for her to talk about them. Evidently it was important for Mrs. Kim to share the depth of her suicidal struggle with someone who she trusted would understand and accept her subjective experience as a resolution of her painful past.

Case vignette: Mr. Wu

Mr. Wu, a middle-aged immigrant from China, had been diagnosed with schizoaffective disorder since he was a young adult. When he was referred to Ken, his social worker at the mental health clinic about 12 years ago, he was socially isolated, complaining of feeling hopeless and helpless about his mental illness, and neglecting his health and physical appearance. While he denied having any active suicidal ideations, he would make statements like, "I have no life. Every one of my siblings and friends I know are married." Ken would validate his feelings and say, "Life is not fair. It must be hard for you to think of good reasons to live." Ken, however, noticed that Mr. Wu had keen observation and a wry sense of humor about life. When he shared that with Mr. Wu several times, Mr. Wu appeared to be pleasantly surprised. As Mr. Wu gradually developed a close relationship with Ken and came to trust him, he noticed that Mr. Wu began to dress better and complained less about life. Several years into the relationship, Mr. Wu began to come into session when he was feeling down and made comments like, "I did not kill myself yet. I need to complain about my life." Ken would smile and said, "Indeed! So glad to see you are still alive. Let's talk." As Mr. Wu developed this communication routine with Ken, he was actually comfortable to use suicidal thought as an opener to discuss the level and nuances of his distress.

Case vignette: Mr. Nguyen

Mr. Nguyen, a middle-aged Vietnamese immigrant who suffered from several episodes of psychosis due to his depression, was temporarily assigned to Judy, an Asian practitioner who did not speak his native language. Mr. Nguyen spoke some conversational English and Judy sometimes used an interpreter if she felt the need to explore issues with him. Judy built her rapport with Mr. Nguyen by showing interest in his life and asking detailed questions about his daily routine. Judy had asked Mr. Nguyen to show her pictures of his wife and children who were still in Vietnam. She sat in during his consultation sessions with the Vietnamese-speaking psychiatrist, and learned to use a few Vietnamese phrases to inquire about his well-being. Mr. Nguyen never disclosed any suicidal history, and tended to be reticent about his emotional distress. After a couple of months, Judy again asked for an interpreter to be in the session. As she reviewed Mr. Nguyen's psychiatric history, she asked if she could ask some personal questions now that she and Mr. Nguyen knew each other better. With Mr. Nguyen's permission, she contextualized her suicide assessment question with her knowledge of Mr. Nguyen's struggles with living alone in the US and not able to support his family at home. She also instructed the interpreter to do a verbatim translation of her remarks while she communicated her empathy with her eye contact and facial expression. After a brief silence, Mr. Nguyen disclosed that there were a couple of times that he swallowed a handful of pills but he forced himself to vomit when he thought about his family. Mr. Nguyen also acknowledged that he had never told his family and friends about his attempts, but he felt that it was important to share it with Judy and other staff who "took care of him."

An important theme in these case scenarios was the practitioners' ability to accept their clients' suicidal behavior and help them process their myriad underlying feelings. It was apparent that the opportunity for clients to be able to disclose these dark and troubled thoughts and feelings to "someone who would not be afraid of them," as one practitioner aptly put it, was a therapeutic experience. Such experience of being *with the client* epitomizes the essence of the relational model.

Suicide interventions and assessment as a seamless process

From a relational model perspective, it is difficult to separate suicide assessment from intervention. Clients with suicidal thoughts often feel they have limited options and sense of control in their lives. Thus their being given a voice in the assessment process is a corrective emotional experience. The aforementioned case scenarios also showed that the practitioners' partnership with the clients through their genuine concern for their well-being as well as validation of their struggles are powerful antidotes to their suicidal thoughts.

In the following case discussion we present a more detailed scenario of how a practitioner worked with her client in a crisis with serious suicidal thoughts and plans. The practitioner took a calculated risk to stay with the client's suicidal feelings and explore the triggers and underlying issues. Her deliberations of her intervention are also included in the presentation to offer a more nuanced view of the use of relational approaches and how they made good clinical sense in resolving a suicidal crisis.

Case vignette: Ling

Ling was a Chinese woman in her late twenties who came to the US several years ago when she married someone in a pre-arranged marriage. Shortly after her immigration, her husband found out that she had a history of psychotic episodes and subsequently divorced her. Ling managed to remain in the US and support herself working in a nail salon. A couple of years later, she reunited with a high school friend and married him. It was a good relationship but only lasted a year when her second husband died of sudden illness. Ling became depressed and sought mental health treatment for a while when she had difficulties maintaining her job. A couple of months ago she returned to treatment with Fan, her psychologist who worked with her previously. Ling had been dating someone for a while but was feeling anxious and stressed by the relationship. Ling was not quite able to articulate the troubling aspect of the relationship. She had tried to break up with this boyfriend but he always talked her back into the relationship within a few days.

One day, Ling came into session looking dejected and said to Fan, "I am not happy." Fan tried to explore the precipitant and nature of her distress, using Ling's words, "Why are you not happy? What happened this week?"

Ling shook her head and said, "I don't know." But she went on to talk about how she had gone up to the roof of her apartment building and thought about jumping.

This was the first time Ling disclosed any suicidal ideations to Fan. Previously she had made vague references to death ideation when her second husband passed away. Fan was taken by surprise, and decided to interject a statement of reality, "That sounds serious. You had thoughts about killing yourself and you put them into action."

Ling nodded and after a brief silence, mentioned that she read a newspaper article recently about a man who jumped from a building with a baby in his arms in China, and the article talked about how his head was smashed.

The graphic description unnerved Fan a bit. Fan thought about sending Ling to the psychiatrist for an emergency consultation and assess for the need to hospitalize Ling. She decided against the idea as she noticed that Ling was looking at her and she felt that Ling seemed to be searching for some empathic connection from her.

Fan shared her initial reaction: "That was a scary and horrible story. So suicide seemed to be on your mind a lot. Why is that?"

Ling shook her head again and said: "I don't know."

After some tangential talking about minor squabbles at work with coworkers, Ling went back again to the issue of her suicidal thoughts. She told Fan that she recently tried walking into the middle of the street to see what would happen. But then she quickly walked back to the pedestrian pavement.

Fan decided that Ling seemed to be asking for her input to understand her suicidal thought process, and that perhaps Ling herself was scared by these thoughts. So she decided to probe, "What stopped you from jumping from the roof and getting killed by traffic in the street?"

Ling replied, "I don't want to be like the guy in China. What if I survive the jumping and become handicapped? I also saw that there was only one car in the far distance when I stepped off the curb." Even though Ling did not really answer Fan's question, her answer indicated that she was ambivalent about killing herself. Fan decided that it was important to engage and support Ling in articulating her desires to live. She looked at Ling and said, "I'm glad you did not want to take a chance, even though I think there are many other good reasons for not going through with it." But Fan did not want to come across as patronizing and "lecturing" Ling. So she just gently patted Ling on the shoulder and smiled at Ling.

Fan realized that Ling had been very defended against a lot of painful memories and feelings that possibly contributed to her turning them against herself. So she made another attempt to explore with Ling the underlying issues of her suicidal ideation by starting with the precipitant, "If we were to go back in time, what happened this week that was possibly upsetting to you?"

After thinking for a while, Ling blurted out: "My boyfriend called me and wanted to get together." But she didn't seem to be able to recall or articulate why that was upsetting. Ling just added that she felt so troubled by the call that she had to leave work early.

Fan asked if she was thinking of getting back into a relationship with him.

Ling said "no" emphatically and continued, "I feel very differently about him now and I do not want to be with him anymore." However, Ling was not able to give specifics about why her feelings for her boyfriend had changed.

Fan brought up a recent incident when the boyfriend did not call Ling for a few days after she experienced a psychotic episode, and asked if Ling was upset about that.

This time Ling was able to come up with some insights: "Yes, he reminds me that I am a patient with mental illness when I am with him."

Fan asked if this boyfriend reminded Ling of her first husband. Ling nodded.

Fan asked, "What about your second husband?"

Ling shook her head, "He was a good man, but he died so soon and so sudden."

Fan said gently, "So people close to you either left you or did not appreciate you."

Lin nodded her head and was quiet.

Fan felt she had helped Ling make some connection between her suicidal thoughts, her multiple losses, and strong feelings that she had not allowed herself to get in touch with. While she did not want to delve into those mixed emotions until she got a better sense that Ling was ready, she felt it was important for Ling to leave the session with some understanding and hence a sense of control over those overwhelming urges and feelings.

After a brief silence, Fan said to Lin, "I think I have a better understanding of why you have been thinking about killing yourself. You have gone through a lot since you came to this country. Even though you were strong and tried to move on, it was hard to be disappointed over and over again. So when is it going to end, right?"

Ling smiled a little and nodded. Fan continued the conversation as she recounted how Ling had coped with all the losses and challenges in her life. In highlighting Ling's stressors as well as her resilience, Fan normalized and contextualized her suicidal ideations. Ling's affect lifted as she chimed in and added details and perspectives into Fan's narrative.

Before the session ended, Fan presented Ling with the clinic's safety plan and asked if she would be amenable to looking at it before they discuss it together. Ling agreed and after thinking about the various questions on the form, she was able to come up with suggestions of activity and individuals for support to manage the suicidal ideations in case she experienced them again. Ling also agreed to return to session the same week.

Long-term intervention

- Concrete services to alleviate stressors
- Holding environment to support coping mechanisms and reduce social isolation
- Reinforcement of positive help-seeking behavior
- Empowerment of client.

After the client's imminent risk of suicide is averted or an attempt is aborted, it is important for the practitioner to address the issues underlying the client's suicidal behavior. In working with Asian immigrant clients, this would often entail soliciting essential services to alleviate their common stressors such as homelessness, unemployment, lack of income and medical coverage that severely undermine their quality of life and sense of failure. Practitioners agreed that while their clients' non-adherence to psychotropic medication and subsequent decompensation is a common precipitant to their suicidal behavior, their unresolved stressors and their sense of hopelessness about their lives are often the cause of their diminishing motivation to stay in treatment. Unfortunately it is often a challenge for the practitioners to secure sufficient services and resources for their clients, especially for the undocumented immigrants and those without family support. Oftentimes it is the practitioners' dedication to help their clients and their genuine concern that restored the clients' sense of hope.

Vignette #1

A hospital social worker and a psychiatrist recalled accompanying a young undocumented client from China to a boarding house after his discharge to serve as personal references so he could secure a bed. Even though the landlord eventually evicted the client after he found out that he suffered from mental illness and a dermatological disease, the client developed a trusting relationship with these hospital staff and returned to the hospital several times to seek help when he experienced psychotic symptoms and suicidal ideations.

Vignette #2

A mental health outpatient clinician had been concerned about a middle-aged professional from Japan who was laid off and suffering from depression. The client initially talked a lot about his sense of failure and feelings of shame in regard to his unemployment status, which was reinforced by his wife blaming him for being "lazy" and not accepting menial jobs because of his pride. The client acknowledged some death ideations but indicated that he would not commit suicide because he still had to take care of his elderly mother. As the therapeutic relationship progressed, the client began to develop a positive parental transference toward the clinician and would regularly bring her a cup of tea and small gifts to show his respect and appreciation, a common Japanese ritual toward revered family members. Every so often, he would make reassuring remarks such as, "Please do not worry about me. I will not attempt suicide." It appeared that the client picked up on the clinician's concern and felt empowered when he could offer her verbal reassurance. When the client eventually divorced his wife and decided to return to Japan, he thanked the clinician for her acceptance of his circumstances and her respect for his educational and employment accomplishment. He also shared that his commitment to her in not attempting suicide had sustained him in some of his dark moments.

For many Asian immigrant clients who are socially isolated due to acculturation difficulties and the lack of support systems in their host countries, relationships with the practitioners often become their lifeline in times of distress. As these clients learn over time that they can turn to their practitioners who are supportive and accepting of their circumstances, they will likely be able to modify their learned cognitions from past experiences that viewed suicide as the only option to resolving their problems. As they gain validation of their strengths and resilience as immigrants starting a new life in their host countries, they will be more inclined to accept that cultural values and expectations need to evolve with changes in their environment and assuage their feelings of failure and shame about their life circumstances. These new cognitions and emotions are often reinforced in support groups and family meetings facilitated by the practitioners in mental health settings. Clients are encouraged to seek and reciprocate support among each other and create a holding environment that helps them cope with different negative life events and stressors that emerge over time. Essentially these clients are able to make positive changes in their help-seeking behavior, which is a major protective factor that strengthens their coping capabilities and resources.

Working with suicidal clients presents many challenges to practitioners who work with Asian immigrant clients. The heightened sense of responsibilities for clients who have limited familial support and resources, the seeming conflicts between cultural and professional norms in exploring and discussing suicidal ideations, and the recurrent crises of clients' suicidal behavior can create a tremendous drain on the practitioner's professional capabilities. As practitioners, it is a humbling and frightening thought that there are times we may lose our clients to suicide despite all our earnest efforts. However, this same thought may keep us on a balanced focus that maintaining an empathic connection with the client in the here-and-now relationship is the best we can do for the client and ourselves.

Discussion highlights

Suicide risk factors for Asian immigrants

The varying rates of Asian immigrant groups in different countries need to be examined more closely from the perspective of the interplay of cultural beliefs and the social environment of the host countries. (p. 175)

Suicide assessment

There are no assessment approaches that can accurately predict if and when an individual will kill herself. The complexities of suicidal behavior as impacted by the individual's internal and external forces present tremendous challenges in suicide assessment. (p. 179)

The therapeutic relationship in a suicidal crisis also emphasizes the importance for the practitioner to listen empathically to the client's narratives and understand what it means for the client to be suicidal. (p. 182)

Practitioners agree that Asian clients generally appreciate the direct inquiry on this important issue if it is communicated with concern and respect. (p. 184)

A client will only disclose information about his past and current suicidal behavior if he senses that the practitioner is really trying to help and will not judge him. (p. 186)

The opportunity for clients to be able to disclose their dark and troubled thoughts and feelings to "someone who is not afraid of them" is a therapeutic experience. (p. 188)

Suicide interventions

Suicidality needs to be treated as a central issue of the client and not just a symptom of mental illness that can be managed by psychiatric treatment. (p. 182)

Telling the client that he should not kill himself or remind him of his obligations and responsibilities as "reasons for living" can come across as critical of the client at a time when the client needs unconditional acceptance and support. (p. 185)

Epilog

Looking back

Reconnecting with Asian practitioners: reflections and insights

Reconnecting with practitioners in the Asian community to interview them for this book was a heartwarming, rewarding, and humbling experience. The practitioners we approached were tremendously supportive when we told them that we wanted to write about a practice model for working with Asian immigrant clients that focuses on integrating Asian cultural values and norms in the helping process. Despite their extremely busy schedules the practitioners spent a great deal of time talking with us, often after work hours. We were grateful for the opportunity to learn about their nuanced interactions with their clients. The practitioners' narratives of the way they work with clients went beyond the descriptions found in textbooks, which tend to be conceptual, and gave us insights about how Asian immigrants experience stress, when and how they seek help, and what they perceive as therapeutic communication. The practitioners' account of their work shed light on the enormity and complexities of the challenges that they encounter on a daily basis.

One of the critical challenges is the predominance of clients who, because of their cultural norms and immigrant-related issues, do not disclose personal issues such as suicidal ideation and domestic violence until *after* they feel a sense of safety and acceptance in the helping relationship. This common withholding of crucial psychosocial information by clients can be a huge psychological burden for the practitioners. It made us realize the magnitude of the task that practitioners face.

In reviewing the case vignettes presented by the practitioners, we were impressed with the way they intuitively sensed their clients' needs and focused on the relational nature of their approaches. Indeed, their work with clients was grounded in the centrality of the helping relationship that took into account the cultural context and understanding of the immigrant experience. We gained a clear sense of how the practitioners tactfully worked through the many layers of their clients' implicit communication and reciprocated with therapeutic responses. We were able to discern the clients' affective states and emotional needs, and the empathic bonds that develop between practitioners and their clients. Changing the modes of communication clearly does not diminish the universal human needs of being understood, accepted, and cared for by others. As with individuals from many other ethnic groups, Asian clients may be short on expressing their feelings. But as one practitioner aptly put it, "their emotions run deep." The essential task of practitioners is to help meet client needs by responding in a way that is meaningful to their clients.

Few of the practitioners we interviewed were aware of the relational theory. They described their approaches as the "only way that made sense to our Asian clients." One practitioner remarked that Asians are "socialized to be intuitively relational." The practitioners, by the nature of their cultural upbringing, may indeed be much more attuned to the dynamics of mutuality and the specific sociocultural context of making a connection with clients. At the same time, we believe that the practitioners deserve a great deal of credit for developing skills of the "professional and differential use of self." What appears as "small talk" and "social" conversations and interactions to non-Asian clinicians is actually founded on clinical assumptions and principles with accompanying therapeutic goals and objectives. We believe that "being relational" is a clinical skill that is applied by immersing oneself purposefully in a unique relationship with each client. It is a skill that embodies both elements of art and a science – an integration of theoretical knowledge and the practitioner's creativity in crafting a genuine therapeutic relationship. From this perspective, non-Asian practitioners can transcend the language and cultural barriers and be just as effective in providing a therapeutic experience if they are willing to take some risks, learn from moments of misattunement, and allow the clients to guide them in understanding their subjective realities. From the stance of the relational model, therapeutic outcomes are created in the co-constructed relationship between the practitioner and the client, and depend less on re-construction of the client's past history. Edward T. Hall (1977, p. 57), an American anthropologist specializing in intercultural communication, makes a relevant observation that it is "experience" and not language that is more effective in "transferring thoughts and meanings" between individuals. Likewise, the relational model enables practitioners to avoid what Kleinman (2006, p. 1673) describes as the "major problem with the idea of cultural competency [which] suggests [that] culture can be reduced to a technical skill for which clinicians can be trained to develop expertise." Culture is not a static entity, and practitioners who use a relational framework are able to attune themselves to the evolving beliefs and norms of their immigrant clients who are constantly negotiating between two cultures.

Our subjectivity

We can draw a parallel between the limitations of language that we discussed in this book with the way we presented the practitioners' clinical materials. While we certainly learned a lot from visiting agencies that serve Asian immigrants and interviewing practitioners, we know that our illustrations of the practitioners' work is limited by our subjective experiences, our language, and the linear descriptions in our chapters. Our experiences and the information that we gathered were also shaped by our interest in examining how traditional psychodynamic assessment concepts and intervention skills in the helping process are applied in a relational and Asiacentric context, which are reflected in the dual focus of the book. We discuss the practitioners' conceptualization of the clients' issues from a psychosocial perspective, and highlight their sensitivity to and respect for the clients' individual and cultural defenses. We delineate the relational components that underlie the practitioners' use of cognitive behavioral therapy, narrative therapy, family therapy, supportive counseling, and case management services. However, we are aware that there are dimensions of the fine work of the practitioners that we have neglected.

Research on Asian immigrants

Our attempts to review the literature on Asian immigrants who reside in five different countries ended up being an overly ambitious task. We were pleased to find research on Asian immigrants in all five English-speaking countries. We were also heartened to find an increase in studies that focus on specific national origin groups, rather than lumping the different groups under one umbrella. The studies, for the most part, are based on small-scale convenience samples and it is not possible to make meaningful inferences and comparisons in our discussions. Given the increasing diversity of Asian immigrants and fluid acculturation patterns, capturing this diversity while finding commonality is an emerging challenge for research.

Culture and social change

Culture has been a major focus in our discussion of the case materials as well as our literature review. By definition, culture is a set of internalized collective schemas that shapes the focus of individuals' experience, and at the same time, provides emotional and moral meanings to the experience. However, individuals also shape culture as they actively engage in meaning making, in response to changes in their social, economic, political, and personal environment (Ham, 1993; Kleinman and Benson, 2006; Markus *et al.*, 1997).

The evolvement of culture is evident in Asian societies that have undergone rapid social and economic changes in the last few decades. For example, in China and India, the advancement of modernization has created a boom in urban development and a shift from an agrarian society to a market economy based on industrialization and trade with the Western world. The job growth in urban settings has subsequently altered demographics and the structure of families. The traditional Asian extended families are replaced by nuclear families, with women joining the labor force and many older adults living alone. This trend is also on the rise in other Asian countries, such as South Korea and Japan (Organisation for Economic Co-operation, 2011). The general improvement in economic purchasing power among families in Asian societies, fueled by the expansion of technological information networks and the increase in travel mobility, has led to more exposure and an open attitude to Western values and lifestyle.

There are cultural implications underlying all these changes. While the core cultural emphasis on interdependence, anticipation of others' feelings and needs as well as personal connections is still very much embedded in the collective psyche, there is indeed some erosion of the values of hierarchical collectivism by the influences of Western tenets of individualism (Hou, 2011; Sonawat, 2001). In the Asian immigrant communities, the process of acculturation is also heavily moderated by the individuals' socioeconomic background. Those who migrated from a rural setting with limited education, economic means, and proficiency of the English language tend to adhere more to their traditional values. Nevertheless it appears from our literature review and the case vignettes that similar patterns of cultural changes are evolving in varying degrees. For example, there is apparently some decline in the quality of care for the older generation, a weakening of the patriarchal family structure due to women's financial gains in the labor market, an increase in divorce rates among couples, and a growing interest among Asian parents to modify their parenting practice and communication style with their children. Inherent in these shifting patterns of roles and relationships is a gradual adaptation of values and norms in the realities of immigrants in a Western industrialized society.

Looking ahead

What are the implications for practice with the evolving cultural changes in this global era? We think it is increasingly a challenge to describe cultural characteristics of any ethnic group and use culture-specific knowledge to inform practice. Roland (2011, p. 222) discusses the concept of a "complex layering of the self" for individuals who straddle multiple cultures and environments. He postulates that these individuals acquire new dimensions of their multicultural identity and personality while maintaining some indigenous aspects of their childhood self. We believe this is an apt characterization of our Asian immigrant population and even the second and third generation as well. Our own experience and those of our Asian peers affirm that there are always aspects of us that are uniquely Asian regardless of how much we identify with the Western culture.

We believe that the relational theory offers a viable model to address the challenge of evolving cultures. Its emphasis on mutuality and the contextualization of the client's issues and needs on a here-and-now basis will facilitate an ongoing cultural exploration of beliefs and perceptions between the practitioner and the client.

When we conceptualized the practitioners' approaches using the relational theory during our interviews, the practitioners agreed that this could be a framework to help them describe, analyze, and enhance their work with Asian immigrants. We would like to see further exploration and documentation of these relational approaches in Asian communities in different regions in the US and other English-speaking countries. The client population described in our case materials is primarily from an urban setting and of low socioeconomic background. It would be helpful to understand *if* and *how* practitioners in other settings modify their approaches. For example, in what ways will the helping relationship be different if the immigrant client population is more acculturated in terms of English proficiency and lifestyle? How does that "acculturated layering of self" modify the core Asian values such as communication of thoughts and feelings? The additional information will further illuminate the value of the relational model in the appreciation of the clients' different belief systems. Our objective in applying the relational model in an Asiacentric context is to document that Asian clients can participate in and benefit from a purposeful helping relationship. We also believe that it is important to validate the clinical skills of the practitioners in the Asian community and demonstrate that the "indigenous" approaches are rooted in a sound theoretical base. While these approaches may evolve in time, we think the relational framework can always be a guide in developing cultural competent practice.

With the current emphasis on empirically supported treatment (EST) modalities, the effectiveness and efficacy of the relational model will undoubtedly be questioned. During the past decade, researchers have begun to examine the effectiveness of cultural adaptations of ESTs for Asian American populations. Because ESTs are manualized, researchers can delineate specific aspects of treatments that they have adapted for Asians. Whereas cultural competence is associated with the overall helping process, cultural adaptations are often tied to specific treatments (Bernal *et al.*, 2009). Some of the research studies on cultural adaptations of ESTs include CBT for Chinese patients with depression (Hwang *et al.*, 2006), CBT for Cambodian refugees with PTSD (Otto and Hinton, 2006), and CBT for Vietnamese refugees with PTSD and combined panic attacks (Hinton *et al.*, 2006). While these studies are promising and offer possibilities of developing research-informed practices for Asian immigrants, there are limitations in applying the treatment models to practice. Oftentimes, practitioners are not able to limit their practice to a specific intervention modality because their clients present with a host of problems that are interrelated. Even when clients present with depression or PTSD or severe mental illness, practitioners in community settings need to address the client's entire system including the family, and living conditions affected by low-income status, unemployment, domestic violence, and lack of housing.

We believe, however, that the relational approach can complement specific ESTs in working with Asians. Recent neuroscience research has demonstrated the curative values of a supportive and interactive relationship in addressing maladaptive coping mechanisms. It would be important to augment the findings with specific measurements of the constructs of the model. For Asian immigrants who have been noted to terminate treatment prematurely, a good place to start would be to revisit the issue using a relational model practice. Self-reports by Asian clients on their perceptions of the therapeutic relationship will also help to identify variables for future studies.

The journey of writing this book has taken us to many places. As we contemplate on our experiences at the completion of the book, we realize that the journey has been more than an intellectual endeavor. We would like to think that we have forged the beginning of a working partnership with the Asian practitioners that we have gotten to know, and that we can utilize our skills as members of the academy to give the Asian professional community a voice in multicultural practice, and perhaps take the lead in exploring the way Asian culture adds depth to the relational framework.

Finally, conducting research about Asians immigrants in five different English-speaking countries has made us aware of the global nature of clinical practice with Asians. As sociologists consider the possibility of a global culture in the making, we may also consider a global practice where Asian cultural values and norms are recognized and integrated.

Bibliography

Preface

Chung, I. W. (2006). "Bridging professional and cultural values and norms: A study of Asian American social work students." *Journal of Teaching in Social Work*, 26(1–2), 93–110.

Council on Social Work Education (2009). *Advanced Social Work Practice in Clinical Social Work*. Retrieved 2 December 2012 from www.cswe.org/File.aspx?id=26685.

Hardy, K. V. (2008). "On becoming a GEMM therapist: Work harder, be smarter, and never discuss race." In M. McGoldrick and K. V. Hardy (eds), *Revisioning Family Therapy: Race, Culture, and Gender in Clinical Practice* (pp. 461–68). New York, NY: Guilford Press.

Chapter 1

Ananth, J. (1984). "Treatment of immigrant Indian patients." *Canadian Journal of Psychiatry*, 29, 490–93.

Anderson, H. (2005). "Myths about knowing." *Family Process*, 44(4), 497–504.

Applegate, J. S. (2000). "Theory as story: A postmodern tale." *Clinical Social Work Journal*, 28(2), 141–53.

Berzoff, J., Flanagan, L., and Hertz, P. (2011). *Inside Out and Outside In: Psychodynamic Clinical Theory and Practice in Contemporary Multicultural Contexts*, 3rd Edition. Lanham, Maryland: Rowman & Littlefield Publishers.

Bhela, A. (2010). "Globalization, Hinduism and cultural change in India." *Asia Journal of Global Studies*, 4(2), 93–102.

Blau, J. with Abramovitz, M. (2010). *The Dynamics of Social Welfare Policy*, 3rd Edition, New York: Oxford University Press.

Bonner, C. (2002). "Psychoanalytic theory and diverse populations: Reflections on old practices and new understandings." *Psychoanalytic Social Work*, 9(2), 61–70.

Borden, W. (2009). "Sigmund Freud and the classical psychoanalytic tradition." In W. Borden, *Contemporary Psychodynamic Theory and Practice* (pp. 10–22). Chicago, Illinois: Lyceum Books, Inc.

Bowlby, J. (1969). *Attachment and Loss, Vol. 1: Attachment*. New York: Basic Books.

Bronfenbrenner, U. (1979). *The Ecology of Human Development*. Cambridge, MA: Harvard University Press.

Cappas, N. M., Andres-Hyman, R., and Davidson, L. (2005). "What psychotherapists can begin to learn from neuroscience: Seven principles of a brain-based psychotherapy." *Psychotherapy: Theory, Research, Practice, Training*, 42(3), 374–83.

Chen, G. A. and Kim, S. C. (2009). "Sexuality." In Nita Tewari and Alvin Alvarez (eds), *Asian American Psychology: Current Perspectives* (pp. 247–71). New York: Routledge/Taylor & Francis Group.

Cheung, F. (1995). "Facts and myths about somatization among the Chinese." In T. Y. Lin, W. S. Tseng, E. K. Yeh (eds), *Chinese Societies and Mental Health* (pp. 141–80). Hong Kong: Oxford University Press.

Choi, K. M. and Kim, C. (2012). "Psychodynamic approaches from transcultural perspectives in working with Korean American women." *Families in Society*, 93(4), 279–86.

Choi, M. and Yeom, H. (2011). "Identifying and treating the culture-bound syndrome of Hwa-Byung among older Korean immigrant women: Recommendations for practitioners." *Journal of the American Academy of Nurse Practitioners*, 23(5), 226–32.

Choi, Y. K. (2006). "A transcultural model of Hwa-Byung: A grounded theory." *Journal of Korean Academy of Psychiatric and Mental Health Nursing*, 15(4), 508–12.

Chung, I. (2006). "A cultural perspective on emotions and behavior: An empathic pathway to examine intergenerational conflicts in Chinese immigrant families." *Families in Society*, 87 (3), 367–76.

——(2012). "Sociocultural study of immigrant suicide attempters: An ecological perspective." *Journal of Social Work*, 12 (6), 614–29.

Cooper, M. G. and Lesser, J. G. (2002). "Object relations theory: A relational psychodynamic model." In M. G. Cooper and J. G. Lesser, *Clinical Social Work Practice: An Integrated Approach* (pp. 95–109). Needham Heights, MA: Allyn & Bacon.

Damasio, A. (2001). "Fundamental feelings." *Nature*, 413(6858), 781.

Delhiwala, N. and Sawant, M. Personal communication with author, 5 June 2012.

Devji, M. S. (1999). "The paradoxes of the Kama Sutra and the veil: Asian-Indian women and marital sexuality." In S. R. Gupta (ed.), *Emerging Voices: South Asian American Women Redefine Self, Family, and Community* (pp. 169–92). Walnut Creek, CA: Alta Mira Press.

Erikson, E. (1959). *Identity and the Life Cycle*. New York: International Universities Press.

Flanagan, L. M. (2011). "Object relations theory." In J. Berzoff, L. Flanagan, and P. Hertz (eds), *Inside Out and Outside In: Psychodynamic Clinical Theory and Practice in Contemporary Multicultural Contexts*, 3rd Edition (pp. 118–57). Lanham, Maryland: Rowman & Littlefield Publishers.

Fraser, N., and Gordon, L. (1994). "A genealogy of dependency: Tracing a keyword of the U.S. welfare state." *Signs: Journal of Women in Culture & Society*, 19(2), 309–36.

Freeman, D. (1998). "Emotional refueling in development, mythology, and cosmology: The Japanese Separation-individuation experience." In S. Akhtar and S. Kramer (eds), *The Colors of Childhood: Separation-individuation across Cultural, Racial, and Ethnic Differences* (pp.17–60). Northvale, New Jersey: Jason Aronson, Inc.

Freud, A. (1936). *The Ego and the Mechanisms of Defense*. New York: International Universities Press.

Freud, S. (1911). "Formulations on two principles of mental functioning." *Standard Edition*, 12, 213–27. London: Hogarth Press.

——(1915). "Repression." *Standard Edition*, 14, 141–58. London: Hogarth Press.

Goldstein, E. G. (1995a). "The ego and its defenses." In E. G. Goldstein, *Ego Psychology and Social Work Practice*, 2nd Edition (pp. 72–85). New York: The Free Press.

——(1995b). *Ego Psychology and Social Work Practice*. New York: The Free Press.

——(2001). "Object relations theory: Major concepts." In E. G. Goldstein, *Object Relations Theory and Self Psychology in Social Work Practice* (pp. 53–78). New York: The Free Press.

Greenberg, J. R. and Mitchell, S. A. (1983). *Object Relations in Psychoanalytic Theory*. Cambridge, MA: Harvard University Press.

Greene, R. (1999). "Ecological perspective: An eclectic theoretical framework for social work practice." In R. Greene (ed.), *Human Behavior Theory and Social Work Practice* (pp. 251–59). New York: Aldine De Gruyter.

Hall, E. T. (1977). *Beyond Culture*. Garden City: New York: Anchor Books.

Herron, W. G. (1995). "Development of the ethnic unconscious." *Psychoanalytic Psychology*, 12 (4), 521–31.

Ho, E. Personal communication with author, 14 April 2012.

Hodge, D. R. and Nadir, A. (2008). "Moving toward culturally competent practice with Muslims: Modifying cognitive therapy with Islamic tenets." *Social Work*, 53(1), 31–41.

Hughes, C. C. (1993). "Culture in clinical psychiatry." In A. Gaw (ed.), *Culture, Ethnicity and Mental Illness* (pp. 3–42). Washington, DC: American Psychiatric Press.

Johnson, F. A. (1993). *Dependency and Japanese Socialization*. New York: New York University Press.

Kagitcibasi, C. (1997). "Individuals and collectivism." In J. Berry, M. Segall, and C. Kagitcibasi (eds), *Handbook of Cross-cultural Psychology: Social Behavior and Applications*, vol. 3 (pp. 1–50). Needham Heights, MA: Allyn & Bacon.

Karger, H. J. (2003). "Ending public assistance: The transformation of US public assistance policy into labour policy." *Journal of Social Policy*, 32(3), 383–401.

Kim, J. L. (2009). "Asian American women's retrospective reports of their sexual socialization." *Psychology of Women Quarterly*, 33, 334–50.

Kirmayer, L. J. (2007). "Psychotherapy and the cultural concept of the person." *Transcultural Psychiatry*, 44(2), 232–57.

Kleinman, A. (1988). *The Illness Narratives: Suffering, Healing and the Human Condition*. New York: Basic Books.

——(2004). "Culture and Depression." *New England Journal of Medicine*, 351(10), 951–53.

Le Doux, J. (1997). *The Emotional Brain*. New York: Simon & Schuster.

Le Espiritu, Y. (2001). "'We don't sleep around like White girls do': Family, culture, and gender in Filipina American lives." *Signs: Journal of Women in Culture and Society*, 26(2), 415–40.

Lee, B. (2006). "Teaching justice and living peace: Body, sexuality, and religious education in Asian American communities." *Religious Education*, 101(3), 402–19.

Lee, D. T. S., Kleinman, J., and Kleinman, A. (2007). "Rethinking depression: An ethnographic study of the experiences of depression among Chinese." *Harvard Review Psychiatry*, 15(1), 1–8.

Lokken, J. M. and Twohey, D. (2004). "American Indian perspectives of Euro-American counseling behavior." *Journal of Multicultural Counseling and Development*, 32, 320–31.

McWhinney, I. R., Epstein, R. M., and Freeman, T. (2001). "Rethinking somatization." *Advances in Mind-Body Medicine*, 17(4), 235–39.

Manning, C., Cornelius, L., and Okundaye, J. (2004). "Empowering African Americans through social work practice: Integrating an Afrocentric perspective, ego psychology and spirituality." *Families in Society*, 85(2), 229–35.

Markus, H. R. and Kitayama, S. (1994). "The cultural shaping of emotion: A conceptual framework." In S. Kitayama and H. R. Markus (eds), *Emotion and Culture* (pp. 339–51). Washington, DC: American Psychological Association.

Maslow, A. H. (1954). *Motivation and Personality*. New York: Harper & Row Publishers.

Mahler, M., Pine, F., and Bergman, A. (1975). *Psychological Birth of the Human Infant*. New York: Basic Books.

Nagai, C. (2007). "Culturally based spiritual phenomena: Eastern and western theories and practices." *Psychoanalytic Social Work*, 14(1), 1–22.

Neimeyer, R. A. and Bridges, S. K. (2003). "Postmodern approaches to psychotherapy". In A. S. Gurman and S. B. Messer, *Essential Psychotherapies: Theory and Practice*, 2nd Edition (pp. 272–316). New York: The Guilford Press.

Nye, C. (2005). "Conversations with Suwanrang: The treatment relationship in cultural context." *Clinical Social Work Journal*, 33(1), 37–54.

Ots, T. (1990). "The angry liver, the anxious heart, and the melancholy spleen." *Culture, Medicine and Psychiatry*, 14(1), 21–58.

Pang, K. Y. C. (2000). "Symptom expression and somatization among elderly Korean immigrants." *Journal of Clinical Geropsychology*, 6(3), 199–212.

Parker, G., Gladstone, G., and Chee, K. T. (2001). "Depression in the planet's largest ethnic group: The Chinese." *American Journal of Psychiatry*, 158(6), 857–64.

Robinson, C. (2010). "Harnessing cultural archetypes: Rediscovering the collective cultural unconscious and the stuff Americans are made of." Retrieved 14 December 2012 from *The Journal for Quality & Participation*, www.asq.org/pub/jqp.

Roland, A. (1996). "How universal is the psychoanalytic self?" In A. Roland, *Cultural Pluralism and Psychoanalysis* (pp. 3–21). New York: Routledge.

——(2011). "The familial self revisited." In A. Roland, *Journeys to Foreign Selves: Asians and Asian Americans in a Global Era* (pp. 33–53). New York: Oxford University Press.

Sarri, C. (2008). "The role of the environment in psychoanalytic theory." *Smith College Studies in Social Work*, 78(2–3), 227–42.

Schamess, G. and Shilkret, R. (2011). "Ego psychology." In J. Berzoff, L. Flanagan, and P. Hertz (eds), *Inside Out and Outside In: Psychodynamic Clinical Theory and Practice in Contemporary Multicultural Contexts*, 3rd Edition (pp. 62–96). Lanham, Maryland: Rowman & Littlefield Publishers.

Shweder, R. A., Jensen, L., and Goldstein, W. M. (1995). "Who sleeps by whom revisited: A method for extracting the moral goods implicit in practice." In J. Goodenow, P. Miller, and F. Kessel (eds), *Cultural Practices as Contexts for Development* (pp. 21–39). San Francisco: Jossey-Boss.

Shweder, R. A. (1997). "The surprise of ethnography." *Ethos*, 25(2), 152–63.

Son, H. Personal communication with author, 14 November 2012.

Sue, D. W. and Sue, D. (2003). *Counseling the Culturally Diverse: Theory and Practice*, 4th Edition. New York: John Wiley & Sons.

Tignor, R., Adelman, J., Aron, S., Brown, P., Elman, B., Kotkin, S., Xinru, L., Marchand, S., Pittman, H., Prakash, G., Shaw, B., and Tsin, M. (2008). *Worlds Together, Worlds Apart: A History of the World from the Beginnings of Humankind to the Present*. New York: W. W. Norton & Co.

Tseng, W. C. and Lipson, J. G. (2007). "Fan: An idiom of distress among suicidal patients in Taiwan." *Community Health*, 30(1), 74–83.

Tseng, W. S. (2004). "Culture and psychotherapy: Asian perspectives." *Journal of Mental Health*, 13(2), 151–61.

Vu, M. Personal communication with author, 2 March 2012.

Vu, M. Personal communication with author, 8 June 2012.

Wachtel, P. L. (2008). *Relational Theory and the Practice of Psychotherapy*. New York: The Guilford Press.

Waldman, K. and Rubalcava (2005). "Psychotherapy with intercultural couples: A contemporary psychodynamic approach." *American Journal of Psychotherapy*, 59(3), 227–45.

Winnicott, D. W. (1958). "The capacity to be alone." In D. W. Winnicott, *The Maturational Process and the Facilitating Environment*. London: Hogarth Press and the Institute of Psycho-Analysis, 1965.

——(1960). "Ego distortions in terms of true and false self." In D. W. Winnicott, *The Maturational Process and the Facilitating Environment* (pp.140–52). London: Hogarth Press and the Institute of Psycho-Analysis, 1965.

Wong, G. Personal communication with author, 25 November 2012.

Woods, M. and Hollis, F. (2000). "The psychosocial frame of reference: An overview." In M. Woods and F. Hollis, *Casework: A Psychosocial Therapy*, 5th Edition (pp. 35–76). New York: McGraw-Hill.

Chapter 2

Anderson, H. (2005). "Myths about knowing." *Family Process*, 44 (4), 497–504.

Aron, L. (1996). *A Meeting of Minds: Mutuality in Psychoanalysis*. Hillsdale, NJ: The Analytic Press.

Benjamin, J. (1990). "An outline of intersubjectivity." *Psychoanalytic Psychology*, 7(Suppl), 33–46.

——(1998). *Shadow of the Other: Intersubjectivity and Gender in Psychoanalysis*. New York: Routledge.

Borden, W. (2000). "The relational paradigm in contemporary psychoanalysis: Toward a psychodynamically informed social work perspective." *Social Service Review*, 74(3), 352–79.

——(2009). "Sigmund Freud and the classical psychoanalytic tradition." In W. Borden, *Contemporary Psychodynamic Theory and Practice* (pp. 10–22). Chicago, Illinois: Lyceum Books, Inc.

Bowlby, J. (1969). *Attachment and Loss*, vol. 1. New York: Basic Books.

Bromberg, P. M. (1998). *Standing in the Spaces: Essays on Clinical Process, Trauma, and Dissociation*. Hillsdale, NJ: Analytic Press.

Bronfenbrenner, U. (1979). *The Ecology of Human Development*. Cambridge, MA: Harvard University Press.

Cappas, N. M., Andres-Hyman, R., and Davidson, L. (2005). "What psychotherapists can begin to learn from neuroscience: Seven principles of a brain-based psychotherapy." *Psychotherapy: Theory, Research, Practice, Training*, 42(3), 374–83.

Clark, J. (2006). "Listening for meaning: A research-based model for attending to spirituality, culture and worldview in social work practice." *Critical Social Work*, 7(1). Retrieved 20 March 2012 from http://cronus.uwindsor.ca/units/socialwork/critical.nsf/main/53C5DD5A6144260585257179007 1EFBB?OpenDocument

DeLaCour, E. (1996). "The interpersonal school and its influence on current relational theories." In J. Berzoff, L. Flanagan, and P. Hertz (eds), *Inside Out and Outside In: Psychodynamic Clinical Theory and Practice in Contemporary Multicultural Contexts*, 3rd Edition (pp. 199–217). Lanham, Maryland: Rowman & Littlefield Publishers.

Dewald, P. (1972). *The Psychoanalytic Process*. New York: Basic Books.

Erikson, E. (1959). *Identity and the Life Cycle*. New York: International Universities Press.

Fairbairn, W. R. D. (1952). *An Object Relations Theory of the Personality*. New York: Basic Books.

Flanagan, L. M. (2011). "Object relations theory." In J. Berzoff, L. M. Flanagan, and P. Hertz (eds), *Inside Out and Outside In: Psychodynamic Clinical Theory and Practice in Contemporary Multicultural Contexts*, 3rd Edition (pp. 118–57). Lanham, Maryland: Rowman & Littlefield Publishers.

Floersch, J. E. and Longhofer, J. L. (2004). "Psychodynamic case management." In J. R. Brandell (ed.), *Psychodynamic Social Work*. New York: Columbia University Press.

Fonagy, P. (1998). "Moments of change in psychoanalytic theory: Discussion of a new theory of psychic change." *Infant Mental Health Journal*, 19(3), 346–63.

Freedberg, S. (2009). *Relational Theory for Social Work Practice: A Feminist Perspective*. New York: Routledge.

Freud, S. (1912). "The dynamics of transference." *Standard Edition*, 12, 97–108, London: Hogarth Press, 1958.

Friedman, L. (2002). "What lies beyond interpretation, and is that the right question?" *Psychoanalytic Psychology*, 19(3), 540–51.

Gergen, K. J. (1985). "The social constructionist movement in modern psychology." *American Psychologist*, 40(3), 266–75.

Glicken, M. D. (2004). *Using the Strengths Perspective in Social Work Practice*. New York: Pearson Education, Inc.

Goldstein, E. G. (2001). *Object Relations Theory and Self Psychology in Social Work Practice*. New York: The Free Press.

Goldstein, E. G., Miehls, D., and Ringel, S. (2009). "The relational core of social work practice." In E. G. Goldstein, D. Miehls, and S. Ringel, *Advanced Clinical Social Work Practice: Relational Principles and Techniques* (pp. 1–17). New York: Columbia University Press.

Greenberg, J. (1991). *Oedipus and Beyond: A Clinical Theory*. Cambridge, MA: Harvard University Press.

Greenson, R. (1971). "The 'real' relationship between the patient and the psychoanalyst." In M. Kanzer (ed.), *The Unconscious Today* (pp. 213–32). New York: International University Press.

Hartmann, H. (1939). *Ego Psychology and the Problem of Adaptation*. New York: International Universities Press.

Horvath, A. and Symonds, B. (1991). "Relation between working alliance and outcome in psychotherapy: A meta analysis." *Journal of Counseling and Psychology*, 38(2), 139–49.

Jordan, J. V. (1991). "Empathy, mutuality, and therapeutic change: Clinical implications of a relational model." In J. V. Jordan, A. G. Kaplan, J. B. Miller, I. P. Stiver, and J. L. Surrey (eds), *Women's Growth in Connection: Writings from the Stone Center* (pp. 283–89). New York: Guilford Press.

Kohut, H. (1957). "Introspection, empathy and psychoanalysis: An examination of the relationship between mode of observation and theory." In P. H. Ornstein (ed.), *The Search for the Self: Selected Writings of Heinz Kohut: 1950–1978*, vol. 1 (pp. 205–32). New York: International Universities Press.

——(1971). *The Analysis of the Self*. New York: International Universities Press.

——(1977). *The Restoration of the Self*. New York: International Universities Press.

——(1984). *How Does Analysis Cure?* Chicago: University of Chicago Press.

Lambert, M. J. (1992). "Implications of outcome research for psychotherapy integration." In J. C. Norcross and M. R. Goldfield (eds), *Handbook of Psychotherapy Integration* (pp. 94–129). New York: Basic Books.

Levenson, E. (1985). "The interpersonal (Sullivanian) model." In A. Rothstein (ed.), *Models of the Mind* (pp. 49–67). Madison, CT: International Universities Press.

Lyons-Ruth, K. (1998). "Implicit relational knowing: Its role in development and psychoanalytic treatment." *Infant Mental Health Journal*, 19(3), 282–89.

——(2000). "'I sense that you sense that I sense … ': Sander's recognition process and the specificity of relational moves in the psychotherapeutic setting." *Infant Mental Heath Journal*, 21(1–2), 85–98.

McCabe, R. and Priebe, S. (2004). "The therapeutic relationship in the treatment of severe mental illness: A review of methods and findings." *International Journal of Social Psychiatry*, 50(2), 115–28.

McNamee, S. and Gergen, K. J. (eds) (1992). *Therapy as Social Construction*. Newbury Park, CA: Sage.

Martin, D., Garske, J., and Davis, M. (2000). "Relation of the therapeutic alliance with outcome and other variables: A meta-analytic review." *Journal of Consulting Clinical Psychology*, 68(3), 438–50.

Mattei, L. (1999). "A Latina space. Ethnicity as an intersubjective third." *Smith College Studies in Social Work*, 69(2), 255–67.

Meissner, W. W. (1996). "Empathy in the therapeutic alliance." *Psychological Inquiry*, 16(1), 39–53.

Miller, J. B. and Stiver, I. P. (1991). *A Relational Reframing of Therapy* (Working Paper Series, Work in Progress, No. 52). Wellesley, MA: Stone Center.

——(1995). *Relational Images and their Meaning in Psychotherapy* (Working Paper Series, Work in Progress, No. 74). Wellesley, MA: Stone Center.

Miller, W. R. and Rollnick, S. (2002). *Motivational Interviewing: Preparing People for Change*, 2nd Edition. New York: Guilford Press.

Mitchell, S. A. (1988). *Relational Concepts in Psychoanalysis*. Cambridge, MA: Harvard University Press.

Ogden, T. H. (1994). "The analytic third: Working with intersubjective clinical facts." *International Journal of Psycho-Analysis*, 75(1), 3–20.

Patterson, C. H. (1984). "Empathy, warmth, and genuineness: A review of reviews." *Psychotherapy*, 21(4), 431–38.

Perlman, F. T. and Brandell, J. R. (2011). "Psychoanalytic theory." In J. R. Brandell (ed.), *Theory and Practice in Clinical Social Work*, 2nd Edition (pp. 41–79). Thousand Oaks, California: SAGE Publications.

Rogers, C. (1951). *Client-centered Therapy*. New York: Houghton Mifflin.

Saleeby, D. (2006). *The Strengths Perspective in Social Work Practice*, 4th Edition. New York: Longman.

Sander, L. W. (1962). "Issues in early mother-child interaction." *Journal of the American Academy of Child Psychiatry*, 1, 141–66.

——(1995). *Thinking about Developmental Process: Wholeness, Specifity, and the Organization of Conscious Experiencing*. New York: American Psychological Association.

Sarri, C. (1986). "The created relationship: Transference, countertransference and the therapeutic culture." *Clinical Social Work Journal*, 14(1), 39–51.

Scaer, R. (2005). *The Trauma Spectrum: Hidden Wounds and Human Resiliency*. New York: W. W. Norton.

Schore, J. R. and Schore, A. N. (2008). "Modern attachment theory: The central role of affect regulation in development and treatment." *Clinical Social Work Journal*, 36(1), 9–20.

Siegel, D. J. (2012). *The Developing Mind*, 2nd Edition. New York: Guilford Publications, Inc.

Stern, D. (1985). *The Interpersonal World of the Human Infant: A View from Psychoanalysis and Developmental Psychology*. New York: Basic Books.

Stolorow, R. D. and Atwood, G. E. (1992). *Contexts of Being: The Intersubjective Foundations of Psychological Life*. Hillsdale, NJ: Analytic Press.

——(1997). "Deconstructing the myth of the neutral analyst: An alternative from intersubjective systems theory." *Psychoanalytic Quarterly*, 66, 431–49.

Stolorow, R. D., Atwood, G. E., and Brandchaft, B. (1994). *The Intersubjective Perspective*. Northdale, NJ: Jasaon Aronson.

Stolorow, R. D., Brandchaft, B., and Atwood, G. E. (1987). *Psychoanalytic Treatment: An Intersubjective Approach*. Hillsdale, NJ: Analytic Press.

Sullivan, H. S. (1953). *The Interpersonal Theory of Psychiatry*. New York: Norton.

Teitelbaum, S. (1991). "A developmental approach to resistance." *Clinical Social Work Journal*, 19(9), 119–130.

Tronick, E. (2007). "Implicit relational knowing: Its role in development and psycho-analytic treatment." In E. Tronick, *The Neurobehavioral and Social-emotional Development of Infants and Children* (pp. 412–17). New York: Norton.

Wachtel, P. L. (2008). *Relational Theory and the Practice of Psychotherapy*. New York: The Guilford Press.

Winnicott, D. W. (1960). "Ego distortions in terms of true and false Self." In D. W. Winnicott, *The Maturational Process and the Facilitating Environment* (pp. 140–52). London: Hogarth Press and the Institute of Psycho-Analysis, 1965.

——(1965). *The Maturational Processes and the Facilitating Environment*. New York: International Universities Press.

——(1971). *Playing and Reality*. London: Burns & Oates.

Woods, M. and Hollis, F. (2000). "The client-worker relationship." In M. Woods and F. Hollis, *Casework: A Psychosocial Therapy*, 5th Edition (pp. 229–61). New York: McGraw-Hill.

Zepf, S. (2007). "The relationship between the unconscious and consciousness – a comparison of psychoanalysis and historical materialism." *Psychoanalysis, Culture and Society*, 12 (2), 105–23.

Chapter 3

Bae, S.-W., and Kung, W. W.-M. (2000). "Family intervention for Asian Americans with a schizophrenia patient in the family." *American Journal of Orthopsychiatry*, 70(4), 532–41.

Bernstein, K. S., Lee, J. S., Park, S. Y., and Jyoung, J. P. (2008). "Symptom manifestations and expressions among Korean immigrant women suffering from depression." *Journal of Advanced Nursing*, 61(4), 393–402.

Bhugra, D. (2003). "Migration and depression." *Acta Psychiatrica Scandinavaca*, 108 (Suppl. 418), 67–72.

Chen, C.-M. (2006). "Asian communication studies: What and where to now." *Review of Communication*, 6(4), 295–311.

Chin, J. L. (1993). "Transference." In J. L. Chin, J. H. Liem, M. A. Domokos-Cheng Ham, and G. K. Hong (eds), *Transference and Empathy in Asian American Psychotherapy: Cultural Values and Treatment Needs* (pp. 15 –33). Westport, CT: Praeger Publishers.

Chung, I. W. (2008). "Affective lexicons and indigenous responses: Therapeutic interventions in social work practice with Chinese immigrant elders." *China Social Work Journal*, 1(3), 237–47.

Comas-Díaz, L. and Jacobsen, F. M. (1991). "Ethnocultural transference and countertransference in the therapeutic dyad." *American Journal of Orthopsychiatry*, 61(3), 392–402.

Delhiwala, N. and Sawant, M. Personal communication with author, 5 June 2012.

Gibbons, S. B. (2011). "Understanding empathy as a complex construct: A review of the literature." *Clinical Social Work Journal*, 39(3), 243–52.

Greene, G., Jensen, C., and Jones, D. (1996). "A constructivist perspective on clinical social work practice with ethnically diverse clients." *Social Work*, 41(2), 172–79.

Fonagy, P. (1998). "Moments of change in psychoanalytic theory: Discussion of a new theory of psychic change." *Infant Mental Health Journal*, 19(3), 346–53.

Hall, E. T. (1977). *Beyond Culture*. Garden City, NY: Anchor Books.

Ham, M. D. C. (1993). "Empathy." In J. L. Chin, J. H. Liem, M. D. C. Ham, and G. K. Hong (eds). *Transference and Empathy in Asian American Psychotherapy: Cultural Values and Treatment Needs* (pp. 35–58). Westport, CT: Praeger Publishers.

Ho, E. Personal communication with author, 21 April 2012.

Hwang, W., Myers, H., Abe-Kim, J., and Ting, J. (2008) "A conceptual paradigm for understanding culture's impact on mental health: The cultural influences on mental health (CIMH) model." *Clinical Psychology Review*, 28(2), 211–27.

Ino, S. M. and Glicken, M. D. (1999). "Treating Asian American clients in crisis: A collectivist approach." *Smith College Studies in Social Work*, 69(3), 525–42.

Ishii, S. (2004). "Proposing a Buddhist consciousness-only epistemological model for intra-personal communication research." *Journal of Intercultural Communication Research*, 33(2), 63–76.

Ito, K. L. and Maramba, G. G. (2002). "Therapeutic beliefs of Asian American Therapists: Views from an ethnic-specific clinic." *Transcultural Psychiatry*, 39(1), 33–73.

Kadushin, A. and Kadushin, G. (1997). *The Social Work Interview*, 4th Edition. New York: Columbia University Press.

Kim, J. M. (2005). "Culture specific psychoeducational induction talk as an intervention to increase service utilization among minority populations: The case of Korean Americans." In G. R. Waltz and R. Yep (eds), *Vistas: Compelling Perspectives on Counseling* (pp. 129–32). Alexandria, VA: American Counseling Association.

Kim, S. H. (2003). "Korean cultural codes and communication." *International Area Review*, 6 (1), 93–114.

Kim, S. W. Personal communication with author, 23 April 2012.

Leong, F. and Lee, S. H. (2006). "A cultural accommodation model for cross-cultural psychotherapy: Illustrated with the case of Asian Americans." *Psychotherapy*, 43 (4), 410–23.

Li, J. Personal communication with author, 6 June 2012.

Markus, H. R. and Kitayama, S. (1994). "The cultural shaping of emotion: A conceptual framework." In S. Kitayama and H. R. Markus (eds), *Emotion and Culture* (pp. 339–51). Washington DC: American Psychological Association.

Miike, Y. (2007). "An Asiacentric reflection on Eurocentric bias in communication theory." *Communication Monographs*, 74(2), 272–78.

Oatley, K. (1993). "Social construction in emotion." In M. Lewis and J. M. Haviland (eds), *Handbook of Emotions* (pp. 29–40). New York: Guilford Press.

Ots, T. (1990). "The angry liver, the anxious heart, and the melancholy spleen." *Culture, Medicine and Psychiatry*, 14(1), 21–58.

Pedersen, P. B., Crethar, H. C., and Carlson, J. (2008). *Inclusive Cultural Empathy: Making Relationships Central in Counseling and Psychotherapy*. Washington DC: American Psychological Association.

Raith, F. and Shim H. J. Personal communication with author, 13 July 2012.

Rogers, C. (1951). *Client-centered Therapy*. New York: Houghton Mifflin.

Roland, A. (1996). *Cultural Pluralism and Psychoanalysis*. New York: Routledge.

——(2011). *Journeys to Foreign Selves: Asians and Asian Americans in a Global Era*. New York: Oxford University Press.

Saleeby, D. (1994). "Culture, theory and narratives." *Social Work*, 39(4), 351–59.

Saral, T. B. (1983). "Hindu philosophy of communication." *Communication*, 8(1), 47–58.

Sarri, C. (1991). *The Creation of Meaning in Social Work*. New York: Guilford Press.

Scaer, R. (2005). *The Trauma Spectrum: Hidden Wounds and Human Resiliency*. New York: W. W. Norton.

Shonfeld-Ringel, S. (2001). "A re-conceptualization of the working alliance in cross-cultural practice with non-western clients: Integrating relational perspectives and multicultural theories." *Clinical Social Work Journal*, 29(1), 53–63.

Simpao, E. Personal communication with author, 25 September 2012.

Son, H. Personal communication with author, 27 November 2012.

Sue, D. W., and Sue, D. (2003). *Counseling the Culturally Diverse: Theory and Practice*, 4th Edition. New York: John Wiley & Sons.

Tronick, E. (2007). "Implicit relational knowing: Its role in development and psycho-analytic treatment." In E. Tronick, *The Neurobehavioral and Social-emotional Development of Infants and Children* (pp. 412–17). New York: Norton.

Tseng, W. S. (2004). "Culture and psychotherapy: Asian perspectives." *Journal of Mental Health*, 13(2), 151–61.

Vu, M. Personal communication with author, 6 July 2012.

Wachtel, P. L. (1998). *Therapeutic Communication: Knowing What to Say When*. New York: The Guilford Press.

Wong, N. Y. and Bagozzi, R. P. (2005). "Emotional intensity as a function of psychological distance and cultural orientation." *Journal of Business Research*, 58(4), 533–42.

Woods, M. and Hollis, F. (2000). *Casework: A Psychosocial Therapy*, 5th Edition. New York: McGraw-Hill.

Yew-Schwartz, P. Personal communication with author, 24 November 2012.

Zhou, S. Personal communication with author, 18 June 2012.

Chapter 4

Aroian, K. J., and Norris, A. E. (2000). "Resilience, stress, and depression among Russian immigrants to Israel." *Western Journal of Nursing Research*, 22(1), 54–67.

Australian Government Department of Immigration and Citizenship (2011). *2010–11 Migration Program Report*: Program Year to 30 June 2011. Retrieved 23 February 2012 from www.immi.gov.au/media/statistics/pdf/report-on-migration-program-2010-11.pdf.

——(2012). *Fact Sheet 4 – More than 60 Years of Post-war Migration*. Retrieved 25 February 2012 from www.immi.gov.au/media/fact-sheets/04fifty.htm.

Australian Institute of Health and Welfare (2011). *Adoptions Australia 2010–11*. Child welfare series no. 52. Cat. no. CWS 40. Retrieved 4 March 2012 from www.aihw.gov.au/publication-detail/?id=10737420776&tab=2.

Ayers, J. W., Hofstetter, C. R., Usita, P., Irvin, V. L., Kang, S., and Hovell, M. F. (2009). "Sorting out the competing effects of acculturation, immigrant stress, and social support on depression." *Journal of Nervous and Mental Disease*, 197(10), 742–47.

Beiser, M., Hou, F., Hyman, I., and Tousignant, M. (2002). "Poverty, family process, and the mental health of immigrant children in Canada." *American Journal of Public Health*, 92(2), 220–27.

Berry, J. W. (2003). "Conceptual approaches to acculturation." In K. M. Chun, P. B. Organista, and G. Marin (eds), *Acculturation: Advance in Theory, Measurement, and Applied Research* (pp. 17–38). Washington, DC: American Psychological Association.

Berry, J. W., and Sam, D. L. (1997). "Acculturation and adaptation." In J. W. Berry, Y. H. Poortinga, and J. Pandey (eds), *Handbook of Cross-cultural Psychology*, vol. 3 (pp. 291–326). Boston: Allyn & Bacon.

Betts, K. (1996). "Immigration and public opinion in Australia." *People and Place*, 4(3), 9–20.

Boehnlein, J. K., Tran, H. D., Riley, C., Vu, K. C., Tan, S., and Leung, P. K. (1995). "A comparative study of family functioning among Vietnamese and Cambodian refugees." *Journal of Nervous and Mental Diseases*, 183(12), 768–73.

Brown, T. N. (2003). "Critical race theory speaks to the sociology of mental health." *Journal of Health & Social Behavior*, 44(3), 292–301.

Campbell-Sills, L., Cohan, S. L., and Stein, M. B. (2006). "Relationship of resilience to personality, coping, and psychiatric symptoms in young adults." *Behaviour Research and Therapy*, 44(4), 585–99.

Child Exploitation and Online Protection Centre (2011). *Child Trafficking Update*. Retrieved 15 November 2012 from www.aic.gov.au/documents/D/8/6/%7bD868274B-2F97–45DB-BA32–33DBB7290A7C4%7dtandi401.pdf.

Cho, E. and Shin, S. (2008). "Survival, adjustment, and acculturation of newly immigrated families with school-age children: Stories of four Korean families." *Diaspora, Indigenous, and Minority Education*, 2(1), 4–24.

Chung, R. C.-Y. and Kagawa-Singer, M. (1993). "Predictors of psychological distress among southeast Asian refugees." *Social Science & Medicine*, 36(5), 631–39.

Citizenship and Immigration Canada. (2011). *Immigration Overview: Permanent and Temporary Residents*. Retrieved 3 March 2012 from www.cic.gc.ca/english/pdf/research-stats/facts2010.pdf.

Colebatch, T. (2011). "Asian migration a tour de force." *The Age*. Retrieved 3 March 2012 from www.theage.com.au/national/asian-migration-a-tour-de-force-20110616-1g62x.html.

Collins, J. (1995). "Asian immigration to Australia." In R. Cohen (ed.), *The Cambridge Survey of World Migration* (pp. 376–79). New York: Cambridge University Press.

Coughlan, J. E. (1997). "Korean immigrants in Australia." In J. E. Coughlan and D. J. McNamara (eds), *Asians in Australia: Patterns of Migration and Settlement* (pp. 171–97). South Melbourne: McMillan Education.

Falicov, C. J. (2012). "Immigrant family processes: A multidimensional framework." In F. Walsh (ed.), *Normal Family Processes: Growing Diversity and Complexity*. New York, NY: Guilford Press.

Fujimoto, Y. (2004). "The experience of Asian expatriates in Australia." *Journal of Doing Business Across Borders*, 3(1), 24–32.

Gee, G. C. and Ponce, N. (2010). "Associations between racial discrimination, limited English proficiency, and health-related quality of life among 6 Asian ethnic groups in California." *American Journal of Public Health*, 100(5), 888–95.

Gee, G. C., Ro, A., Shariff-Marco, S., and Chae, D. (2009). "Racial discrimination and health among Asian Americans: Evidence, assessment, and directions for future research." *Epidemiologic Reviews*, 31(1), 130–51.

Gee, G. C., Spencer, M. S., Chen, J., and Takeuchi, D. (2007). "A nationwide study of discrimination and chronic health conditions among Asian Americans." *American Journal of Public Health*, 97(7), 1275–282.

Gijsbert, O. (2007). "Global Indian diasporas: Exploring trajectories of migration and theory." In O. Gijsbert (ed.), *Global Indian Diasporas: Exploring Trajectories of Migration and Theory* (pp. 9–30). Amsterdam: University of Amsterdam.

Gordon, M. (1964). *Assimilation in American Life*. New York, NY: Oxford University Press.

Government of Canada (2012). *National Action Plan to Combat Human Trafficking*. Retrieved 15 November 2012 from www.publicsafety.gc.ca/prg/le/_fl/cmbt-trffkng-eng.pdf.

Guo, X. (2005). *Immigrating to and Ageing in Australia: Chinese Experiences*. PhD Dissertation, Murdoch University.

Han, G.-S. (2002). "From overt to covert racial discrimination in Australia: The experiences of Korean migrants." *Korean Social Science Journal*, 29(2), 1–13.

Heim, D., Hunter, S. C., and Jones, R. (2011). "Perceived discrimination, identification, social capital, and well-being: Relationships with physical health and psychological distress in a U.K. minority ethnic community sample." *Journal of Cross-Cultural Psychology*, 42(7), 1145–164.

Ho, E. and Bedford, R. (2008). "Asian transnational families in New Zealand: Dynamics and challenges." *International Migration*, 46(4), 41–62.

Ho, E. S. (2002). "Multi-local residence, transnational networks: Chinese 'astronaut' families in New Zealand." *Asian Pacific Migration Journal*, 11(1), 145–64.

Hugo, G. (2005a). "Asian experiences with remittances." In D. F. Terry and S. R. Wilson (eds), *Beyond Small Change: Making Migrant Remittances Count* (pp. 375–95). Washington, DC: Inter-American Development Bank.

——(2005b). "The new international migration in Asia: Challenges for population research." *Asian Population Studies*, 1(1), 93–120.

Huh, N. S. and Reid, W. J. (2000). "Intercountry, transracial adoption and ethnic identity: A Korean example." *International Social Work*, 43(1), 75–87.

Human Resources and Skills Development Canada (2011). *Intercountry Adoption Services*. Retrieved 25 February 2012 from www.hrsdc.gc.ca/eng/community_partnerships/international_adoption/publications/2006/canadian_issues.shtml.

Hwang, W.-C., and Ting, J. Y. (2008). "Disaggregating the effects of acculturation and acculturative stress on the mental health of Asian Americans." *Cultural Diversity and Ethnic Minority Psychology*, 14(2), 147–54.

Ip, M. (2000). "Beyond the 'settler' and 'astronaut' paradigms: a new approach to the study of the new Chinese immigrants to New Zealand." In M. Ip, S. H. Kang, and S. Page (eds), *Migration and Travel Between Asia and New Zealand* (pp. 3–17). Auckland, New Zealand: Asia-Pacific Migration Research Network.

Kessler, R. C., Berglund, P., Demler, O., Jin, R., Koretz, D., and Merikangas, K. (2003). "The epidemiology of major depressive disorder: Results from the National Comorbidity Survey Replication (NCS-R)." *Journal of the American Medical Association*, 40(3), 208–30.

Khan, Z. (2006). "Attitudes toward counseling and alternative support among Muslims in Toledo, Ohio." *Journal of Muslim Mental Health*, 1(1), 21–42.

Kim, U., and Choi, S. (1994). "Individualism, collectivism, and child development: A Korean perspective." In P. M. Greenfield and R. R. Cocking (eds), *Cross-cultural Roots of Minority Child Development* (pp. 227–57). Hillsdale, NJ: Lawrence Erlbaum.

Kroll, J., Habenicht, M., Mackenzie, T., Yang, M., Chan, S., Vang, T., Nguyen, T., Ly, M., Phommasovanh, B., Nguyen, H., Vang, Y., Sovannasoth, L., and Cabugao, R. (1989). "Depression and posttraumatic stress disorder in Southeast Asian refugees." *American Journal of Psychiatry*, 146(12), 1592–597.

Kwong, P. (1997). *Forbidden Workers: Illegal Chinese Immigrants and American Labor*. New York: New Press.

Larsen, J. J. (2010). "Migration and people trafficking in southeast Asia." *Trends and Issues in Crime and Criminal Justice, 401*. Retrieved 3 December 2012 from www.aic.gov.au/documents/D/8/6/%7bD868274B-2F97–45DB-BA32–33DBB7290A7C4%7dtandi401.pdf.

Laszloffy, T. and Hardy, K. (2000). "Uncommon strategies for a common problem: Addressing racism in family therapy." *Family Process*, 39 (1), 35–50.

Law, S., Hutton, M., and Chan, D. (2003). "Clinical, social, and service use characteristics of Fuzhounese undocumented immigrant patients." *Psychiatric Services*, 54(7), 1034–37.

Lee, H.-S., Brown, S. L., Mitchell, M. M., and Schiraldi, G. R. (2008). "Correlates of resilience in the face of adversity for Korean women immigrating to the US." *Journal of Immigrant and Minority Health*, 10, 415–22.

Lee, J. (2007). "Striving for the American dream: Struggle, success, and intergroup conflict among Korean immigrant entreprenuers." In M. Zhou and J. V. Gatewood (eds), *Contemporary Asian America: A Multidisciplinary Reader* (pp. 243–58). New York: New York University Press.

Levitt, P. and Jaworsky, B. N. (2007). "Transnational migration studies: Past developments and future trends." *Annual Review of Sociology*, 33, 129–56.

Loue, S. (2009). "Migration and mental health." In S. Loue and M. Sajatovic (eds), *Determinants of Minority Mental Health* (pp. 57–72). New York: Springer.

Luthar, S. S., Cicchetti, D., and Becker, B. (2000). "The construct of resilience: A critical evaluation and guidelines for future work." *Child Development*, 71(3), 543–62.

McLaughlin, A. A., Doane, L. S., Costiuc, A. L., and Feeny, N. C. (2009). "Stress and resilience." In S. Loue and M. Sajatovic (eds), *Determinants of Minority Mental Health* (pp. 349–64). New York: Springer.

McNamara, D. J. and Coughlan, J. E. (1997). "Asians in Australia: An introduction." In J. E. Coughlan and D. J. McNamara (eds), *Asians in Australia: Patterns of Migration and Settlement* (pp. 1–9). South Melbourne: MacMillan Education Australia.

Mak, A. S. and Nesdale, D. (2001). "Migrant distress: The role of perceived racial discrimination and coping resources." *Journal of Applied Social Psychology*, 31(12), 2632–647.

Martin, P. and Widgren, J. (2002). "International migration: Facing the challenge." *Population Bulletin*, 57(1), 3–43.

Miko, F. T. (2003). "Trafficking in women and children: The U.S. and international response." *CRS Report for Congress*. Retrieved 15 November 2012 from http://fpc.state.gov/documents/organization/31990.pdf.

Miller, M. J., Yang, M., Farrell, J. A., and Lin, L.-L. (2011). "Racial and cultural factors affecting the mental health of Asian Americans." *American Journal of Orthopsychiatry*, 81(4), 489–97.

Mishra, V. (2007). *The Literature of the Indian Diaspora: Theorizing the Diasporic Imagery*. London: Routledge.

New Zealand Department of Labour (2012). *Migration Trends Key Indicators Report: July 2010– June 2011*. Retrieved 25 February 2012 from www.dol.govt.nz/publications/general/monthly-migration-trends/11jun.

Office for National Statistics (2012). *Ethnicity and National Identity in England and Wales 2011*. Retrieved 29 March 2013 from www.ons.gov.uk/ons/dcp171776_290558.pdf.

Oishi, N. (2008). "Family without borders? Asian women in migration and the transformation of family life." *Asian Journal of Women's Studies*, 14(4), 54–79.

Pandey, A., Aggarwal, A., Devane, R., and Kuznetsov, Y. (2006). "The Indian Diaspora: A unique case?" In Y. Kuznetsov (ed.), *Diaspora Networks and the International Migration of Skills: How Countries Can Draw on their Talent Abroad*. Washington, DC: The World Bank.

Papademetriou, D. G., Sumption, M., Terrazas, A., Burkert, C., Loyal, S., and Ferrero-Turrion, R. (2010). "Migration and immigrants two years after the financial collapse: Where do we stand?" Retrieved 25 February 2012 from www.migrationpolicy.org/pubs/MPI-BBCreport-2010.pdf.

Paradies, Y. (2006). "A systematic review of empirical research on self-reported racism and health." *International Journal of Epidemiology*, 35(4), 888–901.

Parrenas, R. S. (2005). *Children of Global Migration: Transnational Families and Gendered Woes*. Palo Alto, CA: Stanford University Press.

Potocky-Tripodi, M. (2002). *Best Practices for Social Work with Refugees and Immigrants*. New York: Columbia University Press.

Rangaswamy, P. (2005). "South Asian diaspora." In M. Ember, C. Ember, and I. Skoggrad (eds), *Encyclopedia of the Diasporas: Immigrants and Refugees around the World*. New York: Springer.

Rasanathan, K., Craig, D., and Perkins, R. (2006). "The novel use of 'Asian' as an ethnic category in the New Zealand health sector." *Ethnicity and Health*, 11(3), 211–27.

Rastogi, M. (2007). "Coping with transitions in Asian Indian families: Systemic clinical interventions with immigrants." *Journal of Systemic Therapies*, 26(2), 55–67.

Ross-Sheriff, F. (2011). "Global migration and gender." *Affilia-Journal of Women and Social Work*, 26(3), 233–38.

Rudmin, F. W. (2003). "Critical history of the acculturation psychology of assimilation, separation, integration, and marginalization." *Review of General Psychology*, 7(1), 3–37.

Ryan, J. (2002). "Chinese women as transnational migrants: Gender and class in global migration narratives." *International Migration*, 40(2), 93–114.

Schwartz, S. J., Unger, J. B., Zamboanga, B. L., and Szapoczik, J. (2010). "Rethinking the concept of acculturation." *American Psychologist*, 65(4), 237–51.

Selman, P. (2009a). "Intercountry adoption in Europe 1998–2007: Patterns, trends, and issues." In K. Rummary, I. Greener, and C. Holden (eds), *Social Policy Review 21: Analysis and Debate in Social Policy* (pp. 133–65). Bristol: Social Policy Press.

——(2009b). "The rise and fall of intercountry adoption in the 21st century." *International Social Work*, 52(5), 575–94.

Shibusawa, T. (2004). "La practica clinica con le famiglie di immigrati asiatici. (Clinical practice with Asian immigrant families)" In M. Andolfi (ed.), *Famiglie immigrate e psicoterapia transculturale (Immigrant Families and Transcultural Psychotherapy)* (pp. 102–15). Milan, Italy: Franco Angeli.

——(2008). "Living up to the American dream: The price of being the model immigrants." *Psychotherapy Networker*, May/June, 41–57.

Subramanian, A. (2007). "Indians in North Carolina: Race, class, culture in the making of immigrant identity." In M. Zhou and J. V. Gatewood (eds), *Contemporary Asian America: A Mulitidisciplinary Reader* (pp. 158–75). New York: New York University Press.

Takei, I., and Sakamoto, A. (2011). "Poverty among Asian Americans in the 21st century." *Sociological Perspectives*, 54(2), 251–76.

Taylor, S. E. (1995). *Health Psychology*. New York: McGraw Hill.

Thompson, S., Manderson, L., Woelz-Stirling, N. Cahill, A., and Kelaher, M. (2002). "The social and cultural context of the mental health of Filipinas in Queensland." *Australian and New Zealand Journal of Psychiatry*, 36(5), 681–87.

Trickett, E. J., and Jones, C. J. (2007). "Adolescent culture brokering and family functioning: A study of families from Vietnam." *Cultural Diversity and Ethnic Minority Psychology*, 13(2), 143–50.

Tummala-Narra, P., Alegria, M., and Chen, C.-N. (2011). "Perceived discrimination, acculturative stress, and depression among South Asians: Mixed findings." *Asian American Journal of Psychology*, 2(3), 205–18.

US Census Bureau (2008). *An Older and Modern Nation by Midcentury*. Retrieved 15 October 2012 from www.census.gov/newsroom/releases/archives/population/cb08-123.html.

——(2012). *The Asian Population: 2010*. Retrieved 15 October 2012 from www.census.gov/prod/cen2010/briefs/c2010br-11.pdf.

United Nations Department of Economic and Social Affairs (2008). *International Migration Stock*. Retrieved 20 February 2012 from http://esa.un.org/migration/index.asp?panel=1.

——(2011). *International Migration Report 2009: A Global Assessment*. Retrieved 20 February 2012 from www.un.org/esa/population/publications/migration/WorldMigrationReport2009.pdf.

Walsh, F. (2010). "Family resilience." In F. Walsh (ed.), *Normal Family Process: Growing Diversity and Complexity* (pp. 399–427). New York, NY: Guilford Press.

Wang, S., and Lo, L. (2004). "Chinese immigrants in Canada: Their changing composition and economic performance." *CERIS Working Paper No. 30*. Retrieved 25 February 2012 from http://ceris.metropolis.net/wp-content/uploads/pdf/research_publication/working_papers/wp30.pdf.

——(2005). "Chinese immigrants in Canada: Their changing economic composition and economic performance." *International Migration Journal*, 43(3), 36–71.

Ward, C. (2009). "Acculturation and social cohesion: Emerging issues for Asian immigrants in New Zealand." In C.-H. Leong and J. W. Berry (eds), *Intercultural Relations in Asia: Migration and Work Effectiveness* (pp. 3–24). Singapore: World Scientific Publishing.

Ward, C. and Masgoret, A. M. (2008). "Attitudes towards immigrants, immigration and multiculturalism in New Zealand: A social psychological analysis." *International Migration Review*, 42(1), 222–43.

Xie, X., Xia, Y., and Zhou, Z. (2004). "Strengths and stress in Chinese immigrant families: A qualitative study." *Great Plain Research*, 14(2), 203–18.

Yoo, H. C., Gee, G. C., Lowthrop, C. K., and Robertson, J. (2010). "Self-reported racial discriminiation and substance use among Asian Americans in Arizona." *Journal of Immigrant and Minority Health*, 12(5), 683–90.

Yoon, I.-J. (2005). "Korean diaspora." In M. Ember, C. Ember, and I. Skoggrad (eds), *Encyclopedia of Diasporas: Immigrants and Refugees around the World* (pp. 201–13). New York: Springer.

Zhou, M. and Gatewood, J. V. (2007). "Transforming Asian America: Globalization and contemporary immigration to the United States." In M. Zhou and J. V. Gatewood (eds), *Contemporary Asian America: A Multidisciplinary Reader*, 2nd Edition (pp. 115–38). New York: New York University Press.

Chapter 5

Agbayani-Siewert, P. (1994). "Filipino American culture and family: Guidelines for practitioners." *Families in Society*, 75(7), 429–38.

Ahn, A. J., Kim, B. S. K., and Park, Y. S. (2008). "Asian cultural values gap, cognitive flexibility, coping strategies, and parent-child conflicts among Korean Americans." *Cultural Diversity and Ethnic Minority Psychology*, 14(4), 353–63.

Baumrind, D. (1991). "Parenting styles and adolescent development." In J. Brooks-Gunn, R. Lerner, and A. C. Petersen (eds), *The Encyclopedia on Adolescence* (pp. 746–658). New York: Garland.

Bond, M. H. and Hwang, K. K. (1986). "The social psychology of Chinese people." In M. H. Bond (ed.), *The Psychology of the Chinese People* (pp. 213–64). Hong Kong: Oxford Univeristy Press.

Bui, H. N. (2009). "Parent-child conflicts, school troubles, and differences in delinquency across immigration generations." *Crime and Delinquency*, 55(3), 412–41.

Chae, M. H. and Foley, P. F. (2010). "Relationship of ethnic identity, acculturation, and psychological well-being among Chinese, Japanese, and Korean Americans." *Journal of Counseling and Development*, 88(4), 466–76.

Chang, J. and Le, T. N. (2005). "Influence of parents, peer delinquency, and school attitudes on academic achievement in Chinese, Cambodian, Laotian or Mien, and Vietnamese youth." *Crime & Delinquency*, 51(2), 238–64.

Chang, J., Rhee, S., and Weaver, D. (2006). "Characteristics of child abuse in immigrant Korean families and correlates of placement decisions." *Child Abuse & Neglect*, 30(8), 881–91.

Chao, R. K. (1994). "Beyond parental control and authoritarian parenting style: Under-standing Chinese parenting through the cultural notion of training." *Child Development*, 65(4), 1111–19.

——(2001). "Extending research on the consequences of parenting style for Chinese Americans and European Americans." *Child Development*, 72(6), 1832–43.

Chao, R. K. and Kaeochinda, K. F. (2010). "Parental sacrifice and acceptance as distinct dimensions of parental support among Chinese and Filipino American adolescents." In S. T. Russell, L. J. Crockett, and R. K. Chao (eds), *Asian American Parenting and Parent-adolescent Relationships* (pp. 61–77). New York, NY: Springer.

Choi, Y. (2007). "Academic achievement and problem behaviors among Asian Pacific Islander American adolescents." *Journal of Youth and Adolescence*, 36(4), 403–15.

Choi, Y., He, M., and Harachi, T. W. (2008). "Intergenerational cultural dissonance, parent-child conflict and bonding, and youth problem behaviors among Vietnamese and Cambodian immigrant families." *Journal of Youth and Adolescence*, 37(1), 85–96.

Chuang, S. S., and Su, Y. (2009). "Do we see eye to eye? Chinese mothers' and fathers' parenting beliefs and values for toddlers in Canada and China." *Journal of Family Psychology*, 23(3), 331–41.

Chung, D. K. (1992). "Asian cultural commonalities: A comparison with mainstream American culture." In S. Furuto, R. Biswas, D. Chung, K. Murase, and E. Ross-Seriff (eds), *Social Work Practice with Asian Americans* (pp. 27–44). Newbury Park, CA: Sage.

Chung, I. W. (2006). "A cultural perspective on emotions and behavior: An empathic pathway to examine intergenerational conflicts in Chinese immigrant families." *Families in Society*, 87(3), 367–76.

——(2012). "Practice with Asian families and intergenerational issues." In E. Congress and M. Gonzales (eds), *Multicultural Perspectives in Social Work Practice with Families* (pp. 157–70). New York, NY: Springer.

Chung, R. C.-Y. and Bemak, F. (2002). "The relationship of culture and empathy in cross-cultural understanding." *Journal of Counseling & Development*, 80(2), 154–59.

Constantine, M. G., Alleyene, V. L., Caldwell, L. D., McRae, M. B., and Suzuki, M. B. (2005). "Coping responses of Asian, Black, and Latino/Latina New York City residents following the September 11, 2001 terrorist attacks against the United States." *Cultural Diversity and Ethnic Minority Psychology*, 11(4), 293–308.

Dosanjh, J. S. and Ghuman, P. A. S. (1998). "Child-rearing practices of two generations of Punjabis: Development of personality and independence." *Children & Society*, 12(1), 25–37.

Dugsin, R. (2001). "Conflict and healing in family experience of second-generation emigrants from India living in North America." *Family Process*, 40(2), 233–41.

Dwalry, M. A. (2008). "Parental inconsistency versus parental authoritarianism: Associations with symptoms of psychological disorders." *Journal of Youth and Adolescence*, 37(5), 616–26.

Erikson, E. H. (1980). *Identity and the Life Cycle*. New York: Norton.

Eyou, M. L., Adair, V., and Dixon, R. (2000). "Cultural identity and psychological adjustment of adolescent Chinese immigrants in New Zealand." *Journal of Adolescence*, 23 (5), 531–43.

Falicov, C. J. (2011). "Migration and the life cycle." In M. McGoldrick, B. Carter, and N. Garcia-Preto (eds), *The Expanded Family Life Cycle: Individual, Family and Social Perspectives*, 4th Edition) (pp. 336–47). Boston: Pearson Allyn & Bacon.

Farver, J. A. M., Narang, S. K., and Bhada, B. R. (2002). "East meets West: Ethnic iden-tity, acculturation and conflict in Asian Indian families." *Journal of Family Psychotherapy*, 16 (3), 338–50.

Fong, R. (1997). "Child welfare practice with Chinese families: Assessment issues for immigrants from the People's Republic of China." *Journal of Family Social Work*, 2(1), 33–47.

Fong, T. P. (2002). *The Contemporary Asian American Experience: Beyond the Model Minority*, 2nd Edition. New Jersey: Prentice Hall.

Fuligini, A. J., Tseng, V., and Lam, M. (1999). "Attitudes toward family obligations among American adolescents with Asian, Latin American, and European backgrounds." *Child Development*, 70(4), 1030–44.

Garcia-Preto, N. (2010). "Transformation of the Family System During Adolescence." In M. McGoldrick, B. Carter, and N. Garcia-Preto (eds), *The Expanded Family Life Cycle: Individual, Family, and Social Perspectives*, 4th edition (pp. 232–46). Boston, MA: Allyn & Bacon.

Gershoff, E. T. (2002). "Corporal punishment by parents and associated child behaviors and experiences: A meta-analytic and theoretical review." *Psychological Bulletin*, 128(4), 539–79.

Goodman, R. (2002). "Child abuse in Japan: 'Discovering' and the development of policy." In R. Goodman (ed.), *Family and Social Policy in Japan: Anthropological Approaches* (pp. 131–55). Cambridge: University of Cambridge.

Goyette, K. and Xie, Y. (1999). "Educational expectations of Asian American youths: Determinants of ethnic differences." *Sociology of Education*, 72(1), 22–36.

Hackett, L. and Hackett, R. (1994). "Child-rearing practices and psychiatric disorders in Gujarati and British children." *British Journal of Social Work*, 24(2), 191–202.

Harrington, D. and Dubowitz, H. (1999). "Preventing child maltreatment." In R. L. Hampton (ed.), *Family Violence, Prevention & Treatment* (pp. 122–47). Thousand Oaks, CA: Sage Publishers.

Hiles, M. and Luger, C. (2006). "The resolutions approach: Working with denial in child protection cases." *Journal of Systemic Therapies*, 25(2), 24–37.

Hindin, M. J. (2005). "Family dynamics, gender differences and educational attainment in Filipino adolescents." *Journal of Adolescence*, 28(3), 299–316.

Ho, Y. F. (1994). "Filial piety, authoritarian moralism, and cognitive conservatism in Chinese societies." *Genetic, Social, and General Psychology Monographs*, 120(3), 347–65.

Hong, J. S. (2010). "Understanding Vietnamese youth gangs in America: An ecological systems analysis." *Aggression and Violent Behavior*, 15(4), 253–60.

Huang, K.-Y., Calzalda, E., Cheng, S., and Brotman, L. M. (2012). "Physical and mental health disparities among young children of Asian immigrants." *The Journal of Pediatrics*, 160(2), 331–36.

Humphreys, C., Atkar, S., and Balwin, N. (1999). "Discrimination in child protection work: Recurring themes in work with Asian families." *Child & Family Social Work*, 4(4), 283–91.

Hwang, W.-C. (2006). "Acculturative family distancing: Theory, research, and clinical practice". *Psychotherapy: Theory, Research, Practice, Training*, 43(4), 397–409.

Hwang, W.-C., Wood, J. J., and Fujimoto, K. (2010). "Acculturative family distancing (AFD) and depression in Chinese American families." *Journal of Consulting and Clinical Psychology*, 78(5), 655–67.

Irfan, S. (2008). "Childrearing practice among South Asian Muslims in Britain: The cultural context of physical punishment." *Journal of Muslim Minority Affairs*, 28(1), 147–61.

Jambunathan, S., and Counselman, K. P. (2002). "Parenting attitudes of Asian Indian mothers living in the United States and in India." *Early Child Development and Care*, 172(6), 657–62.

Jin, M. K., Jacobvitz, D., and Hazen, N. (2010). "A cross-cultural study of attachment in Korea and the United States: Infant and maternal behavior during the strange situation." In P. Erdman and K.-M. Ng (eds), *Attachment: Expanding the Cultural Connections* (pp. 143–56). New York, NY: Routledge.

Johnson, F. A. (1993). *Dependency and Japanese Socialization*. New York: New York University Press.

Kacker, L., Vacadar, S., and Kumar, P. (2007). *A Study of Child Abuse: India 2007*. Retrieved 7 May 2012 from http://wcd.nic.in/childabuse.pdf.

Kang, H., Okazaki, S., Abelmann, N., Kim-Prieto, C., and Lan, Shanshan. (2010). "Redeeming immigrant parents: How Korean American emerging adults reinterpret their childhood." *Journal of Adolescent Research*, 25(3), 441–64.

Kim, S. Y. and Ge, X. (2000). "Parenting practices and adolescent depressive symptoms in Chinese American families." *Journal of Family Psychology*, 14(3), 420–35.

Kim, U. and Choi, S. (1994). "Individualism, collectivism, and child development: A Korean perspective." In P. M. Greenfield and R. R. Cocking (eds), *Cross-cultural Roots of Minority Child Development* (pp. 227–57). Hillsdale, NJ: Lawrence Erlbaum.

Kuo, B. C. H. (2011). "Culture's consequences on coping: Theories, evidences and dimensionalities." *Journal of Cross-Cultural Psychology*, 42(6), 1084–1100.

Kwok, S.-M., and Tam, D. M. Y. (2005). "Child abuse in Chinese families in Canada: Implications for child protection practice." *International Social Work*, 48(3), 341–48.

Landale, N. S., Thomas, K. J. A., and Van Hook, J. (2011). "The living arrangements of children of immigrants." *Future of Children*, 21(1), 43–70.

Larsen, S., Kim-Goh, M., and Nguyen, T. D. (2008). "Asian American immigrant families and child abuse: Cultural considerations." *Journal of Systemic Therapies*, 27(1), 16–29.

Lau, A. S., Takeuchi, D. T., and Alegria, M. (2006). "Parent-to-child aggression among Asian American parents: Culture, context, and vulnerability." *Journal of Marriage and Family*, 68(5), 1261–74.

Le, T. N., Monfared, G., and Stockdale, G. D. (2005). "The relationship of school, parents, and peer contextual factors with self-reported delinquency for Chinese, Cambodian, Lao/Mien, and Vietnamese youths." *Crime & Delinquency*, 51(2), 192–219.

Lee, E. and Mock, M. R. (2005). "Asian families: An overview." In M. McGoldrick, J. Giordano, and N. Garcia-Preto (eds), *Ethnicity and Family Therapy*, 3rd Edition. (pp. 269–89). New York: Guilford Press.

Lee, R. M., Su, J., and Yoshida, E. (2005). "Coping with intergenerational family conflict among Asian American college students." *Journal of Counseling Psychology*, 52(4), 389–99.

Leong, R. (1994). "Unfurling pleasure, embracing race." In G. Kundaka (ed.), *On a Bed of Rice: An Asian American Erotic Feast* (pp. xi–xxx). New York, NY: Anchor Books.

Lin, C. C. and Fu, V. R. (1990). "A comparison of child-rearing practices among Chinese, immigrant Chinese, and Caucasian-American parents." *Child Development*, 61(2), 429–33.

Long, P. D. P. (1997). "Cultural and social factors and Vietnamese gangs." *Journal of Contemporary Criminal Justice*, 13(4), 331–39.

Maiter, S. and George, U. (2003). "Understanding context and culture in the parenting approaches of immigrant South Asian mothers." *Affilia-Journal of Women and Social Work*, 18(4), 411–28.

Maker, A. H., Shah, P. V., and Agha, Z. (2005). "Child physical abuse: Prevalence, characteristics, predictors, and beliefs about parent-child violence in South Asian, Middle Easter, East Asian, and Latina women in the United States." *Journal of Interpersonal Violence*, 20(11), 1406–28.

Mason, K. O. (1992). "Family change and support of the elderly in Asia: What do we know?" *Asia-Pacific Population Journal*, 7(3), 12–23.

Mathews, B., and Kenny, M. C. (2008). "Mandatory reporting legislation in the United States, Canada, and Australia: A cross-jurisdictional review of key features, differences, and issues." *Child Maltreatment*, 13(1), 50–63.

Min, P. (1998). *Change and Conflicts: Korean Immigrant Families in New York*. New York: Allyn & Bacon.

Mulatti, L. (1995). "Families in India: Beliefs and realities." *Journal of Comparative Family Studies*, 26(1), 11–25.

Ngo, H. M. and Le, T. N. (2007). "Stressful life events, culture, and violence." *Journal of Immigrant Health*, 9, 75–84.

Nguyen, L., Arganza, G. F., Huang, L. N., Liao, Q., Nguyen, H. T., and Santiago, R. (2004). "Psychiatric diagnoses and clinical characteristics of Asian American youth in children's services." *Journal of Child and Family Studies*, 13(4), 483–95.

Noh, S., Beiser, M., Kaspar, V., Hou, F., and Rummens, J. (1999). "Perceived racial discrimination, depression, and coping: A study of Southeast Asian refugees in Canada." *Journal of Health and Social Behavior*, 40(3), 193–207.

Noh, S., and Kaspar, V. (2003). "Perceived discrimination and depression: Moderating effects of coping, acculturation, and ethnic support." *American Journal of Public Health*, 93 (2), 232–38.

O'Brian, C., and Lau, L. S. W. (1995). "Defining child abuse in Hong Kong." *Child Abuse Review*, 4(1), 38–46.

Office of Minority Health (2007). *Health status of Asian American and Pacific Islander Women*. Retrieved 28 August 2011 from http://minorityhealth.hhs.gov/templates/content.aspx?ID=3721.

Pang, V. O., Mizokawa, D. T., Morishima, J. K., and Olstad, R. G. (1985). "Self-concepts of Japanese-American children." *Journal of Cross-Cultural Psychology*, 16(1), 99–109.

Pelczarski, Y. and Kemp, S. P. (2006). "Patterns of child maltreatment referrals among Asian and Pacific Islander Families." *Child Welfare*, 85(1), 5–31.

Pettys, G. L. and Balgopal, P. R. (1998). "Multigenerational conflicts and new immigrants: An Indo-American experience." *Families in Society*, 79(4), 410–24.

Phinney, J. S. (2003). "Ethnic identity and acculturation." In K. M. Chun, P. Balls Organista, and G. Marin (eds), *Acculturation: Advances in Theory, Measurement, and Applied Research* (pp. 63–81). Washington, DC: American Psychological Association.

Phinney, J. S. and Ong, A. D. (2007). "Conceptualization and measurement of ethnic identity: Current status and future directions." *Journal of Counseling Psychology*, 54(3), 271–81.

Phinney, J. S., Lochner, B. T., and Murphy, R. (1990). "Ethnic identity development and psychological adjustment in adolescence." In A. R. Stiffman and L. E. Davis (eds), *Ethnic Issues in Adolescent Mental Health* (pp. 53–72). Thousand Oaks, CA: Sage Publications.

Pillari, V. (2005). "Indian Hindu families." In M. McGoldrick, J. Giordano, and N. Garcia-Preto (eds), *Ethnicity & Family Therapy* (pp. 395–406). New York: Guilford.

Pyke, K. (2000). "'The normal American family' as an interpretive structure of family life among grown children of Korean and Vietnamese immigrants." *Journal of Marriage and the Family*, 62(1), 240–55.

Qin, D. B. (2008). "Doing well vs. feeling well: Understanding family dynamics and the psychological adjustment of Chinese immigrant adolescents." *Journal of Youth and Adolescence*, 37(1), 22–35.

Rastogi, M. (2007). "Coping with transitions in Asian Indian families: Systemic clinical interventions with immigrants." *Journal of Systemic Therapies*, 26(2), 55–67.

Rhee, S., Chang, J., and Rhee, J. (2003). "Acculturation, communication patterns, and self-esteem among Asian and Caucasian American adolescents." *Adolescence*, 3(152), 749–68.

Roland, A. (1996). *Cultural Pluralism and Psychoanalysis: The Asian and North American Experience*. New York: Routledge.

Root, M. P. P. (2005). "Filipino families." In M. McGoldrick, J. Giordano, and N. Garcia-Preto (eds), *Ethnicity & Family Therapy*, 3rd Edition (pp. 313–31). New York, NY: Guilford.

Rosenbloom, S. and Way, N. (2004). "Experiences of discrimination among African Americans, Asian American, and Latino Adolescents in an urban high school." *Journal of Youth and Society*, 35, 420–51.

Schwartz, S. J., Unger, J. B., Zamboanga, B. L., and Szapoczik, J. (2010). "Rethinking the concept of acculturation." *American Psychologist*, 65(4), 237–51.

Segal, U. (1991). "Cultural variables in Asian Indian families." *Families in Society*, 72(4), 233–41.

Shek, D. T. and Chan, L. K. (1999). "Hong Kong's Chinese parents' perceptions of the ideal child." *The Journal of Psychology*, 133(3), 291–302.

Shibusawa, T. (2001). "Japanese American parenting." In N. B. Webb (ed.), *Culturally Diverse Parent–Child and Family Relationships: A Guide for Social Workers and Other Practitioners* (pp. 283–303). New York: Columbia University Press.

Sonuga-Barke, E. J. S. and Mistry, M. (2000). "The effect of extended family living on the mental health of three generations within two Asian communities." *British Journal of Clinical Psychiatry*, 39(2), 129–41.

Spencer, J. H. and Le, T. N. (2006). "Parent refugee status, immigration stressors, and Southeast Asian youth violence." *Journal of Immigrant Health*, 8, 359–68.

Steinberg, L., Blatt-Eisengart, I., and Cauffman, E. (2006). "Patterns of competence and adjustment among adolescents from authoritative, authoritarian, indulgent, and neglectful homes: A replication in a sample of serious juvenile offenders." *Journal of Research on Adolescence*, 16(1), 47–58.

Stewart, S. M., Bond, M. H., Kennard, B. D., Ho, L. M., and Zaman, R. M. (2002). "Does the Chinese construct of *guan* export to the West?" *International Journal of Psychology*, 37(2), 74–82.

Tajima, E. A. and Harachi, T. W. (2010). "Parenting beliefs and physical discipline practices among Southeast Asian immigrants: Parenting in the context of cultural adaptation to the United States." *Journal of Cross-Cultural Psychology*, 41(2), 212–35.

The Commonwealth Fund (1998). *The Commonwealth Fund Survey of the Health of Adolescent Girls*. New York: Commonwealth Fund.

Tomita, S. K. (1998). "The consequences of belonging: Conflict management techniques among Japanese Americans." *Journal of Elder Abuse & Neglect*, 9(3), 41–68.

Tompar-Tiu, A. and Sustento-Seneriches, S. (1995). *Depression and other Mental Health Issues: The Filipino American Experience*. San Francisico: Jossey-Bass.

Tweed, R. G., White, K., and Lehman, D. R. (2004). "Culture, stress, and coping: Internally- and externally-targeted control strategies of European Canadians, East Asian Canadians, and Japanese." *Journal of Cross-Cultural Psychology*, 35(6), 652–68.

Woelz-Stirling, N., Manderson, L., Kelaher, M., and Benedicto, A.-M. (2001). "Young women in conflict: Filipinas growing up in Australia." *Journal of Intercultural Studies*, 22(3), 295–306.

Wolf, D. A. (1997). "Family secrets: Transnational struggles among Children of Filipino immigrants." *Sociological Perspectives*, 40(3), 457–82.

Wu, C. and Chao, R. K. (2011). "Intergenerational cultural dissonance in parent–adolescent relationships among Chinese and European Americans." *Developmental Psychology*, 47(2), 493–508.

Wu, S.-J. (2001). "Parenting in Chinese American families." In N. B. Webb (ed.), *Culturally Diverse Parent–Child and Family Relationships: A Guide for Social Workers and Other Practitioners* (pp. 235–60). New York: Columbia University Press.

Xiong, Z. B., Eliason, P. A., Detzner, D. F., and Cleveland, M. (2005). "Southeast Asian immigrants' perceptions of good adolescents and good parents." *Journal of Psychology*, 139 (2), 159–75.

Yang, S. (2009). "Cane of love: Parental attitudes towards corporal punishment in Korea." *British Journal of Social Work*, 39(8), 1540–555.

Yap, J. (1986). "Philippine ethnoculture and human sexuality." *Journal of Social Work and Human Sexuality*, 4(3), 121–34.

Yee, B. W. K., Huang, L. N., and Lew, A. (1998). "Families: Life-span socialization in a cultural context." In L. C. Lee and N. W. S. Zane (eds), *Handbook of Asian American Psychology* (pp. 83–135). Thousand Oaks, CA: Sage Publications.

Yeh, C. J., Kim, A. B., Pituc, S. T., and Atkins, M. (2008). "Poverty, loss and resilience: The story of Chinese immigrant youth." *Journal of Counseling Psychology*, 55(1), 34–48.

Ying, Y.-W., and Han, M. (2007). "The longitudinal effect of intergenerational gap in acculturation on conflict and mental health in Southeast Asian American adolescents." *American Journal of Orthopsychiatry*, 77(1), 61–66.

Yip, T., Gee, G. C., and Takeuchi, D. T. (2008). "Racial discrimination and psychological distress: The impact of ethnic identity and age among immigrant and United States-born Asian adults." *Developmental Psychology*, 44(3), 787–800.

Yoshihama, M. (2002). "Battered women's coping strategies and psychological distress: Differences by immigrant status." *American Journal of Community Psychology*, 30(3), 429–52.

Yurgelun-Todd, D. A. and Killgore, W. D. S. (2006). "Fear-related activity in the prefrontal cortex increases with age during adolescence: A preliminary fMRI study." *Neuroscience Letters*, 406(3), 194–99.

Chapter 6

Abe-Kim, J., Takeuchi, D., and Hwang, W.-C. (2002). "Predictors of help-seeking for emotional distress among Chinese Americans: Family matters." *Journal of Counseling and Clinical Psychology*, 70(5), 1186–190.

Abraham, M. (2000). *Speaking the Unspeakable: Marital Violence among the South Asian Community in the United States*. New Brunswick, New Jersey: Rutgers University Press.

Ahmad, F., Driver, N., McNally, M. J., and Stewart, D. E. (2009). "'Why doesn't she seek help for partner abuse?': An exploratory study with South Asian immigrant women." *Social Science & Medicine*, 69(4), 613–22.

Anitha, S. (2010). "No recourse, no support: State policy and practice towards South Asian women facing domestic violence in the UK." *British Journal of Social Work*, 40(2), 462–79.

Asian & Pacific Islander Institute on Domestic Violence (2010). *Innovative Strategies to Address Domestic Violence in Asian and Pacific Islander Communities: Examining Themes, Models, and Interventions*. San Francisco, CA: Asian & Pacific Islander Institute on Domestic Violence.

——(2012). *Fact sheet: Domestic Violence in South Asian Communities*. Retrieved 23 June 2012 from www.apiidv.org/files/DVFactSheet-SouthAsian-APIIDV-2012.pdf.

Australian Domestic and Family Violence Clearing House. Retrieved 25 June 2012 from www.austdvclearinghouse.unsw.edu.au/good_practice.html.

Babin, E. A., Palazzolo, K. E., and Rivera, K. D. (2012). "Communication skills, social support, and burnout among advocates in a domestic violence agency." *Journal of Applied Communication Research*, 40(2), 147–66.

Bell, K. M. and Naugle, A. E. (2008). "Intimate partner violence theoretical considerations: Moving towards a contextual framework." *Clinical Psychology Review*, 28(7), 1096–1107.

Bennett, L., Riger, S., Schewe, P., Howard, A., and Wasco, S. (2004). "Effectiveness of hotline, advocacy, counseling and shelter services for victims of domestic violence." *Journal of Interpersonal Violence*, 19(7), 815–29.

Bhuyan, R., Mell, M., Senturia, K., Sullivan, M., and Shiu-Thornton, S. (2005). "'Women must endure according to their karma': Cambodian immigrant women talk about domestic violence." *Journal of Interpersonal Violence*, 20(8), 902–21.

Bonomi, A. E., Anderson, M. L., Reid, R. J., Rivara, F. P., and Thompson, R. S. (2009). "Medical and psychosocial diagnoses in women with a history of intimate partner violence." *Archives of Internal Medicine*, 169(18), 1692–97.

Brown, C. and O'Brien, K. M. (1998). "Understanding stress and burnout in shelter workers." *Professional Psychology: Research and Practice*, 29(4), 383–85.

Bui, H. N. (2003). "Help-seeking behavior among abused immigrant women." *Violence Against Women*, 9(2), 207–39.

Bui, H. N. and Morash, M. (1999). "Domestic violence in Vietnamese immigrant community." *Violence Against Women*, 5(7), 765–95.

Bybee, D. I. and Sullivan, C. M. (2002). "The process through which an advocacy intervention resulted in positive change for battered women over time." *American Journal of Community Psychology*, 30(1), 103–32.

——(2005). "Predicting re-victimization of battered women 3 years after exiting a shelter program." *American Journal of Community Psychology*, 36(1), 85–96.

Cabinet Office Japan (2009). *Research Regarding Violence between Men and Women*. Retrieved 21 June 2012 from www.gender.go.jp/e-vaw/chousa/images/pdf/chousagaiyou.pdf.

Cavanaugh, M. M. and Gelles, R. J. (2005). "The utility of male domestic violence offender typologies: New directions for research, policy, and practice." *Journal of Interpersonal Violence*, 20(2), 155–66.

Cho, H. (2012). "Intimate partner violence among Asian Americans: Risk factor differences across ethnic subgroups." *Journal of Family Violence*, 27(3), 215–24.

Cunradi, C. B., Caetano, R., and Schafer, J. (2002). "Alcohol-related problems, drug use, and male intimate partner violence severity among US couples." *Alcoholism: Clinical and Experimental Research*, 26(4), 493–500.

Dasgupta, S. D. (2000). "Charting the course: An overview of domestic violence in the South Asian community in the United States." *Journal of Social Distress and the Homeless*, 9 (3), 173–85.

Dunn, L. J. and Powell-Williams, M. (2007). "Everyone makes choices: Victim advocates and the social construction of battered women's victimization and agency." *Violence Against Women*, 13(10), 977–1001.

Dutton, D. (1994). "The origin and structure of the abusive personality." *Journal of Personality Disorder*, 8(3), 181–91.

EACH (2009). *Asian Women, Domestic Violence and Mental Health: A Toolkit for Health Professionals*. Retrieved 23 June 2012 from www.ndvf.org.uk/files/document/889/original.pdf.

Garcia-Moreno, C., Jansen, H. A., Ellsberg, M., Heise, L., and Watts, C. H. (2006). "Prevalence of intimate partner violence: findings from the WHO multi-country study on women's health and domestic violence." *Lancet*, 368(9543), 1260–69.

Gibbons, D., Lichtenberg, P., and van Beusekom, J. (1994). "Working with victims: Being empathic helpers." *Clinical Social Work Journal*, 22(2), 211–22.

Gill, A. (2004). "Voicing the silent fear: South Asian women's experiences of domestic violence." *The Howard Journal of Criminal Justice*, 43(5), 465–83.

Goodman, L. A., Smyth, K. F., Borges, A. M., and Singer, R. (2009). "When crises collide: How intimate partner violence and poverty intersect to shape women's mental health and coping." *Trauma, Violence, & Abuse*, 10(4), 306–29.

Hamel, J. (2007). "Domestic violence: A gender-inclusive conception." In J. Hamel and T. L. Nicholls (eds), *Family Interventions in Domestic Violence: A Handbook for Gender-inclusive Theory and Treatment* (pp. 3–26). New York, NY: Springer

Hattendorf, J. and Tollerud, T. R. (1997). "Domestic violence: Counseling strategies that minimize the impact of secondary victimization." *Perspectives in Psychiatric Care*, 33(1), 14–23.

Hicks, M. H.-R. (2006). "The prevalence and characteristics of intimate partner violence in a community study of Chinese American women." *Journal of Interpersonal Violence*, 21(10), 1249–69.

Jenkins, S. R. and Baird, S. (2002). "Secondary traumatic stress and vicarious trauma: A validational study." *Journal of Traumatic Stress*, 15(5), 423–32.

Jin, X. and Keat, J. E. (2010). "The effects of change in spousal power on intimate partner violence among Chinese immigrants." *Journal of Interpersonal Violence*, 25(4), 610–25.

Johnson, M. P. (1995). "Patriarchal terrorism and common couple violence: Two forms of violence against women." *Journal of Marriage and the Family*, 57(2), 283–94.

Johnson, M. P. and Ferraro, K., J. (2000). "Research on domestic violence in the 1990s: Making distinctions." *Journal of Marriage and the Family*, 62(4), 948–63.

Jordan, C. E., Campbell, R., and Follingstad, D. (2010). "Violence and women's mental health: The impact of physical, sexual, and psychological aggression." *Annual Review of Clinical Psychology*, 6, 607–28.

Kaliivayalil, D. (2010). "Narratives of suffering of South Asian immigrant survivors of domestic violence." *Violence Against Women*, 16(7), 789–811.

Kim, H. and Kahng, S. K. (2011). "Examining the relationship between domestic violence and depression among Koreans: The role of self-esteem and social support as mediators." *Asian Social Work and Policy Review*, 5(3), 181–97.

Kim, I. J. and Zane, N. (2004). "Ethnic and cultural variations in anger regulation and attachment patterns among Korean American and European American male batterers." *Cultural Diversity and Ethnic Minority Psychology*, 10(2), 151–68.

Kim, J. Y. and Sung, K. (2000). "Conjugal violence in Korean American families: A residue of the cultural tradition." *Journal of Family Violence*, 15(4), 331–45.

Lee, M. Y. (2000). "Understanding Chinese battered women in North America: A review of the literature and practice implications." *Journal of Multicultural Social Work*, 8(3–4), 215–41.

Lee, Y.-S. and Hadeed, L. (2009). "Intimate partner violence among Asian immigrant communities." *Trauma, Violence, & Abuse*, 10(2), 143–70.

McCann, L. and Pearlman, L. (1990). "Vicarious traumatization: A framework for understanding the psychological effects of working with victims." *Journal of Tramatic Stress*, 3(1), 131–49.

Panchandadeswaran, S. and McCloskey, L. A. (2007). "Predicting the timing of women's departure from abusive relationships." *Journal of Interpersonal Violence*, 22(1), 50–65.

Papp, A. (2010). "Culturally driven violence against women: A growing problem in Canada's immigrant communities." *FCCP Policy Series No. 92*. Retrieved 25 June 2012 from www.fcpp.org/files/1/Culturally-Driven Violence Against Women.pdf.

Pillai, S. (2001). "Domestic violence in New Zealand: An Asian immigrant perspective." *Economic and Political Weekly*, 38(11), 965–74.

Preisser, A. (1999). "Domestic violence in South Asian communities in America." *Violence Against Women*, 5(6), 684–99.

Raj, A. and Silverman, J. G. (2003). "Immigrant South Asian women at greater risk for injury from intimate partner violence." *American Journal of Public Health*, 93(3), 435–38.

Raj, A., Livramento, K. N., Santana, M. C., Gupta, J., and Silverman, J. G. (2008). "Victims of intimate partner violence more likely to report abuse from in-laws." *Violence Against Women*, 12(10), 936–49.

Saroca, C. (2007). "Filipino women, migration, and violence in Australia: Lived reality and media image." *Kasarinlan: Journal of Third World Studies*, 21(1), 75–110.

Shirwadakar, S. (2004). "Canadian domestic violence policy and Indian immigrant women." *Violence Against Women*, 10(8), 860–79.

Shiu-Thornton, S., Senturia, K., and Sullivan, M. (2005). "'Like a bird in a cage': Vietnamese women survivors talk about domestic violence." *Journal of Interpersonal Violence*, 20(8), 959–76

Sokoloff, N. J. and Dupont, I. (2005). "Domestic violence at the intersections of race, class, and gender: Challenges and contributions to understanding violence against marginalized women in diverse communities." *Violence Against Women*, 11(1), 38–64.

Song, L.-Y. and Shih, C.-Y. (2010). "Recovery from partner abuse: The application of a strengths perspective." *International Journal of Social Welfare*, 19(1), 23–32.

Song, Y. I. (1996). *Battered Korean Women in Korean Immigrant Families: The Silent Scream.* New York: Garland.

Sullivan, C. M. (2006). "Interventions to address intimate partner violence: The current state of the field." In J. R. Lutzker (ed.), *Preventing Partner Violence: Research and Evidence-based Intervention Strategies* (pp. 195–212). Washington, DC: American Psychological Association.

Tjaden, P. and Thoennes, N. (2000). *Extent, Nature, and Consequences of Intimate Partner Violence: Findings from the National Violence Against Women Survey.* Retrieved 25 June 2012 from www.ncjrs.gov/pdffiles1/nij/181867.pdf.

Tse, S. (2007). "Family violence in Asian communities, combining research and community development." *Social Policy Journal of New Zealand*, 31, 170–94.

Wang, Hao. Personal communication with author, 9 May 2012.

Wang, J.-Y., Probst, J. C., Moore, C. G., Martin, A. B., and Bennett, K. J. (2011). "Place of origin and violent disagreement among Asian American families: Analysis across five States." *Journal of Immigrant Minority Health*, 13, 635–46.

Women's Aid. Retrieved 25 June 2012 from www.womensaid.org.uk/landing_page.asp?section=000100010024&sectionTitle=Find+a+local+service.

Wong, F. Y., DiGangi, J., Young, D., Huang, J. Z., Smith, B. D., and John, D. (2011). "Intimate partner violence, depression, and alcohol use among a sample of foreign-born Southeast Asian women in an urban setting in the United States." *Journal of Interpersonal Violence*, 26(2), 211–29.

World Health Organization. (2002). *World Report on Violence and Health.* Retrieved 25 June 2012 from http://whqlibdoc.who.int/publications/2002/9241545615_eng.pdf.

Xu, X., Campbell, J. C., and Zhu, F.-C. (2001). "Intimate partner violence against Chinese women: The past, present, and future." *Trauma, Violence, & Abuse*, 4(2), 296–315.

Yick, A. G. and Oomen-Early, J. A. (2008). "A 16-year examination of domestic violence among Asians and Asian Americans in the empirical knowledge base: A content analysis." *Journal of Interpersonal Violence*, 23(8), 1075–94.

Yoshioka, M. and Dang, Q. (2000). *Asian Family Violence Report: A Study of Cambodian, Chinese, Korean, South Asian, and Vietnamese Communities in Massachusetts.* Retrieved 25 June 2012 from www.atask.org/site/images/pdf/asianfamilyviolencereport.pdf.

Yoshioka, M., DiNoia, J., and Ullah, K. (2001). "Attitudes toward marital violence: An examination of four Asian communities." *Violence Against Women*, 7(8), 900–926.

Zlotnick, C., Johnson, D. M., and Kohn, R. (2006). "Intimate partner violence and long-term psychosocial functioning in a national sample of American Women." *Journal of Interpersonal Violence*, 21(2), 262–75.

Chapter 7

AARP Public Policy Institute (2004). *Sources of Income for Persons in 2002*. Retrieved 15 April 2010 from www.aarp.org/research/socialsecurity/benefits/sources_of_income_for _older_persons_in_2002.html.

Allers, C. T., Benjack, K. J., and Allers, N. T. (1992). "Unresolved childhood sexual abuse: Are older adults affected?" *Journal of Counseling and Development*, 71(1), 14–17.

American Association for Retired Persons (2001). *A Report on Multicultural Boomers Coping with Family and Aging Issues* Washington, DC: American Association for Retired Persons.

Anderson, G. and Hovarth, J. (2004). "The growing burden of chronic disease in America." *Public Health Reports*, 119(3), 263–70.

Angel, R. J., Angel, J. L., Kee, G.-Y., and Markides, K. S. (1999). "Age at migration and family dependency among older Mexican immigrants: Recent evidence from the Mexican American EPESE." *Gerontologist*, 39(1), 59–65.

Area Agency on Aging. (2008). *Older Americans Act*. Retrieved 30 September 2007, from www.aoa.gov/about/legbudg/oaa/legbudg_oaa.asp.

Arnsberger, P. (2005). "Best practices in care management for Asian American elders: The case of Alzheimer's disease." *Care Management Journals*, 6(4), 171–77.

Baer, R. (ed.). (2006). *Mindfulness-based Approaches: A Clinican's Guide to Evidence Base and Applications*. Burlington, MA: Academic Press.

Bellomo, A., Altamura, M., Ventriglio, A., Rella, A., Quartesan, R., and Elisei, S. (2007). "Psychological factors affecting medical conditions in consultation-liaison psychiatry." *Advances in Psychosomatic Medicine*, 28, 127–40.

Bhatnagar, K. and Frank, J. (1997). "Psychiatric disorders in the elderly from the Indian sub-continent living in Bradford." *International Journal of Geriatric Psychiatry*, 12(9), 907–12.

Blazer, D. G. (2002). "The prevalence of depressive symptoms." *Journals of Gerontology*, 57(3), M150–M151.

Braun, K. L. and Nichols, R. (1997). "Death and dying in four Asian American cultures: A descriptive study." *Death Studies*, 21(4), 327–59.

Braun, K. L., Onaka, A. T., and Horiuchi, B. Y. (2001). "Advance directive completion rates and end-of-life preferences in Hawaii." *Journal of the American Geriatrics Society*, 49(12), 1708–13.

Brodaty, H., Luscombe, G., Parker, G., Wilhelm, K., Hickie, I., Austine, M.-P., and Mitchell, P. (2001). "Early and late onset depression in old age: Different aetiologies, same phenomenology." *Journal of Affective Disorders*, 66 (2–3), 225–36.

Busuttil, W. (2004). "Presentations and management of Post Traumatic Stress Disorder and the elderly: A need for investigation." *International Journal of Geriatric Psychiatry*, 19(5), 429–39.

Byers, A. L., Yaffe, K., Covinsky, K. E., Friedman, M. B., and Bruce, M. L. (2010). "High occurence of mood and anxiety disorders among older adults." *Archives of General Psychiatry*, 67(5), 489–96.

Centers of Disease Control and Prevention National Center for Injury Prevention and Control. Web-Based Injury Statistics Query and Reporting System (WISQARS). Retrieved 20 December 2007 from www.cdc.gov/ncipc/wisqars.

Chao, S. Z., Lai, N. B., Tse, M. M., Ho, R. J., Kong, J. P., Matthews, B. R., Miller, B. L., and Rosen, H. J. (2011). "Recruitment of Chinese American elders into dementia research: The UCSF ADRC experience." *The Gerontologist*, 51(SI), S125–S133.

Chen, S., Sullivan, N. Y., Lu, Y. E., and Shibusawa, T. (2003). "Asian Americans and mental health services: A study of utilization patterns in the 1990s." *Journal of Ethnic & Cultural Diversity in Social Work*, 12(2), 19–42.

Cheuk, J. T. Y., Chang, Q. K. N., and Ungvari, G. S. (2009). "Demoralization as a diagnostic conundrum: Case reports." *Hong Kong Journal of Psychiatry*, 19(4), 159–63.

Chow, H. P. H. (2010). "Growing old in Canada: Physical and psychological well-being among elderly Chinese immigrants." *Ethnicity & Health*, 15(1), 61–72.

Chow, J. C., Jaffee, K., and Snowden, L. R. (2003). "Racial/ethnic disparities in the use of mental health services in poverty areas." *American Journal of Public Health*, 93(5), 792–97.

Chung, H. (2002). "The challenges of providing behavioral treatment to Asian Americans." *Western Journal of Medicine*, 176(4), 222–23.

Clarke, D. M., Cook, K. E., Coleman, K. J., and Smith, G. C. (2006). "A Qualitative Examination of the Experience of "Depression" in Hospitalized Medically Ill Patients." *Psychopathology*, 39(6), 303–12.

Cook, J. M. (2001). "Post-traumatic disorder in older adults." *PTSD Research Quarterly*, 12(3), 1–3.

de Figueiredo, J. M. (1993). "Depression and demoralization: Phenomenologic differences and research perspectives." *Comprehensive Psychiatry*, 34(5), 308–11.

Diwan, S., Jonnalagadda, S. S., and Gupta, R. (2004). "Differences in the structure of depression among older Asian Immigrants in the United States." *Journal of Applied Gerontology*, 23(4), 370–84.

Dong, X., Chang, E.-S., Wong, E., and Simon, M. (2011). "The Perceptions, Social Determinants, and Negative Health Outcomes Associated With Depressive Symptoms Among U.S. Chinese Older Adults." *The Gerontologist*, 52(5), 650–63.

Elder, G. H. J., Johnson, M. K., and Crosnoe, R. (2003). "The emergence and development of life course theory." In J. T. Mortimer and M. J. Shanahan (eds), *Handbook of the Life Course* (pp. 3–22). New York: Kluwer Academic/Plenum Publishers.

Evandrou, M. (2000). "Ethnic inequality in later life." *Health Statistics Quarterly*, 8, 20–28.

Federal Interagency Forum on Aging-related Statistics (2012). *Older Americans 2012: Key Indicators of Well-being*. Retrieved 5 December 2012 from www.agingstats.gov/agingstatsdotnet/ Main_Site/Data/2010_Documents/Docs/OA_2010.pdf.

Fiske, A., Wetherhill, J. L., and Gatz, M. (2009). "Depression in older adults." *Annual Review of Clinical Psychology*, 5, 363–89.

Gallagher-Thompson, D., Steffen, A. M., and Thompson, L. W. (eds). (2008). *Behavioral and Cognitive Therapies with Older Adults*. New York, NY: Springer.

Gerber, L., Nguyen, Q., and Bounkea, P. K. (1999). "Working with Southeast Asian people who have migrated to the United States." In K. Nader, N. Dubrow and B. H. Stamm (eds), *Honoring Differences: Cultural Issues in the Treatment of Trauma and Loss* (pp. 98–118). Philadelphia, PA: Brunner/Mazel.

Goncalves, D. C., Albuquerque, P. B., Byrne, G. J., and Pachana, N. A. (2009). "Assessment of depression in aging contexts: General considerations when working with older adults." *Professional Psychology: Research and Practice*, 40(6), 609–16.

Gupta, R. and Chaudhuri, A. (2008). "Elder Abuse in a Cross-Cultural Context: Assessment, Policy and Practice." *Indian Journal of Gerontology*, 22(3), 148–71.

Hall, G. C. N., Hong, J. J., Zane, N. W. S., and Meyer, O. L. (2011). "Culturally competent treatments for Asian Americans: The relevance of mindfulness and acceptance-based psychotherapies." *Clinical Psychology: Science and Practice*, 18(3), 215–31.

Hasnain, R. and Rana, S. (2010). "Unveiling Muslim voices: Aging parents with disabilities and their adult children and family caregivers in the United States." *Topics in Geriatric Rehabilitiation*, 26(1), 46–61.

Hertzman, C. (2004). "The life-course contribution to ethnic disparities in health." In N. B. Anderson, R. A. Bulatao, and B. Cohen (eds), *Critical Perspectives on Racial and Ethnic Differences in Health in Late Life* (pp. 145–70). Washington, DC: The National Academies Press.

Hooyman, N. R. and Kiyak, H. A. (2002). *Social Gerontology: A Multidisciplinary Perspective*, 6th Edition. Boston, MA: Allyn & Bacon.

Hu, T. W., Snowden, L. R., Jerrell, J. M., and Kang, S. H. (1993). "Public mental health services to Asian American ethnic groups in two California counties." *Asian American and Pacific Islander Journal of Health*, 1(1), 79–90.

Iwamasa, G. and Hilliard, K. M. (1999). "Depression and anxiety among Asian American elders: a review of the literature." *Clinical Psychology Review*, 19(3), 343–57.

Jang, M., Lee, E., and Woo, K. (1998). "Income, language, and citizenship status: Factors affecting the health care access and utilization of Chinese Americans." *Health & Social Work*, 23(2), 136–45.

Jenkins, C. N. H., Le, T., McPhee, S. J., Stewart, S., and Ha, N. T. (1996). "Health care access and preventive care among Vietnamese immigrants: Do traditional beliefs and practices pose barriers?" *Social Science & Medicine*, 43(7), 1049–56.

Kellerman, N. P. F. (2001). "The long-term psychological effects and treatment of holocaust trauma." *Journal of Loss and Trauma*, 3(19), 197–218.

Kim, H. S., Sherman, D. K., and Taylor, S. E. (2008). "Culture and social support." *American Psychologist*, 63(6), 518–26.

Kim, K. C., Kim, S., and Hurh, W. M. (1991). "Filial piety and intergenerational relationship in Korean immigrant families." *International Journal on Aging and Human Development*, 33(3), 233–45.

Kim, W. and Chen, Y.-L. (2011). "The social determinants of depression in elderly Korean immigrants in Canada: Does acculturation matter?" *International Journal of Aging and Human Development*, 73(4), 283–98.

Kissane, D. W. (2001). "Demoralisation – A useful conceptualisation of existential distress in elderly." *Australian Journal on Ageing*, 20(3), 110–11.

Kleinman, A. (1988). *The Illness Narrative: Suffering, Healing, and the Human Condition*. New York, NY: Basic Books.

Kogan, J. N., Edelstein, B. A., and McKee, D. R. (2000). "Assessment of anxiety in older adults: Current status." *Journal of Anxiety Disorders*, 14(2), 109–32.

Kuo, B. C. H. (2011). "Culture's consequences on coping: Theories, evidences and dimensionalities." *Journal of Cross-Cultural Psychology*, 42(6), 1084–100.

Kuo, B. C. H., Chong, V., and Joseph, J. (2008). "Depression and its psychosocial correlates among older Asian immigrants in North America." *Journal of Aging and Health*, 20(6), 615–52.

Lai, D. (2004). "Health status of older Chinese in Canada: Findings from the SF36 Health Survey." *Canadian Journal of Public Health*, 95(3), 193–97.

Lai, D. and Surood, S. (2008). "Predictors of depression in aging South Asian Canadians." *Journal of Cross-Cultural Gerontology*, 23(1), 57–75.

Larson, E. B. and Imai, Y. (1996). "An overview of dementia and ethnicity with special emphasis on the epidemiology of dementia." In G. Yeo and D. Gallagher-Thompson (eds), *Ethnicity & the Dementias* (pp. 9–20). Washington, DC: Taylor & Francis.

Lauderdale, D. S., Kuohung, V., Chang, S.-L., and Chin, M. H. (2003). "Identifying older Chinese immigrants at high risk for osteoporosis." *Journal of General Internal Medicine*, 18(7), 508–15.

Le, Q. K. (1997). "Mistreatment of Vietnamese elderly by their families in the United States." *Journal of Elder Abuse & Neglect*, 9(2), 51–62.

Lee, E. (1996). "Chinese American families." In E. Lee (ed.), *Working with Asian Americans: A Guide for Clinicians* (pp. 46–78). New York: Guilford Press.

Lee, M. M., Lin, S. S., Wrensch, M. R., Adler, S. R., and Eisenberg, D. (2000). "Alternative therapies used by women with breast cancer in four ethnic populations." *Journal of National Cancer Institute*, 92(1), 42–47.

Lee, S. E., Diwan, S., and Yeo, G. (2010). "What do Korean American immigrants know about Alzheimer's disease (AD)? The impact of acculturation and exposure to the disease on AD knowledge." *International Journal of Geriatric Psychiatry*, 25(1), 66–73.

Lee, S. M., Lin, X., Haralambous, B., Dow, B., Vrantsidis, F., Tinney, J., Blackberry, I., Lautenschlager, N., and Giudice, D. L. (2011). "Factors impacting on early detection of dementia in older people of Asian background in primary healthcare." *Asia-Pacific Psychiatry*, 3(3), 120–27.

Leung, J. P. (1998). "Emotions and mental health in Chinese people." *Journal of Child and Family Studies*, 7(2), 115–28.

Levkoff, S., Levy, B., and Weitzman, P. F. (1999). "The role of religion and ethnicity in the help-seeking of family caregivers of elders with Alzheimer's disease and related disorders." *Journal of Cross-Cultural Gerontology*, 14(4), 335–56.

Li, W. W. and Chong, M. D. (2012). "Transnationalism, social wellbeing and older Chinese migrants." *Graduate Journal of Asia-Pacific Studies*, 8(1), 29–44.

Lindbloom, E. J., Hough, L. D., and Urban, K. R. E. (2012). "Elder abuse." In J. Holroyd-Leduc and M. Reddy (eds), *Evidence-based Geriatric Medicine* (pp. 166–74). West Sussex, UK: Wiley-Blackwell.

Liu, D., Hinton, L., Tran, C., Hinton, D., and Barker, J. (2008). "Re-examining the Relationships Among Dementia, Stigma, and Aging in Immigrant Chinese and Vietnamese Family Caregivers." *Journal of Cross-Cultural Gerontology*, 23(3), 283–99.

Lynch, T. R., Morse, J. Q., Mendelson, T., and Robins, C. J. (2003). "Dialectical behavior therapy for depressed older adults: A randomized pilot study." *American Journal of Geriatric Psychiatry*, 11(1), 33–45.

Ma, G. X. (1999). "Between two worlds: The use of traditional and Western health services by Chinese immigrants." *Journal of Community Health*, 24(6), 421–37.

McBride, M. R. and Parreno, H. (1996). "Filipino-American families and caregiving." In G. Yeo and D. Gallagher-Thompson (eds), *Ethnicity & the Dementias* (pp. 123–35). Washington, DC: Taylor & Francis.

McCormick, W. C., Uomoto, J., Young, H., Graves, A. B., Vitaliano, P., Mortimer, J. A., Edland, S. D., and Larson, E. B. (1996). "Attitudes toward use of nursing homes and home care in older Japanese-Americans." *Journal of the American Geriatric Society*, 44(7), 769–77.

McGarry, J., Simpson, C., and Hinchliff-Smith, K. (2011). "The impact of domestic abuse for older women: a review of the literature." *Health & Social Care in the Community*, 19(1), 3–14.

McInnis-Dittrich, K. (2005). *Social Work with Elders: A Biopsychosocial Approach to Assessment and Intervention*. Boston, MA: Pearson.

Milne, A. and Chryssanthopoulou, C. (2005). "Dementia care-giving in black and Asian populations: reviewing and refining the research agenda." *Journal of Community & Applied Social Psychology*, 15(5), 319–37.

Mittelman, M. S., Roth, D. L., Coon, D. W., and Haley, W. E. (2004). "Sustained benefit of supportive intervention for depressive symptoms in caregivers of patients with Alzheimer's Disease." *American Journal of Psychiatry*, 161(5), 850–56.

Mui, A. C. (1993). "Self-reported depressive symptoms among Black and Hispanic frail elders: A sociocultural perpsective." *Journal of Applied Gerontology*, 12(2), 170–87.

Mui, A. C. and Shibusawa, T. (2008). *Asian American Elders in the 21st Century: Key Indicators of Psychosocial Well-being*. New York: Columbia University Press.

Mutchler, J. E., Prakash, A., and Burr, J. A. (2000). "The demography of disability and the effects of immigrant history: Older Asians in the United States." *Demography*, 44(2), 251–63.

Ngo, D., Tran, T. V., Gibbons, J. L., and Oliver, J. M. (2001). "Acculturation, pre-migration traumatic experiences, and depression among Vietnamese Americans." *Journal of Human Behavior in the Social Environment*, 3(3/4), 225–42.

Pang, E. C., Jordan-Marsh, M., Silverstein, M., and Cody, M. (2003). Health-Seeking Behaviors of Elderly Chinese Americans: Shifts in Expectations *The Gerontologist*, 43(6), 864–75.

Pang, K.-Y. C. (1991). *Korean Elderly Women in America: Everyday Life, Health and Illness*. New York: AMS Press, Inc.

——(1995). "A cross-cultural understanding of depression among Korean immigrants: Prevalence, symptoms, and diagnosis." *Clinical Gerontologist*, 15(4), 3–20.

Pearson, D. M., Kim, H. S., and Sherman, D. K. (2009). "Culture, social support and coping with bereavement for Asians and Asian Americans." *The Forum*, 35(2), 7–8.

Phua, V. C., Kaufman, G., and Park, K. S. (2001). "Strategic adjustments of elderly Asian Americans: Living arrangements and headship." *Journal of Comparative Family Studies*, 32 (2), 263–81.

Pinquart, M., Duberstein, P. R., and Lyness, J. M. (2006). "Treatments for later-life depressive conditions: a meta-analytic comparison of pharmacotherapy and psychotherapy." *American Journal of Psychiatry*, 163(9), 1493–501.

Ranguram, R., Weiss, M. G., Channabasavann, S. M., and Devins, G. M. (1996). "Stigma, depression, and somatization in South India." *American Journal of Psychiatry*, 153 (8), 1043–49.

Saint Arnault, D. (2009). "Cultural determinants of help-seeking: A model for research and practice." *Research and Theory for Nursing Practice: An International Journal*, 23(4), 259–78.

Schnurr, P. P., Spiro, A., III, Vielhauer, M. J., Findler, M. N., and Hamblen, J. L. (2002). "Trauma in the lives of older men: Findings from the normative aging study." *Journal of Clinical Geropsychology*, 8(3), 175–87.

Shiang, J., Blinn, R., Bongar, B., Stephens, B., Allison, D., and Shactzberg, A. (1997). "A comparison of Caucasian and Asian groups 1987–94." In A. Leenaars, R. Moris, and Y. Takahashi (eds), *Suicide: Individual, Culture, and International Perspectives* (pp. 80–91). New York: Guilford Press.

Shibusawa, T. and Chung, I. (2009). "Wrapping and unwrapping emotions: Clinical practice with East Asian immigrant elders." *Clinical Social Work Journal*, 37(4), 312–19.

Shibusawa, T., and Mui, A. C. (2002). "Stress, Coping, and Depression Among Japanese American Elders." *Journal of Gerontological Social Work*, 36(1–2), 63–81.

Silveira, E. R. T., and Shah, E. (1998). "Social determinants of psychiatric morbidity and well-being in immigrant elders and Whites in east London." *International Journal of Geriatric Psychiatry*, 13(11), 801–12.

Sorkin, D., Nguyen, H., and Ngo-Metzger, Q. (2011). "Assessing the mental health needs and barriers to care among a diverse sample of Asian American older adults." *Journal of General Internal Medicine*, 26(6), 595–602.

Statistics New Zealand (2006). *Demographic Aspects of New Zealand's Ageing Population*. Wellington: Statistics New Zealand.

Tam, S. and Neysmith, S. (2006). "Disrespect and isolation: Elder abuse in Chinese communities." *Canadian Journal on Aging*, 25(2), 141–51.

Tang, M. (2011). "Can cultural values help explain the positive aspects of caregiving among Chinese American caregiver?" *Journal of Gerontological Social Work*, 54(6), 551–69.

Tsai, D. T. and Lopez, R. A. (1997). "The use of social supports by elderly Chinese immigrants." *Journal of Gerontological Social Work*, 29(1), 77–94.

Turner, S., Christie, A., and Haworth, E. (2005). "South Asian and white people an dementia: A qualitative study of knowledge and attitudes." *Diversity in Health and Social Care*, 2(3), 197–209.

Turvey, C., Carney, C., Arndt, S., Wallace, R. B., and Herzog, A. R. (1999). "Conjugal loss and syndromal depression in a sample of elders aged 70 years or older." *American Journal of Psychiatry*, 156(10), 1596–1601.

VanItallie, T. B. (2005). "Subsyndromal depression in the elderly: Underdiagnosed and undertreated." *Metabolism: Clinical and Experimental*, 54(Suppl. 1), 39–44.

Walker, M. D., Babbar, B., Opotowsky, A. R., Rohira, A., Nabizadeh, F., Badia, M. D., Chung, W., Chiang, J., Medratta, A., McMahon, D., Liu, G., and Bilezikian, J. P. (2006). "A referent bone mineral density database for Chinese American women." *Osteoporosis International*, 17(6), 878–87.

Worth, A., Irshad, T., Bhopal, R., Brown, D., Lawton, J., Grant, E., Murray, S., Kendall, M., Asam, J., Gardee, R., and Sheikh, A. (2009). "Vulnerability and access to care for South Asian Sikh and Muslim patients with life limiting illness in Scotland: Prospective longitudinal qualitative study." *British Medical Journal*, 338:b183doi:10.1136/bmj.b183.

Yamashiro, G., and Matsuoka, J. K. (1997). "Help-seeking among Asian and Pacific Americans: A Multiperspective analysis." *Social Work*, 42(2), 176–86.

Yee, B. W. K. (1997). "The social and cultural context of adpative aging among Southeast Asian elders." In J. Sokolovsky (ed.), *The Cultural Context of Aging* (pp. 293–303). Westport, CT: Greenwood.

Chapter 8

Abe-Kim, J., Takeuchi, D. T., Hong, S., Zane, N., Sue, S., Spencer, M. S., Appel, H., Nicdao, E., and Algeria, M. (2007). "Use of mental health-related services among immigrant and US-born Asian Americans: Results from the National Latino and Asian American study." *American Journal of Public Health*, 97(1), 91–98.

Akutsu, P. D. and Chu, J. P. (2006). "Clinical problems that initiate professional help-seeking behaviors from Asian Americans." *Professional Psychology: Research and Practice*, 37 (4), 407–15.

Apter, A., Horesh, D., Ggothelf, D., Graffi, H., and Lepkifker, E. (2001). "Relationship between self-disclosure and serious suicidal behavior." *Comprehensive Psychiatry*, 42, 70–75.

Baldessarini, R. J., Pompili, M., and Tondo, L. (2006). "Suicidal risk in antidepressant drug trials." *Archives of General Psychiatry*, 63(3), 246–48.

Bartels, S. J., Coakley, E., Oxman, T. E., Constantino, G., Oslin, D., Chen, H., and Sanchez, H. (2002). "Suicidal and death ideation in older primary care patients with depression, anxiety and at-risk alcohol use." *American Journal of Geriatric Psychiatry*, 10(4), 417–417.

Beautrais, A. L. (2006). "Suicide in Asia." *Crisis*, 27(2), 55–57.

Beck, A. T., Brown, G., and Steer, R. A. (1997). "Psychometric characteristics of the scale for suicide ideation with psychiatric outpatients." *Behavior Research and Therapy*, 35(11), 1039–46.

Beck, A. T., Brown, G., Berchick, R. J., Stewart, B. L., and Steer, R. A. (1990). "Relationship between hopelessness and ultimate suicide: A replication with psychiatric outpatients." *American Journal of Psychiatry*, 147(2), 190–95.

Beck, A. T., Brown, G., Steer, R. A., Dahlsgaard, K., and Grisham, J. R. (1999). "Suicide ideation at its worst point: A predictor of eventual suicide in psychiatric outpatients." *Suicide and Life-Threatening Behavior*, 29(1), 1–9.

Bhugra, D. (2002). "Suicidal behavior in South Asians in the U.K." *Crisis*, 23(3), 108–13.

Bhugra, D. and Desai, M. (2002). "Attempted suicide in South Asian women." *Advances in Psychiatric Treatment*, 8(6), 418–23.

Bird, S. (2011). "How to complete a death certificate: A guide for GPs." *Australian Family Physcian*, 40(6), 446–49.

Blair-West, G. W., Cantr, C. H., Mellsop, G. W., and Eyeson-Annan, M. L. (1999). "Lifetime suicide risk in major depression: Sex and age determinants." *Journal of Affective Disorders*, 55(2), 171–78.

Brewin, C. R., Andrews, B., and Valentine, J. D. (2000). "Meta-analysis of risk factors for post traumatic stress disorder in trauma-exposed adults." *Journal of Consulting and Clinical Psychology*, 68(5), 748–66.

Burr, J. (2002). "Cultural stereotypes of women from South Asian communities: Mental health care professionals' explanations for patterns of suicide and depression." *Social Science & Medicine*, 55(5), 835–45.

Callahan, J. (1994). "Defining crisis and emergency." *Crisis*, 15, 164–71.

Canadian Vital Statistics System. *Death Database*. Retrieved 20 August 2012 from www23. statcan.gc.ca/imdb/p2SV.pl?Function=getSurvey&sdds=3233&lang=en&db=imdb& adm=8&dis=2.

Cavanagh, J. T. O., Carson, A. J., Sharpe, M., and Lawrie, S. M. (2003). "Psychological autopsy studies of suicide: A systemic review." *Psychological Medicine*, 33(3), 395–405.

Centers for Disease Control and Prevention (2011). *National Vital Statistics Reports Deaths: Final Data for 2009*, (60)6. Retrieved 12 August 2012 from www.cdc.gov/nchs/data/ nvsr/nvsr60/nvsr60_03.pdf.

———(2012). *National Vital Statistics Report Deaths: Preliminary Data for 2010*, (60)4. Retrieved 12 August 2012 from www.cdc.gov/nchs/data/nvsr/nvsr60/nvsr60_03.pdf.

———*National Center for Injury Prevention and Control*. Retrieved 20 August 2012 from Web-based Injury Statistics Query and Reporting System (WISQARS): www.cdc.gov/ncipc/ wisqars.

Chan-Yip, A. and Kirmayer, L. (1998). *Health Care Utilization and Child Care Practices among Chinese-Canadian Women in a Pediatric Practice*. Retrieved 10 August 2010 from http:// upload.mcgill.ca/tcpsych/Report7.pdf.

Chandrasekaran, R. and Gnanaselane, J. (2008). "Predictors of repeat suicidal attempts after first-ever attempt: A two-year follow-up study." *Hong Kong Journal of Psychiatry*, 28, 131–35.

Chen, A. W. and Kazanjian, A. (2005). "Rate of mental health service utilization by Chinese immigrants in British Columbia." *Canadian Journal of Public Health*, 96(1), 49–51.

Cheng, J. K., Fancher, T. L., Ratanasen, M., Conner, K. R., Duberstein, P. R., Sue, S., and Takeuchi, D. (2010). "Lifetime suicidal ideation and suicide attempts in Asian Americans." *Asian American Journal of Psychology*, 1(1), 18–30.

Chu, J. and Sue, S. (2011). "Asian American mental health: What we know and what we don't know." *Online Readings in Psychology and Culture, Unit 3*. Retrieved 23 August 2012 from http://scholarworks.gvsu.edu/orpc/vol3/iss1/4.

Chung, I. (2010). "Changes in the sociocultural reality of Chinese immigrants: Challenges and opportunities in help-seeking behavior." *International Journal of Social Psychiatry*, 56(4), 436–47.

———(2011). "Sociocultural Study of immigrant suicide attempters: An ecological perspective." *Journal of Social Work*, 12(6), 614–29.

Cipriani, A., Pretty, H., Hawton, K., and Geddes, J. R. (2005). "Lithium in the prevention of suicidal behavior and all-cause mortality in patients with mood disorders: A systematic review of randomized trials." *American Journal of Psychiatry*, 162(10), 1805–19.

Community Action on Suicide Prevention Education and Research (2011). *Chief Coroner Statistics 2011*. Retrieved 23 August 2012 from www.casper.org.nz/sites/default/files/Chief Coroner Stats 2011.pdf.

Conwell, Y., Duberstein, P.R., Cox, C., Herrman, J. H., Forbes, N. T., and Caine, E. D. (1996). "Relationships of age and axis I diagnoses in victims of completed suicide: A psychological autopsy study." *American Journal of Psychiatry*, 153(8), 1001–8.

Daniel, S. S. and Goldston, D. B. (2012). "Helplessness and lack of connectedness to others as risk factors for suicidal behavior across the lifespan: Implications for cognitive-behavioral treatment." *Cognitive and Behavioral Practice*, 19(2), 288–300.

Daigle, M. S. (2005). "Suicide prevention through means restriction: Assessing the risk of substitution. A critical review and synthesis." *Accident Analysis and Prevention*, 37, 625–32.

De Leo, D. (2002). "Struggling against suicide: The need for an integrative approach." *Crisis*, 23(1), 23–31.

Duldulao, A. A., Takeuchi, D. T., and Hong, S. (2009). "Correlates of suicidal behaviors among Asian Americans." *Archives of Suicide Research*, 13(3), 277–90.

Durkheim, E. (1897) *Le Suicide*. Trans. J. H. Spalding and G. Simpton (1951). New York: Free Press.

Eaton, W. and Harrison, G. (2000). "Ethnic disadvantage and schizophrenia." *Acta Psychiatrica Scandinavica*, 407(Suppl. 1), 38–43.

Ellis, T. E. and Goldston, D. B. (2012). "Working with suicidal clients: Not business as usual." *Cognitive and Behavioral Practice*, 19(2), 205–8.

Ellis, T. E. and Patel, A. (2012). "Client suicide: What now?" *Cognitive and Behavioral Practice*, 19(2), 277–87.

Ellis, T. E. and Rutherford, B. (2008). "Cognition and suicide: Two decades of progress." *International Journal of Cognitive Therapy*, 1(1), 47–68.

Fazel, M., Wheeler, J., and Danesh, J. (2005). "Prevalence of serious mental disorder in 7000 refugees settled in Western countries: A systemic review." *Lancet*, 365(9467), 1309–14.

Freedenthal, S. (2007). "Challenges in assessing intent to die: Can suicide attempters be trusted?" *Omega: Journal of Death and Dying*, 55(1), 57–70.

Freud, S. (1916). "Mourning and Melancholia." *Standard Edition*, 14. London: Hogarth Press.

Gipson, P. and King, C. (2012). "Health behavior theories and research: Implications for suicidal individuals' treatment linkage adherence." *Cognitive and Behavioral Practice*, 19(2), 209–17.

Glover, G., Marks, F., and Nowers, M. (1989). "Parasuicide in young Asian women." *British Journal of Psychiatry*, 154, 271–72.

Goldney, R. D. (2010). "A note on the reliability and validity of suicide statistics." *Psychiatry, Psychology and Law*, 17(1), 52–56.

Granello, D. H. and Granello, P. F. (2007). *Suicide: An Essential Guide for Helping Professionals and Educators*. New York: Pearson Education, Inc.

Gupta, S. (1991). "Psychosis in migrants from the Indian subcontinent and English-born controls." *British Journal of Psychiatry*, 159(2), 222–25.

Haynes, R. (1987). "Suicide and social response in Fiji." *British Journal of Psychiatry*, 151(1), 21–26.

Hendin, H. (1978). "Suicide: The psychosocial dimension." *Journal of Suicide and Life Threatening Behavior*, 8(2), 99–117.

Hendin, H., Phillips, M. R., Vijaykumar, L., Pirkis, J., Wang, H., Yip, P., Wasserman, D., Bertolote, J. M., Fleischmann, A. (2008). "Epidemiology of suicide in Asia." In H. Hendin, L. Vijayuakumar, J. M. Bertolote, H. Wang, M. R. Phillips, and J. Pirkis (eds), *Suicide and Suicide Prevention in Asia* (pp. 7–18). Geneva, Switzerland: WHO Press.

Heron, M. (2011). "Deaths: Leading causes for 2007." *National Vital Statistics Reports*, 59, 8.

Hicks, M. H. and Bhugra, D. (2003). "Perceived causes of suicide attempts by U.K. South Asian women." *American Journal of Orthopsychiatry*, 73 (4): 455–62.

Hjern, A. and Allebeck, P. (2002). "Suicide in first- and second-generation immigrants in Sweden: A comparative study." *Social Psychiatry and Psychiatric Epidemiology*, 37(9), 423–29.

Ide, N., Kõlves, K., Cassaniti, M., and De Leo, D. (2012). "Suicide of first-generation immigrants in Australia, 1974–2006." *Social Psychiatry and Psychiatric Epidemiology*, 47(12), 1–11.

Ineichen, B. (2008). "Suicide and attempted suicide among South Asians in England: Who's at risk?" *Mental Health and Family Medicine*, 5(3), 135–38.

Jang, Y., Chiriboga, D. A., and Okazaki, S. (2009). "Attitudes toward mental health services: Age group differences in Korean American adults." *Aging & Mental Health*, 13(1), 127–34.

Ji, J. (2000). "Suicide rates and mental health services in modern China." *The Journal of Crisis Intervention and Suicide Prevention*, 21(3), 118–21.

Jobes, D. A. (2000). "Collaborating to prevent suicide: A clinical-research perspective." *Suicide and Life-threatening Behavior*, 30(1), 8–17.

Jobes, D. A. and Drozd, J. F. (2004). "The CAMS approach to working with suicidal patients." *Journal of Contemporary Psychotherapy*, 14(1), 73–85.

Joiner, T. E. (2002). "The trajectory of suicidal behavior over time." *Suicide and Life-Threatening Behavior*, 32(1), 33–41.

——(2005). *Why People Die by Suicide*. Cambridge, MA: Harvard University Press.

Kahn, M. M. and Reza, H. (2000). "The pattern of suicide in Pakistan." *Crisis*, 21(1), 31–35.

Kamal, Z. and Loewenthal, K. M. (2002). "Suicide beliefs and behaviour among young Muslims and Hindus in UK." *Mental Health, Religion and Culture*, 5(2),111–18.

Kelly, K. T. and Knudson, M. P. (2000). "Are no-suicide contracts effective in preventing suicide in suicidal patients seen by primary care physicians?" *Archives of Family Medicine*, 9 (10), 1119–21.

Kennedy, M. A., Parhar, K. K., Samra, J., and Gorzalka, B. (2005). "Suicide ideation in different generations of immigrants." *Canadian Journal of Psychiatry*, 50(6), 353–56.

Kreyenbuhl, J. A., Kelly, D. L., and Conley, R. R. (2002). "Circumstances of suicide among individuals with schizophrenia." *Schizophrenia Research*, 58 (2–3), 253–61.

Kroll, J. (2000). "Use of no-suicide contracts by psychiatrists in Minnesota." *The American Journal of Psychiatry*, 157(10), 1684–686.

Kuo, W. H., Tsai, Y.-M. (1986). "Social networking, hardiness and immigrant's mental health." *Journal of Health and Social Behavior*, 27, 133–49.

Leenaars, A. A. (2008). "Suicide: A cross-cultural theory." In F. T. L. Leong and M. M. Leach (eds), *Suicide among Racial and Ethnic Minority Groups: Theory, Research, and Practice* (pp. 13–37). New York: Routledge.

Leong, F. T. L., Leach, M. M., and Gupta, A. (2008). "Suicide among Asian Americans: A critical review with research recommendations." In F. T. L. Leong and M. M. Leach (eds), *Suicide among Racial and Ethnic Minority Groups: Theory, Research, and Practice* (pp. 117–41). New York: Routledge.

Lester, D. (2008). "Theories of suicide." In F. T. L. Leong and M. M. Leach (eds), *Suicide among Racial and Ethnic Minority Groups: Theory, Research, and Practice* (pp. 39–53). New York: Routledge.

Li, Y., Li, Y., and Cao, J. (2012). "Factors associated with suicidal behaviors in Mainland China: A meta-analysis." *BMC Public Health*, 12(1), doi: 10.1186/1471-2458-12-524.

Lim, J. Personal communication with author, 15 August 2012.

Linehan, M. M., Comtois, K. A., and Ward-Ciesielski, E. F. (2012). "Assessing and managing risks with suicidal individuals." *Cognitive and Behavioral Practice*, 19(2), 218–32.

Linehan, M. M., Goodstein, J. L., Nielsen, S. L., and Chiles, J. A. (1983). "Reasons for staying alive when you are thinking of killing yourself: The Reasons for Living Inventory." *Journal of Consulting and Clinical Psychology*, 51(2), 276–86.

Luo, T. Personal communication with author, 30 July 2012.

McKenzie, K., Serfaty, M., and Crawford, M. (2003). "Suicide in ethnic minority groups." *British Journal of Psychiatry*, 183(2), 100–101.

Mann, J. (1998). "The neurobiology of suicide." *Nature Medicine*, 4(1), 25–30.

Meltzer, H. Y., Alphs, L., Green, A. I., Altamura, A. C., Anand, R., Bertoldi, A., Bourgeois, M., Chouinard, G., Islam, M. Z., Kane, J.; Krishnan, R., Lindenmayer, J.-P., Potkin, S., and InterSePT Study Group (2003). "Clozapine treatment for suicidality in schizophrenia: International suicide prevention trial (InterSePT)." *Archives of General Psychiatry*, 60(1), 82–91.

Menninger, K. (1938). *Man Against Himself*. New York: Harcourt, Brace & Co.

Meyer, O. L., Zane, N., Cho, Y., and Takeuchi, D. T. (2009). "Use of specialty mental health services by Asian Americans with psychiatric disorders." *Journal of Consulting and Clinical Psychology*, 77(5), 1000–1005.

Mullen, B. and Smyth, J. M. (2004). "Immigrant suicide rates as a function of ethnophaulisms: Hate speech predicts death." *Psychosomatic Medicine*, 66(3), 343–48.

National Crime Records Bureau. Government of India, Ministry of Home Affairs (2010). *Accidental Deaths and Suicides in India, 2010*. Retrieved 20 August 2012 from http://ncrb.nic.in/ADSI2010/ADSI2010-full-report.pdf.

National Institute of Mental Health (2010). *Suicide in the US: Statistics and Prevention*. Retrieved 8 September 2012 from www.nimh.nih.gov/health/publications/suicide-in-the-us-statistics-and-prevention/index.shtml#CDC-Web-Tool.

Neeleman, J. and Wessely, S. (1999). "Ethnic minority suicide: a small area geographical study in south London." *Psychological Medicine*, 29(2), 429–36.

New York City Department of Health and Mental Hygiene (2012). *New York City Vital Signs*, February 2012, 11(1).

Oquendo, M. A., Waternaux, C., Brodsky, B., Parsons, B., Haas, G. L., Malone, K. M., and Mann, J. J. (2000). "Suicidal behavior in bipolar mood disorder: Clinical characteristics of attempters and nonattempters." *Journal of Affective Disorders*, 59(2), 107–17.

Phillips, M. R., Yang, C., Zhang, Y., Wang, L., Ji, H., and Zhou, M. (2002). "Risk factors for suicide in China: A national case-control psychological autopsy study." *Lancet*, 360 (9347), 1728–36.

Pilkington, A., Masetfi, R. M., and Watson, R. (2011). "Factors affecting intentions to access psychiatric services amongst British Muslims of South Asian Origin." *Mental Health, Religion and Culture*, 15(1), 1–22.

Qin, P. and Mortensen, P. B. (2001). "Specific characteristics of suicide in China." *Acta Psychiatrica Scandinavica*, 103(2), 117–21.

Redaniel, M. R., Lebanan-Dalida, M. A., and Gunell, D. (2011). "Suicide in the Philippines: Time trend analysis (1974–2005) and literature review." *BMC Public Health*, 11(1), 536.

Reeves, T. J. and Bennett, C. E. (2004). "We the people: Asians in the United States." *Census 2000 Special Reports*, CENSR-17, US Department of Commerce.

Rudd, M. D., (2008). "Suicide warning signs in clinical practice." *Current Psychiatry Reports*, 10(1), 87–90.

Rudd, M. D., Berman, A. L., Joiner, T. E., Jr., Nock, M. K., Silverman, M. M., Mandrusiak, M., Van Orden, K., and Witte, T. (2006). "Warning signs for suicide: Theory, research, and clinical applications." *Suicide and Life-threatening Behavior*, 36(3), 255–62.

Ruddell, P. and Curwen, B. (2002). "Understanding suicidal ideation and assessing for risk." *British Journal of Guidance and Counselling*, 30(4), 363–72.

Sanchez, F. and Gaw, A. (2007). "Mental health care of Filipino Americans." *Psychiatric Services*, 58(6), 810–15.

Schneidman, E. S. (1993). *Suicide as Psychache: A clinical approach to self-destructive behavior.* Northvale, NJ: Aronson.

Scowcroft, E. (2012). *Suicide Statistics Report 2012: Data for 2008–12.* Retrieved 28 August 2012 from www.samaritans.org/sites/default/files/kcfinder/files/suicide%20Statistics%20 Report%202012.pdf

Shah, A., Lindesay, J., and Dennis, M. (2011). "Suicides by country of birth groupings in England and Wales: Age associated trends and standardized mortality ratios." *Social Psychiatry Psychiatric Epidemiology*, 46(3), 197–206.

Silveira, E. R. and Ebrahim, S. (1998). "Social determinants of psychiatric morbidity and well-being in immigrant elders and whites in East London." *International Journal of Geriatric Psychiatry*, 13(11), 801–12.

Skogman, K., Alsen, M., and Ojehagen, A. (2004). "Sex differences in risk factors for suicide after attempted suicide: A follow-up study of 1052 suicide attempters." *Social Psychiatry Psychiatric Epidemiology*, 39(2), 113–20.

Soni Raleigh, V. and Balarajan, R. (1992). "Suicide and self-burning among Indians and West Indians in England and Wales." *British Journal of Psychiatry*, 161(3), 365–68.

Stanley, B. and Brown, G. K. (2012). "Safety planning intervention: A brief intervention to mitigate suicide risk." *Cognitive and Behavioral Practice*, 19(2), 256–64.

Stuart, G. W., Minas, I. H., Klimidis, S., and O'Connell, S. (1996). "English language ability and mental health service utilization: A census." *Australian and New Zealand Journal of Psychiatry*, 30(2), 270–77.

Sundaram, V., Qin, P., and Zollner, L. (2006). "Suicide risk among persons with foreign background in Denmark." *Suicide and Life-Threatening Behavior*, 36(4), 481–89.

Thompson, S., Manderson, L., Woelz-Stirling, N., Cahill, A., and Kelaher, M. (2002). "The social and cultural context of the mental health of Filipinas in Queensland." *Australian and New Zealand Journal of Psychiatry*, 36(5), 681–87.

US Census Bureau (2012). *Table 10, Resident Population by Race, Hispanic Origin, and Age 2000 and 2009: August 2012.* Retrieved 8 September 2012 from www.census.gov/compendia/ statab/2012/tables/12s0010.pdf.

Varnik, P. (2012). "Suicides in the World." *Int. J. Environ. Res. Public Health*, 9(3), 760–71.

Vijayakumar, L. (2004). "Suicide prevention: The urgent need in developing countries." *World Psychiatry*, 3(3), 158–59.

Yan Cheng, J. K., Fancher, T. L., Ratanasen, M., Conner, K. R., Duberstein, P. R., Sue, S., and Takeuchi, D. (2010). "Lifetime suicidal ideation and suicide attempts in Asian Americans." *Asian American Journal of Psychology*, 1(1), 18–30.

Yip, P., Callanan, C., and Yuen, H. (2000). "Urban/rural and gender differentials in suicide rates: East and West." *Journal of Affective Disorders*, 57(1–3), 99–106.

Wang, A. G. and Mortensen, G. (2006). "Core features of repeated suicidal behavior: A long-term follow-up after suicide attempts in a low-suicide-incidence population." *Social Psychiatry Psychiatric Epidemiology*, 41(2), 103–7.

Wang, P. S., Lane, M., Olfson, M., Pincus, H. A., Wells, K. B., and Kessler, R. C. (2005). "Twelve-month use of mental health services in the United States: Results from the National Comorbidity Survey Replication." *Archives of General Psychiatry*, 62(6), 629–40.

Westefeld, J. S., Lillian, M. R., Rogers, J. R., Maples, M. R., Bromley, J. L., and Alcorn, J. (2000). "Suicide: An overview." *The Counseling Psychologist*, 28(4), 445–510.

World Health Organization (2008). *WHO Statement, 10 September 2008*. Retrieved 4 September 2012 from www.who.int/mental_health/prevention/suicide/wspd_2008_statement.pdf.

——(2012). *SUPRE Suicide Prevention: Country Reports and Charts*. Retrieved 23 August 2012 from www.who.int/mental_health/prevention/suicide/country_reports/en/index.html.

Xu, J., Kochanek, K. D., Murphy, S. L., and Tejada-Vera, B. (2010). "Deaths: Final data for 2007." *National Vital Statistics Reports*, 58(19), 10.

Zane, N. and Mak, W (2003). "Major approaches to the measurement of acculturation among ethnic minority populations: A content analysis and an alternative empirical strategy." In K. M. Chun, P. Balls Organista, and G. Marin (eds), *Acculturation: Advances in Theory, Measurement, and Applied Research* (pp. 39–60). Washington, DC: American Psychological Association.

Zhang, J., Conwell, Y., Zhou, L., and Jiang, C. (2004). "Culture, risk factors and suicide in rural China: A psychological autopsy case control study." *Acta Psychiatrica Scandinavica*, 110(6), 430–37

Epilog

Bernal, G., Jiménez-Chafey, M. I., and Domenech Rodríguez, M. M. (2009). "Cultural adaptation of treatments: A resource for considering culture in evidence-based practice." *Professional Psychology: Research and Practice*, 40(4), 361–68.

Hall, E. T. (1977). *Beyond Culture*. Anchor Books: Garden City, New York.

Ham, M. D. C. (1993). "Empathy." In J. L. Chin, J. H. Liem, M. D. C. Ham, and G. K. Hong (eds). *Transference and Empathy in Asian American Psychotherapy: Cultural Values and Treatment Need* (pp. 35–58). Westport, CT: Praeger Publishers.

Hinton, D. E., Safren, S. A., Pollack, M. H., and Tran, M. (2006). "Cognitive-behavior therapy for Vietnamese refugees With PTSD and comorbid panic attacks." *Cognitive and Behavioral Practice*, 13(4), 271–81.

Hou, X. (2011). "From Mao to the market: Community capitalism in rural China." *Theory, Culture and Society*, 28(2), 46–68.

Hwang, W.-C., Wood, J. J., Lin, K. M., and Cheung, F. (2006). "Cognitive-behavioral therapy with Chinese Americans: Research, theory, and clinical practice." *Cognitive and Behavioral Practice*, 13(4), 293–303.

Kleinman, A. (1994). "Culture and depression," *New England Journal of Medicine*, 351(10), 951–53.

Kleinman, A. and Benson, P. (2006). "Anthropology in the clinic: The problem of cultural competency and how to fix it." *PLOS Medicine*, 3(10), 1673–676.

Markus, H., Mullally, P., and Kitayama, S. (1997). "Selfways: Diversity in modes of cultural participation." In U. Neisser and D. Joplin (eds), *The Conceptual Self in Context: Culture* (pp. 13–61). Cambridge, New York: Cambridge University Press.

Organisation for Economic Co-operation (2011). *Families are changing.* Retrieved 1 December 2012 from www.oecd.org/els/familiesandchildren/47701118.pdf.

Otto, M. W. and Hinton, D. E. (2006). "Modifying exposure-based CBT for Cambodian refugees with post traumatic stress disorder." *Cognitive and Behavioral Practice*, 13(4), 261–270.

Roland, A. (2011). *Journeys to Foreign Selves: Asians and Asian Americans in a Global Era.* New York: Oxford University Press.

Sonawat, R. (2001). "Understanding families in India: A reflection of societal changes." *Psicologia: Teoria e Pesquisa*, 17(2), 177–86. Retrieved 1 December 2012 from www.scielo.br/pdf/ptp/v17n2/7878.pdf.

Index

acculturation 52, 84, 86, 97, 98–99, 103, 105, 108, 110, 134, 161, 176–77, 183, 193, 197–98
acculturative family distancing (AFD) 105
acculturative stress: risk factors 84, 87 *see* migration: adaptation challenges; *see also* immigration-related stressors; protective factors against 87–88
adolescence: in Asian cultures 103, 105; in Western cultures 102–3, 105
adoptees from Asia 80
aggression and sexuality in Asian hierarchical culture 14
Alzheimer's Disease 156, 160–61; *see* dementia
anxiety among elders 154, 158; among Asian elders 158
Asian and Western cultural differences in parental expectations 90, 94, 96–97
Asian authoritarian parenting style 95, 106
Asian communication style 51–52, 55; affective lexicons 52, 60, 62; generational differences 110, 115, 198; high-context 52; indirect ix, x, 55, 108; intuitive sensing 58–59, 115, 142; *see also* intersubjectivity; minimizing of emotions in conversations 52; vocabulary in Asian languages 17, 52
Asian families: core values and structures of 91; parent–child communication 90, 94–95, 105, 108–10, 115, 120, 198; discipline and punishment 90, 97–99, 110–11, 123, 127
Asian immigrant populations in English-speaking countries, history and growth of xiv; in Australia and New Zealand 81; in Canada 81–82; in UK 82; in USA 82

Asian immigrants' ties with their families in home countries: financial support from Bangladeshi, Filipino and *Viet kieu* 78
Asian parenting practice 90, 92, 94–95, 99, 105–6, 108, 110, 113, 119
Asian psyche 23, 198; *see* Asian sense of self
Asian sense of self 22–24, 27, 58, 92–93, 116
Asians living outside their country of birth, 77
assessment, interventions, prevention, 20–24
authoritative parenting style 94–95

Beck, A. 173
bilateral family system in Southeast Asian countries 91
Buddhism 51, 63, 65, 96

"capacity to be alone" 22
case management xvi, 66, 138, 144, 164, 197
child abuse cases, Asian immigrant families 19
child welfare laws in English-speaking countries 100
child-rearing practices and social interaction: of western Europe and North American societies 22; of traditional Asian societies 22–23; *see* Asian parenting practice
Choi, K. M. 23
chronic illness, older adults in the US 154
classical Freudian theory: biological drives of aggression and sexuality 9, 32; interpretation 32, 35, 63–64; intrapsychic conflicts 9, 30, 34; "the

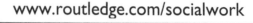

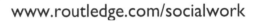

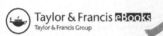